NUCLEAR CARDIOLOGY AND CARDIAC MAGNETIC RESONANCE

PHYSIOLOGY, TECHNIQUES AND APPLICATIONS

ERNST EVERT VAN DER WALL

Kluwer Academic Publishers

Dordrecht / Boston / London

Library of Congress Cataloging-in-Publication Data

```
Wall, E. van der.
    Nuclear cardiology and cardiac magnetic resonance / Ernst Evert
  Van der Wall.
       p.   cm.
    ISBN 0-7923-1780-7 (HB : alk. paper)
    1. Heart--Radionuclide imaging.   I. Title.
    [DNLM: 1. Cardiovascular Diseases--diagnosis.  2. Magnetic
  Resonance Imaging--methods.   WG 141 W187n]
  RC683.5.R33W35  1992
  616.1'207548--dc20
  DNLM/DLC
  for Library of Congress                        92-15313
                                                    CIP
```

ISBN 0-7923-1780-7

Distributed by Kluwer Academic Publishers,
P.O. Box 17, 3300 AA Dordrecht, The Netherlands.

Kluwer Academic Publishers incorporates
the publishing programmes of
D. Reidel, Martinus Nijhoff, Dr W. Junk and MTP Press.

Sold and distributed in the U.S.A. and Canada
by Kluwer Academic Publishers,
101 Philip Drive, Norwell, MA 02061, U.S.A.

In all other countries, sold and distributed
by Kluwer Academic Publishers Group,
P.O. Box 322, 3300 AH Dordrecht, The Netherlands.

Printed on acid-free paper

Printed in the Netherlands by Hans Soto Productions

CONTENTS

Preface

PHYSIOLOGY

TECHNIQUES

APPLICATIONS

Ernst Evert van der Wall M.D.
Department of Cardiology
University of Leiden
Leiden, The Netherlands

4

PREFACE

Cardiovascular nuclear medicine emerged 15 years ago as a new noninvasive technique for the detection of human cardiac disease. It arised from the fields of nuclear medicine and cardiology and the cooperation of both specialties has been very productive. At present, nuclear cardiology techniques belong to the routine armamentarium of the clinical cardiologist. Results obtained by perfusion markers, metabolic tracers, and radionuclide angiography have shown to have important impact on patient management. Although exercise electrocardiography and echocardiography yield the large bulk of necessary data in the cardiac patient, nuclear cardiology provides important data that go far beyond the results obtained by the standard procedures. Magnetic resonance imaging is a relative newcomer in cardiology and has still to prove its value in clinical cardiology. Yet, initial results have been encouraging both in congenital heart disease and in coronary artery disease. This book is based on 16 review publications that have been written throughout the period of 1985 till present time. Most chapters have been published in the period 1989 until 1991; the preceding review papers have been updated as much as possible. Furthermore, Chapter 15 entitled " What's new in cardiac imaging" has been especially written for this book. The Chapters 9, 11 and 13 have been recently written and have not been published yet. The book offers a bird's eye view on the clinical potential of the nuclear cardiology techniques (nuclear and MRI) in the practice of cardiology. It does not address detailed technical considerations or less frequently used imaging modalities; for these the reader is referred to general nuclear medicine texts.

The present book has been grossly divided into three Sections: 1) Physiology, 2) Techniques, and 3) Clinical Applications. The section Physiology deals with the nuclear medicine background of myocardial perfusion, myocardial metabolism, and cardiac function (Chapters 1,2, and 3). The section Techniques discusses the planar techniques, in particular for the perfusion tracer thallium-201, the Single Photon Emission Computed Tomography (SPECT) technique, and the Positron Emission Tomography (PET) technique (Chapters 4,5, and 6). This section also addresses the physical background of Magnetic Resonance Imaging (MRI) (Chapter 7). The section Clinical Applications discusses the value of the nuclear cardiology for a variety of cardiac disease from detection of myocardial infarction to its merits for evaluating cardiomyopathies (Chapters 8-14). Chapter 10 shortly adresses the experimental and clinical value of Magnetic Resonance Spectroscopy (MRS). Chapter 15 describes the latest developments in nuclear cardiology with emphasis on new cardiac imaging agents. Finally, Chapter 16 presents the currently advocated Guidelines in Nuclear Cardiology.

Of course there were co-authors involved in several publications and I am very grateful for their assistance in writing these reviews. I like to acknowledge the following co-authors - in alphabetical order : JW Arndt, CAPL Ascoop, JAK Blokland, HA Bosker, S Braat, AVG Bruschke, PRM van Dijkman, MJPG van Kroonenburgh, GJ Laarman, V Manger Cats, MG Niemeyer, EKJ Pauwels, H Prpic, A de Roos, FC Visser, AE van Voorthuisen, FJTh Wackers.

I hope this book will broaden the knowledge of the nuclear cardiology techniques and will convince the reader of the indispensable value of these techniques in clinical cardiology practice.

Ernst Evert van der Wall, MD

To Barbara, Hein and Sake

1.
Perfusion:
Evaluation of myocardial blood flow by radionuclide imaging

Introduction

In recent years the use of radioactive tracers in clinical cardiology has become a routine procedure in the diagnosis and management of patients of cardiac disease. Radionuclide techniques have achieved a role equal in importance to electrocardiography, echocardiography, and cardiac catheterization. Broadly speaking, radionuclide techniques fall into two major categories: those concerned with the heart as a muscle and those concerned with the heart as a pump. Since this chapter regards the scintigraphic aspects of coronary artery *perfusion*, attention will mainly be focused on the techniques that deal with the heart as a muscle. Before entering these issues, some necessary technical information will be provided.

Cardiac instrumentation

Radionuclide imaging is performed with a gamma camera connected with a computer. The function of the gamma camera is to convert radioactivity into a pictorial representation. After uptake of a radioactive tracer in a specific organ, the gamma rays (photons) of the tracer are detected by the gamma camera, which finally produces electronic signals. The electronic signals are computed as X,Y signals and visualized on an oscilloscope on the camera console as well as sent to a computer for subsequent data analysis. The currently used gamma cameras can grosso modo be divided into 1) the conventional gamma camera, and 2) the positron camera. The conventional gamma camera is a stationary or mobile system with a field of view of 40 cm, which can easily be positioned over the chest cage of the patient. This type of camera is very well suited for routine procedures in large number of patients, because of the wide availability of gamma-emitting radioactive tracers and its relative low cost. A drawback is the difficulty of exactly quantitating radionuclide concentrations in tissue because of attenuation of radioactivity as a function of the distance between organ and camera.

The positron camera is a less widely available and rather expensive type of camera, and is therefore mostly used as a research tool. It employs one or multiple rings of detectors arranged in opposing pairs around the patient. Only positron emitting radioactive tracers can be detected on the basis of positron-electron annihilation. Positrons are positively charged electrons which travel only a very short distance (less than 1 mm) to encounter an electron. When the positron and the electron combine, both are annihilated and the energy of the two particles is converted to two high energy photons (511 kiloelectronVolt) that are emitted 180° apart in opposite directions. Major advantages of this approach include accurate tomographic localization of regional events in organs, adequate correction for photon attenuation and therefore more reliable reflection of the quantity of activity within the heart than is obtained with conventional camera systems.

Radiopharmaceuticals

Radionuclides have three main characteristics:
(1) type of emission, i.e. radiation of alpha, beta, gamma or positron rays, (2) level of energy expressed in kiloelectronVolt (keV), and (3) physical and biological half-life. The ideal radionuclide for cardiac evaluation should have the following properties: (1) a pure gamma-(or positron) emitting tracer with a photon energy of 100-200 keV (positron, 511 keV), (2) a physical half-life of several minutes or hours to permit serial measurements over a short time period, (3) no pharmacologic effects which might affect physiological conditions, and 4) wide availability and low cost. So far, no currently used cardiac imaging agent meets all these requirements.

Methods for measuring blood flow

Many methods for assessing myocardial blood flow have been reported. Most techniques are based on the Fick principle which states that blood flow to an organ is equal to the uptake of any substance divided by the arteriovenous concentration difference of that substance. The principle can be rephrased as:

change of amount/time = flow concentration in - flow concentration out.
In formula:
$$\frac{dq(t)}{dt} = F.(A(t) - B(t)),$$

where the change of quantity in the organ with time dq/dt is related to the flow (F) times the difference in concentration of the input A and output B. Inherent to this principle are the following assumptions: (1) adequate mixing of the substance with the blood, (2) steady state of the system during measurement, (3) no influence of the amount of the substance on transit time, (4) no recirculation of the substance, and (5) unidirectional and steady flow. Myocardial blood flow measurements with radioactive tracers are based on assumptions on tracer kinetics, and these measurements are all directly or indirectly related to the Fick principle. In the following section the evaluation of myocardial blood flow with the use of radioactive tracers will be discussed.

Radionuclide agents for evaluation of blood flow

Radioactive tracers which are extracted from the input network in proportion to flow are known as flow-limited tracers i.e. the amount of tracer which diffuses through the tissue is limited only by the amount delivered. Such tracers are labeled microspheres or labeled macroaggregates. Tracers which are not flow-limited are diffusion-limited i.e. the capillary endothelium or the cellular membranes acts like diffusion barriers. Substances like potassium, thallium, rubidium, ammonia (all monovalent cations) and also inert gases are diffusion-limited tracers. The differences between flow- and diffusion-limited tracers have major consequences for the extraction fraction and net tissue tracer uptake. The extraction fraction is defined as the fraction of activity that is removed by the myocardial tissue between input and output. The net tissue tracer uptake is the product of extraction fraction times flow. For flow-limited tracers the extraction fraction is one (complete extraction) and the net tracer uptake shows a linear response. In case of diffusion-limited tracers the extraction fraction decreases as flow increases and the net tissue tracer uptake shows a nonlinear response (Fig. 1).

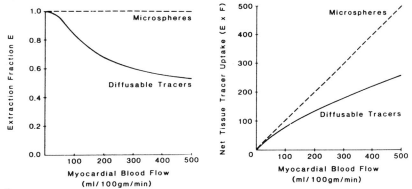

Figure 1
Initial capillary transit extraction fraction (E) and net tissue tracer uptake for microspheres and diffusible tracers of blood flow (F). Extraction fraction and the relationship to blood flow is shown in the left panel. Microspheres are completely extracted during a single capillary transit and the extraction fraction is one. This, however, does not apply to diffusible tracers. Their extraction fraction declines with increasing blood flows because of decreasing capillary residence times with less time for transmembraneous exhange. The right panel shows the net tissue tracer uptake as the product of extraction fraction and blood flow. Note the linear response for microspheres and the nonlinear response for diffusible tracers. The latter response is cause by the flow-dependent decrease in extraction fraction.
From Schelbert HR; Evaluation and quantification of regional myocardial blood flow with positron emission tomography. In: New concepts of cardiac imaging, Eds, Pohost GM, Higgins CB, Morganroth J, Ritchie JL, Schelbert HR, 197, 1987 (with permission).

In practice, however, diffusion-limited tracers can adequately be used for evaluation of relative myocardial perfusion in normal myocardium and in ischemic or infarcted myocardial areas.

A number of agents have been used or investigated for the evaluation of myocardial blood flow. They can be categorized into four different groups, each of which is governed by a different set of tracer kinetic assumptions.(Table 1)

Table 1. Myocardial perfusion agents

	Half-life	keV	Intra-venous	Intra-coronary
1. *Monovalent cations*				
a. Gamma				
Thallium-201	74 h	69, 83	+	
Potassium-43	22.4 h	373, 619	+	
Rubidium-81	4.7 h	511, 190	+	
b. Positron				
Rubidium-82	75 s	511	+	
Nitrogen-13-ammonia	10 min	511	+	
Oxygen-15 labeled water	2 min	511	+	
2. *Inert gases*				
Xenon-133	5.3 days	81, 204		+
Krypton-81m	13 s	190		+
3. *Particulate agents*				
Carbon-11-microspheres	20 min	511		+
Technetium-99m-macroaggregates	6h	140		+
Gallium-68 -macroaggregates or albumin	68 min	511		+
4. *New agents*				
Technetium-99m-Diars	6 h	140	+	
Technetium-99m Tc-isonitriles	6 h	140	+	
Technetium-99m Tc-teboroxime	6 h	140	+	

Diars = diarsenical complex

The extent to which the assumptions concerning the behaviour of a tracer satisfy the mathematical modeling requirements varies between the various classes. The four classes are:

> (1) Monovalent cations,
> (2) Inert gases,
> (3) Particulate agents such as microspheres or macroaggregates,
> (4) New perfusion imaging agents.

(1) Monovalent cations

The initial distribution of radiopharmaceuticals which have a high extraction will be proportional to relative perfusion. This principle was first described by Leon Sapirstein and provides estimates of flow from the relation:

$$q(t) = F.E \int_0^t C(t)dt,$$

which means:
amount present in organ = flow x extraction x concentration.
It is based on the assumption that an intravenously administered tracer is taken up and released by cells throughout the organism in a consistent fashion independent of regional blood flow or metabolic status of the tissue. If a tracer meets these criteria, it will be distributed in proportion to regional perfusion. Most radiopharmaceuticals employed for determinations based on this type of analysis are monovalent cations, which are predominantly potassium analogs. They can be divided into gamma- and positron- emitting agents.

a. Gamma-emitting agents

Thallium-201 is the most common gamma-emitting agent for assessment of myocardial perfusion scintigraphically, although also potassium-43 and rubidium-81 have been used. These agents enter the myocardium by the energy requiring sodium-potassium-ATPase pump mechanisms. They differ in their physical half-lives, gamma emissions, and in myocardial extraction and washout. In a single transit through the coronary bed, the extraction of thallium is 88%, and of potassium and rubidium between 65 and 75%.
Since the myocardial extraction and total body extraction are usually similar, the time course of blood clearance and myocardial concentration will differ for each agent. The most rapid concentration rise in the myocardium occurs with thallium, followed by that of potassium and rubidium. The importance of the time needed for localization stems from the need to maintain a 'steady-state' during the interval of radionuclide concentration rise in the myocardium. Within three circulatory periods, the majority of monovalent cationic myocardial tracer with high extraction fraction (thallium-201, rubidium-81, and potassium-43) has concentrated in the myocardium.
The uptake and distribution of the monovalent cations correlates well with the distribution of myocardial blood flow, whereby uptake is the product of blood flow and extraction fraction. For thallium-201 the extraction fraction is inversely related to flow when coronary flow is in the normal range. At high and low flows, however, the extraction is respectively much less and greater, resulting in underestimation of true flow in high flow states and overestimation of true flow in low flow states. Still thallium-201 is at present the prime radiopharmaceutical for myocardial perfusion

imaging in clinical cardiology.

After intravenous injection of 2 milliCurie (mCi) or 74 MegacBequerel (MBq) thallium-201 about 4 % of tracer localizes in the myocardium and within 10 minutes a myocardial image with a count density of about 2000 counts/cm^2 can be recorded (Fig. 2).

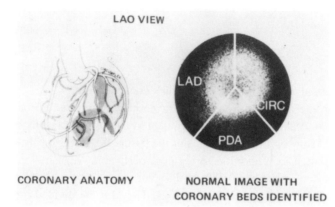

Figure 2

The left anterior oblique (LAO) view best differentiates the major coronary arterial beds, as shown schematically on the left: the LAD supplies the anteroseptal myocardium, the CIRC supplies the posterolateral myocardium, and the PDA supplies the inferior myocardium. In the LAO myocardial image, as shown in a normal study on the right, the anteroseptal myocardium is represented by an anteroseptal wedge of activity, the posterolateral myocardium by a posterolateral wedge, and the inferior myocardium by an inferior wedge.

From Ritchie JL, Hamilton GW, Williams DL, et al: Myocardial imaging with radionuclide-labeled particles: Analysis of the normal image, abnormal image, and technical considerations, Radiology 121:131, 1976 (with permission).

CIRC = left circumflex; PDA = posterior descending artery; LAD = left anterior descending coronary artery.

Myocardial infarction or ischemia may be diagnosed by the visually estimated findings of absent or diminished tracer uptake in regional myocardial areas (Fig. 3).

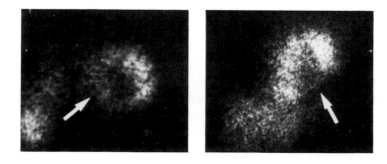

Figure 3

Thallium-201 scintigrams in a patient with anteroseptal myocardial infarction (left) and inferior myocardial infarction (right).

Thallium-201 is particularly useful in conjunction with the electrocardiogram during a standard exercise stress test for the detection of suspected coronary artery disease. The exercise scintigrams may show perfusion defects that are resolved on the rest (redistribution) images taken 4 hours after exercise, indicating reversible ischemia based on a hemodynamic significant stenosis in one of the major coronary arteries. If both the exercise and rest scintigrams have similar defects i.e. show persistence of defects, then this finding is consistent with the presence of tissue necrosis based on a previous myocardial infarction. These observations of reduced myocardial perfusion visualized by thallium-201 have made this tracer a valuable tool in the diagnosis of coronary artery disease. However, thallium-201 has several important shortcomings as an adequate perfusion marker: (1) the low-level gamma emission of 80 keV is not ideal for in vivo imaging since a fair amount of photons will be attenuated by absorption in the body, (2) the extraction of thallium-201 is decreased in high blood flow states, and (3) the physical half-life of 72 hours precludes rapid sequential imaging and may give a relatively high total body exposure. From these observations it can be concluded that absolute measurements of coronary blood flow can not be made with the gamma-emitting monovalent cations. The findings on the thallium-201 scintigrams have to be read as relative intensities of distribution on the images. Since thallium-201 has been used for over 15 years in clinical cardiology, it may be mentioned that absolute measurements of coronary flow may not be required for clinical decision making and that relative determinations of regional distribution may suffice for clinical purposes.

b. Positron emitting radionuclides

Positron-emitting potassium analogs used for tomographic assessment of myocardial perfusion include isotopes of rubidium-82, nitrogen-13-labeled ammonia and oxygen-15 labeled water (Table 1).
Although positron-emitting agents can be imaged with a conventional Anger camera or a modified multicrystal camera, the best images are recorded with positron ring devices. The positron instruments combine high sensitivity and high resolution for myocardial imaging. Recent studies by Gould et al. (1) suggest that reductions of luminal diameter of less than 50% can be detected when these radionuclides are administered in conjunction with dipyridamole vasodilatation. The regional distribution of both ammonia and rubidium have excellent correlations with that of microspheres although they share the limitations of being diffusion-limited tracers (Fig. 4).

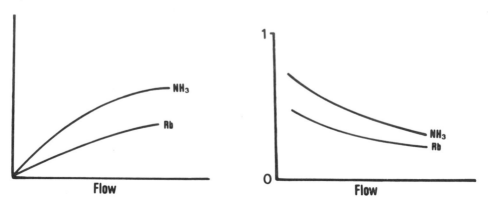

Figure 4

Uptake and extraction fraction of two partially extracted tracers, nitrogen-13 ammonia and rubidium-82, are shown as a function of flow. Extraction of these and similar tracers falls off at higher flows because shortened residence time in the capillary bed reduces uptake across capillary membranes.

From Gould KL, Mullani N, Wong W, Goldstein RA: Positron emission tomography. In: Cardiac imaging and image processing, Eds, Collins SE, Skorton DJ, 330-360, 1986 (with permission).

Rubidium-82

Rubidium-82 (half-life 75 seconds) is daughter of cyclotron-produced strontium-82 (half-life 25 days). The production of the parent strontium-82 requires a high-energy cyclotron, and is accompanied by the production of small quantities of strontium-85 as a radiocontaminant. Since strontium radionuclides localize in bone and have a long biological half-life, the generator system has been refined to minimize the 'breakthrough' of the parent in the eluate. Rubidium-82 (30 to 40 mCi) is eluted from the generator as a monovalent cation and, with a continuous supply from a bedside generator, an intravenous infusion results in an equilibrium in the arterial blood within four half-lives because of the dynamic equilibrium that develops between delivery and decay. The regional myocardial activity can be measured 30 seconds after turning off the intravenous infusion when the arterial activity has dropped to less than 50% of the maximum value in the myocardium. Myocardial imaging with rubidium-82 requires fast acquisition of data. The images recorded during the first 1-2 minutes after intravenous administration depict the blood pool distribution of the radionuclide (if images are recorded with gating, ejection fraction and regional wall motion can be determined), while images recorded after 2 minutes depict regional perfusion. Reasonable quality images can be recorded for 4 to 6 half-lives after infusion, i.e. 1 to 2 half-lives consumed with blood clearance and the remainder for myocardial perfusion.

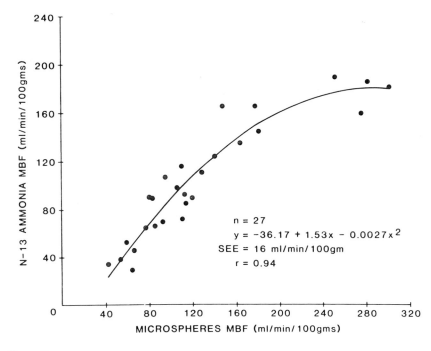

Figure 5

Relation between regional myocardial blood flow (MBF) determined with the microsphere technique and with nitrogen-13 labeled positron emission tomography in 27 dog experiments.
From Shah A, et al: J Am Coll Cardiol 5:92, 1985 (with permission).

Rubidium-82 imaging provides a repeatable and noninvasive measure of regional myocardial perfusion since each patient can be used as his own control. This is a considerable advantage when evaluating the responses of the coronary circulation in various physiologic states. Several studies have shown the value of rubidium-82 for the detection of coronary artery disease by the measurement of coronary flow reserve after dipyridamole-induced vasodilation (1,2). In this way performed, clinical decisions are not only based on arteriographic data but mainly on functional degrees of coronary artery abnormality. Relative disadvantages are 1) the remaining blood activity during the measurement after the infusion, 2) the inverse relation between flow and extraction, which may result in underestimation of increases in regional perfusion, and 3) the independent changes in rubidium uptake that can occur during metabolic abnormalities. However, all the experimental and clinical evidence to date indicates that regional decreases incoronary flow are reflected by changes in uptake of rubidium-82.

Nitrogen-13 ammonia

Nitrogen-13 labeled ammonia serves as a flow marker which concentrates in the myocardium with an extraction fraction of approximately 70%. Similar to rubidium-82, the net uptake of the tracer is related to blood flow in a curvilinear fashion (Fig. 5). This means that the relation between blood flow and myocardial nitrogen-13 ammonia is relatively linear over the physiological range of blood flow, but falls off at higher flows. Moreover, the uptake of nitrogen-13 ammonia by the myocardium is also dependent on metabolic trapping catalysed by glutamine synthetase. However, changes in myocardial blood flow can adequately be recorded by positron emission tomography, since ammonia activity concentrations measured by positron emission tomography have been shown to correlate very well with the standard microsphere technique (3). Accurate quantitation of regional myocardial perfusion with labeled ammonia (and also with rubidium-82) has been elusive, although valuable clinical information has been obtained including determination of extraction of labeled metabolic substrates (labeled glucose) with reference to estimates of perfusion. In addition, like rubidium-82, alterations of perfusion and regional myocardial metabolism in response to pharmacological vasodilator stress may be used to assess the severity of coronary artery disease. The relationship between abnormalities of ammonia extraction and changes in accumulation of labeled glucose may provide a description of viable but transiently ischemic myocardium.

The detection of coronary artery disease by both rubidium-82 and labeled ammonia during exercise or after dipyridamole administration has been improved compared to conventional planar thallium-201 scintigraphy; sensitivity as well as specificity approach 95%.

Radiolabeled water

A third short-lived cyclotron-produced positron emitting radionuclide, oxygen-15, can be used for measurement of coronary blood flow. The tracer can be administered by inhalation of oxygen-15 labeled carbon dioxide, which results in the distribution of oxygen-15 labeled water. It has also been shown that labeled water can be administered as an intravenous bolus.

The myocardial transit is recorded by positron emission tomography, separate blood pool subtraction can be performed with oxygen-15 labeled carbon monoxide, and measurements can then be made of regional myocardial perfusion. This provides another approach to the evaluation of coronary blood flow with negligible contribution from metabolic variables. The utility of this approach has been demonstrated in experimental canine preparations (4). In open chest dogs the single pass extraction of labeled water by the heart averaged 96 ±5% at flows of 80 to 100 ml/100g/min and did not differ significantly over a wide range of flows (from 12 to 300 ml/100 g/min).

Because the extraction fraction was high and consistent, the extraction of tracer appeared to be flow-limited rather than diffusion-limited over the ranges of flow studied. Thus, the tracer should provide a good index of flow in vivo. The underlying assumptions were tested initially in open chest dogs given a 60 seconds intravenous infusion of oxygen-15 labeled water. Labeled water content was measured directly by analysis of tissue.

Regional flow was calculated by direct application of the tissue autoradiographic method. Flows determined in this way correlated closely with flows measured with the radiolabeled microsphere technique (Fig. 6).

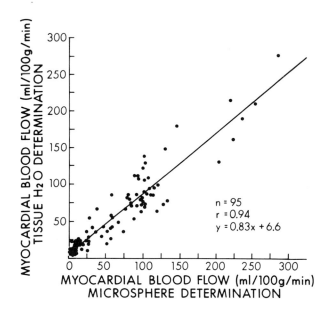

Figure 6
Correspondence between myocardial blood flow assessed with oxygen-15 water and radiolabeled micro-spheres determined invasively. The data, obtained from nine dogs pertain to normal and infarcted myocardium. In four animals flow was augmented with dipyridamole. A close correlation is demonstrated between flow measurements obtained with labeled water and with the microsphere technique.
From Bergmann SR et al: Circulation 70; 724, 1984 (by permission of the American Heart Association, Inc.).

The short physical half-life of oxygen-15 (2 minutes) allows sequential collection of the labeled water and labeled carbon monoxide images within approximately 10 minutes because counts from the first oxygen-15 study approach background after five half-lives.

Results obtained with positron emission tomography indicated that the labeled water determinations of flow correlated closely with those obtained tomographically with gallium-68 macroaggregated albumin microspheres. In subsequent studies, Huang et al. (5) demonstrated the feasibility of determination of myocardial blood flow with a more prolonged infusion of oxygen-15 labeled water tracer. Tomographic determinations of flow in vivo correlated closely with measurements with microspheres. A disadvantage of the labeled water technique is the high tracer activity in blood and lungs, which leads to activity cross-contamination. Nevertheless, it provides another approach for assessment of regional myocardial blood flow and represents therefore an interesting application of positron imaging.

(2) Inert gases

At times it is desirable to define myocardial perfusion in the catheterization laboratory by direct intracoronary injection. Under these circumstances, either the inert gases such as xenon-133 and krypton-81m, or particulate agents such as macroaggregated albumin, can be employed. The use of radioactive inert gases to measure myocardial blood flow requires intracoronary infusion of the gas or inhalation of gas with external detection of the emitted radiation during clearance of dilution of the radioactive gas from the circulation.

Xenon-133

Following intra-arterial administration xenon-133 (half-life 5.3 days) leaves the capillaries and enters tissue in direct proportion to its relative solubility in the tissue compared to that in blood (partition coefficient).
Thereafter, the clearance of the tracer from the tissue is dependent on the rate of perfusion. Measurement of coronary perfusion is based upon an approach developed by Kety and Schmidt described first in 1955 and applied initially to measurement of cerebral blood flow. The mathematical model employed describes the exchange of an inert diffusible tracer across the capillary tissue interface and between vascular and tissue compartments. It represents an extension of the Fick principle. Myocardial blood flow can be calculated from analysis of the clearance of radioactivity from the heart with a corollary of the Kety-Schmidt model.

$$F = KgW/D$$

where: F = myocardial blood flow (ml/100g/min)
K = myocardial tracer disappearance rate constant
g = tracer tissue: blood partition coefficient
W = weight of the myocardium
D = specific gravity of myocardium

Since the myocardial clearance of xenon-133 usually has a half-time of less than 1 minute, a scintillation camera must be present in the catheterization laboratory to measure the myocardial clearance. The rapid clearance of xenon makes it possible to record myocardial perfusion under several different circumstances in rapid succes-

18

sion, with an extremely low radiation burden to the patient (radiation burden of less than 0.1 rads to the myocardium per 0.5 mCi intracoronary injection, usual dose 20 to 30 mCi).

Serial measurements can be performed before, during and after interventions in the catherisation laboratory. Several studies (6,7) have shown the value of xenon-133 in quantitatively determining local perfusion rates in patients with stable angina during atrial pacing or in patients after myocardial infarction or after venous bypass surgery (Fig. 7).

Although the use of xenon-133 allows the measurement of absolute regional flow rates in ml/100g/min, several limitations have to be mentioned. Xenon-133 suffers from significant soft tissue attenuation because of its low gamma emission of 81 keV, which results in variable count statistics depending on uneven thickness of overlying muscle and breast tissue. Moreover and more importantly, xenon-133 shows a high fat solubility in subepicardial myocardial muscle which obscures the myocardial signal and slows the clearance of the tracer from the myocardium. Being a diffusable tracer, xenon-133 also shows a nonlinear correlation between net tissue tracer uptake and myocardial blood flow. Also problems related to streaming of the tracer from the left main stem to one or the other coronary arteries have to be taken into consideration. Despite these drawbacks, recent studies have shown that proper use and interpretation of the xenon technique may allow rapid and accurate asses-sment of regional myocardial perfusion.

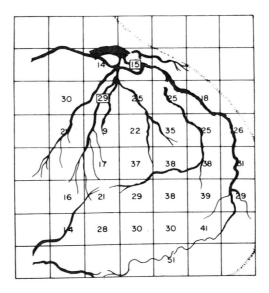

Figure 7
Diffuse reductions of myocardial perfusion are apparent in the left ventricular myocardium of a patient with marked disease of the diagonal and circumflex branches and complete occlusion of the anterior descending branch of the left coronary artery.
From Cannon et al. J Clin Invest 51: 964, 1972 (by copyright permission of the American Society for Clinical Investigation).

Krypton-81m

Ultrashort-lived nuclides have been suggested for the determination of regional myocardial perfusion. After the introduction of the rubidium-81/ krypton-81m generator, it was subsequently shown in animal experiments that krypton-81m (half-life 13 seconds) also had the potential to indicate regional myocardial flow changes. The parent rubidium-81 has a half-life of 4.6 hours, which is unfortunately relatively short. After administration of 20 mCi krypton-81m by continuous infusion directly into the coronary bed, krypton-81m achieves the highest concentration in areas of greatest perfusion. Static images of the distribution of radionuclide are related to the regional distribution. Following an intervention such as pacing, the radionuclide will re-equilibrate in the myocardium dependent on the redistribution of regional perfusion. Approximately three half-lives are required to obtain a new equilibrium state which reflects the regional distribution of perfusion. A second static image recorded under this circumstance can be compared to the image recorded at baseline to identify the change in regional perfusion. Similar to other diffusable tracers, the relationship of regional perfusion to radionuclide distribution with these agents is not linear. The krypton-81m enters the tissue as a result of its high permeability. The combination of short physical half-life and regional perfusion both contribute to the clearance of the radionuclide from the myocardium. As a result, the changes in regional perfusion contribute relatively little to the effective half-life of this agent (e.g., the effective half-life in normal myocardium is approximately 9 seconds, and if flow is doubled, the half-life decreases to 7 seconds, while if flow is halved the half-life increases to 10 seconds). Clinical studies (8) in 25 patients with coronary artery disease have shown that pacing-induced decrease in krypton-81m perfusion was found in all myocardial areas supplied by coronary arteries with more than 70% luminal narrowing. Also, all areas with more than 90% diameter reduction showed early perfusion defects before general signs of ischemia were noticed. Moreover, flow abnormalities persisted after discontinuation of pacing-induced ischemia, indicating an ongoing decrease in regional myocardial blood flow. These findings suggest that the krypton-81m technique has a greater sensitivity for detecting hemodynamically significant lesions than planar thallium-201 imaging.

Limitations of the technique are that only distributional changes can be assessed and not coronary flow changes in absolute quantities. Whether the observed changes really represent a regional decrease in coronary blood flow is impossible to know. A redistribution of radioactivity from areas with limited vasodilatory reserve and diminished increase in flow during pacing to normal areas can result in changes in krypton-81m perfusion as well. Similar to xenon-133, streaming may occur because of improper mixing of the tracer with blood in the left main stem. This may lead to an uneven and unstable distribution pattern. Advantages over xenon-133 are the high energy spectrum, absence of recirculation, and lack of affinity for fat tissue. In conclusion, the krypton-81m technique allows frequent and rapid determination of regional myocardial blood flow changes in patient with coronary artery disease.

(3) Particulate agents

The direct intracoronary administration of particulate radiopharmaceuticals in small quantities (50.000 particles) is safe, and can be particularly useful for defining the amount and the source of collateral perfusion. In this technique either a single radio-labeled microsphere is administered directly into one coronary artery and a second labeled particulate into the other, or the two radiopharmaceuticals can be administered through the same coronary bed before and after an intervention to define the change in myocardial perfusion (dual isotope technique).

Since the particulate radiopharmaceuticals remain in situ following administration, imaging can be performed for several hours after injection. The radiation burden to the myocardium is low, since only 0.1-0.2 mCi of the radiolabel is required to provide a very high quality image in a short interval of imaging. Both gamma- and positron-emitting particles have been used. For instance, macroaggregated albumin particles with a size of 30µ are usually labeled with technetium-99m. Also the positron-emitter gallium-68 has been used to label macroaggregates of albumin somewhat analogous to microspheres for quantification of regional myocardial blood flow in experimental animals. Tomographic measurements of flow corresponds closely with results obtained by quantification of conventional gamma emitting microspheres in samples of tissue assayed in vivo. Recently, carbon-11 has been covalently bound to albumin microspheres and used to measure regional myocardial blood flow tomographically in animals and in man. The limitations of this approach include the need for administration of tracer via left atrium or left ventricle and the potential hazards of administration of particulate material into the coronary circulation supplying myocardium in which perfusion may be compromised already. Nevertheless, adverse effects of such administration have not been evident clinically. Additional potential constraints relate to alterations in the distribution of microspheres with ischemia or when microvascular damage is present as may pertain with ischemia followed by reperfusion.

Direct patient applications have been twofold, 1) to evaluate of the perioperative status of the myocardium, and 2) to assess the physiologic significance of a coronary artery stenosis (9). By injection of different isotopes in each coronary artery, the two coronary beds can be separated which may be useful in preoperative planning. Specifically, the identification of collateral flow from the right coronary artery to the left system, in the presence of prior infarction of the right system, might argue for coronary artery bypass grafting to this artery which would otherwise not be considered since its native bed was infarcted. The second major application of the particle imaging technique is to assess the hemodynamical significance of a given coronary artery stenosis. Particle studies are likely more sensitive than thallium-201 exercise scintigraphy in identifying patients with significant coronary artery disease.

Important limitations are the invasive nature of the technique and the ability to detect only relative differences in flow, reason why the long-range clinical utility of the particle technique is uncertain and still no routine procedure in clinical practice.

(4) New perfusion imaging agents

The relatively poor resolution of thallium-201 has led to a search for a technetium-99m labeled perfusion agent. Efforts to combine technetium-99m into a lipid soluble charged complex appeared to offer the best opportunity for achieving successful myocardial concentration. Several technetium-99m labeled compounds, such as the diarsenical complex of technetium-99m (DiARS) and a dimethyl phospheno-ethane complex (DMPE), and a hexakis complex of technetium were tested in animals and found to have high myocardial uptake. The rapid myocardial concentration of these compounds fulfilled the criteria of Sapirstein tracers and a high correlation with regional perfusion was found. However, when DiARS and DMPE were administered to human subjects, their myocardial concentration was extremely disappointing.

When human studies with the technetium-99m labeled hexakis-isonitrile compound (Tc-99m SestaMIBI) were performed, however, sufficient concentration was observed in the human myocardium to permit high quality planar and tomographic images to be recorded (10). This agent combines the properties of high lipid solubility and technetium chelation. Tc-99m SestaMIBI achieves a localization of up to 2% of the injected dose in the human myocardium. The model of entry of this agent to the myocardium is not fully understood, but may depend primarily on solubility, rather than specific transport, as is the case with the monovalent cations. Following intravenous administration, the isonitrile localizes in the lungs to a sufficient degree that the myocardium cannot be visualized.

The clearance from the lungs is more rapid than that from the heart, which permits myocardial visualization about 1 hour after injection. Serial images recorded after the first hour indicate that myocardial clearance is slow and approximates the physical half-life of technetium-99m. The metabolic fate and the relationship of the distribution of Tc-99m SestaMIBI to regional perfusion are under investigation. It has been shown that, unlike thallium-201, the labeled isonitrile does not redistribute after exercise-induced ischemia (10). This means that an additional injection at rest is necessary for the assessment of transient ischemia. Comparison with thallium-201 did show good correlation in detecting normal and ischemic myocardium in patients with coronary artery disease (See Chapter 15 for current applications of Tc-99m SestaMIBI).

Conclusion

Blood flow measurements are useful in the following clinical situations: 1) detection of coronary artery disease, 2) assessment of pathology after coronary arteriography, 3) pre- and postoperative assessment of coronary artery disease, and 4) detection of acute myocardial infarction. Recent data have demonstrated the utility of applying gamma- and positron-emission tracers for delineation of myocardial ischemia and reperfusion in acute and chronic derangements. In addition, the functional impact of subcritical coronary arterial stenose on myocardial perfusion is definable with the radionuclide approach before and after pharmacologically induced vasodilatory stress.

In contrast to radionuclide techniques, angiographic criteria only define the distribution of the coronary stenoses and collaterals without directly characterizing the functional impact of the summation of these phenomena on myocardial perfusion. Accordingly, clinical assessment of the significance of coronary arterial abnormalities are likely to ultimately require consideration not only of angiographic data but also functional estimates or regional perfusion and factors which potentially modify extraction or clearance of radiolabeled tracers.

It is clear nowadays that the use of radioactive tracers for functional assessment of coronary artery flow has gained a definite role in experimental and clinical cardiology.

References

1. Gould KL, Goldstein RA, Mullani NA, Kirkeeide RL, Wong W-H, Tewson TJ, Berridge MS, Bolomey LA, Hartz RK, Smalling RW, Fuentes F. Noninvasive assessment of coronary stenoses by myocardial perfusion imaging during pharmacologic coronary vasodilation. VIII. Clinical feasibility of positron cardiac imaging without a cyclotron using generator-produced rubidium-82. J Am Coll Cardiol 1986; 4:775- 89.
2. Goldstein RA, Mullani NA, Wong W-H, Hartz RK, Hicks, CH, Fuentes F, Smalling RW, Gould KL: Positron imaging of myocardial infarction with rubidium-82. J Nucl Med 1986; 27:1824-9.
3. Gould KL, Schelbert HR, Phelps ME, Hoffman EJ. Noninvasive assessment of coronary stenoses with myocardial perfusion imaging during pharmacologic coronary vasodilation. V. Detection of 47 percent diameter coronary stenosis with intravenous nitrogen-13 ammonia emisson-computed tomography in intact dogs. Am J Cardiol 1979; 47: 200-8.
4. Bergmann SR, Fox KAA, Rand AL, McElvany KD, Welch MJ, Markham J, Sobel BE. Quantification of regional myocardial blood flow in vivo with H215O. Circulation 1984; 4:724-33.
5. Huang SC, Schwaiger M, Carson RE, Carson J, Hansen H, Selin C, Hoffman EJ, MacDonald N, Schelbert HR, Phelps ME. Quantitative measurement of myocardial blood flow with oxygen-15 water and positron computed tomography: An assessment of potential and problems. J Nucl Med 1980; 26:616-25.
6. Ruddy TD, Yasuda T, Barlai-Kovach M, Nedelman MA, Moore, RH, Alpert NM, Correia JA, Newell JB, Okada RD, Boucher CA, Strauss HW. Measurement of both left ventricular function and regional myocardial perfusion with 133Xe in dogs. Eur J Nucl Med 1987;12:533-41.
7. Korhola O, Valle M, Frick MH. Regional myocardial perfusion abnormalities of xenon-133 imaging in patients with angina pectoris and normal coronary arteries. Am J Cardiol 1977; 39:355-9.
8. Remme WJ, Krauss XH, Van Hoogenhuyze DCA, Cox PH, Storm CJ, Kruyssen DA. Continuous determination of regional myocardial blood flow with intracoronary krypton-81m in coronary artery disease. Am J Cardiol 1985; 56:445-51.

9. Kirk GA, Adams R, Jansen C, Judkins MP. Particulate myocardial perfusion scintigraphy: Its clinical usefulness in evaluation of coronary artery disease. Semin Nucl Med 1977; 7:67-84.
10. Sia STB, Holman BL, McKursick K, Rigo P, Gillis F, Sporn V, Perez-Balino N, Mitta A, Vosberg H, Szabo Z, Schwartzkopff B, Moretti J, Davison A, Lister-James J, Jones A. The utilization of Tc-99m-TBI as a myocardial perfusion agent in exercise studies: Comparison with Tl-201 thallous chloride and examination of its biodistribution in humans. Eur J Nucl Med 1986; 12:333-6.

2.
Metabolism:
Assessment of myocardial metabolism with radiolabeled free fatty acids

Introduction

The regional, noninvasive assessment of myocardial functional integrity with the aim of identifying normal, ischemic and necrotic zones is highly desirable in patients with coronary artery disease (CAD). Therefore attempts have been made to determinate the metabolic integrity of the myocardium quantitatively with radioactively labeled metabolic substrates. Since free fatty acids (FFA) are primary substrates of the normally perfused myocardium, it appears likely that radiolabeled FFA are suitable for the study of myocardial FFA metabolism.

Generally the following requirements for metabolic isotope tracers have to be met:
(a) they should be highly specific indicators of a given metabolic pathway;
(b) they must not alter the physiological behavior of metabolic substrates;
(c) they have to provide an adequate external detection by current imaging devices (gamma or positron camera);
(d) they must be clinically applicable.

These conditions are best fulfilled by radionuclides with chemical identities akin to physiological substrates such as carbon (C), nitrogen (N) and oxygen (O).

C-11, N-13, and O-15 are the isotopes of the constituents of most living matter and of most molecules involved in the majority of metabolic processes. Moreover they are positron-emitting radionuclides (Table 1) and the combined use with positron tomography (PET) offers potential advantages for the assessment of myocardial integrity. An added advantage of these radionuclides is their short half-lives, allowing repeated measurements at short intervals which can be of much importance in intervention procedures.

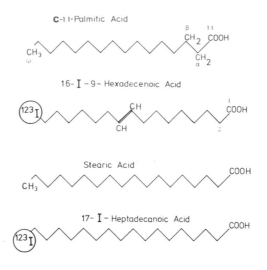

Figure 1

General structure of C-11-palmitate, stearic acid and the most currently used iodinated free fatty acids.

In spite of the advantages of C-11, N-13 and O-15, their use in the assessment of myocardial integrity has been documented only in a limited number of studies. This is due to several factors. Because of the short half-lives the production of these nuclides requires the availability of a cyclotron (or other particle accelerator) in the laboratory where they are to be used. Furthermore, the rapid incorporation of these nuclides into useful molecules is difficult, and the tomographic devices (special positron cameras) necessary for the imaging of these nuclides are complex and expensive. In the recent past, however, the usefulness of this approach has become generally accepted, and the scientific literature contains an increasing number of reports of the use of PET and physiological indicators in the study of the myocardium. Regarding FFA, it would be very convenient to use isotopes of the natural elements of FFA, which are C, O and hydrogen (H), but only C-11 has proven to be adequate as a label to FFA.

Besides metabolic studies with PET, attention has been focused on gamma-emitting radionuclides labeled to FFA, because of potentially wider applicability and lower cost. Moreover, since most suitable gamma-emitting radionuclides have physical half-lives of more than several hours, no in-house cyclotron is required. For instance, iodine-123 (I-123, half-life 13.3 hours) may be very well tagged to FFA and can easily be detected with any commercially available gamma camera.

Table 1
Positron- and gamma-emitting radionuclides potentially used for evaluation of cardiac metabolism

Radionuclide	Emission	Half-life	Production
0-15	positron (511 keV)	2.03 min	requires in-house cyclotron
N-13	positron (511 keV)	9.98 min	requires in-house cyclotron
C-11	positron (511 keV)	20.4 min	requires in-house cyclotron
I-123	gamma (159 keV)	13.3 h	cyclotron-produced
I-131	gamma (364 keV)	8.06 days	reactor-produced
Te-123m	gamma (159 keV)	120 days	cyclotron produced

Although many different labeled fatty acids have been studied, this review will mainly call attention to the most important investigations in this field, i.e. the study of FFA labeled with the physiological tracer C-11 and with I-123 (Figure 1).

We will firstly describe the myocardial FFA metabolism, then consider the metabolism and kinetics of radiolabeled FFA and finally discuss the potential clinical value of radiolabeled FFA.

Myocardial fatty acid metabolism

FFA are preferred myocardial substrates and fatty acid oxidation normally accounts for 60 to 80% of energy production by the heart. Even when moderate ischemia supervenes, FFA liberated from triglycerides are metabolized in preference to glucose. However, under conditions of marked ischemia or severe hypoxia (oxygen delivery less than 20% of normal), anaerobic metabolism provides a substantial proportion of energy via glycolytic mechanisms.

The metabolic pathway of fatty acid has been well clarified (Figure 2). Long-chain fatty acids are synthesized in the liver and adipose tissue, transported in blood bound primarily to albumin, and extracted by myocardium as a function of several factors including: chain length, molarity of both albumin and fatty acid, metabolic integrity of the cell, perfusion (since regional coronary flow determines residence time), and myocardial energy requirements. Both ischemia and hypoxia lead to decreased extraction.

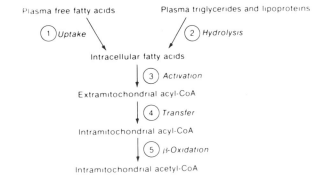

Figure 2
Overall scheme of fatty acid metabolism (From Katz A M, (1977) Physiology of the Heart, New York, Raven Press, with permission).

27

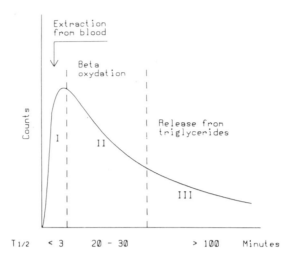

Figure 3
Schematic illustration of the characteristic time-activity curve of clinically used radiolabeled FFA in the myocardium. Three different phases are recognized.

Fatty acids in interstitial or intracellular fluid are bound to soluble proteins, and uptake of fatty acids into the cell appears to depend on competition between cellular binding sites and binding sites on albumin. Intracellular fatty acids are activated and converted to thioester derivatives in the cytosol in reactions requiring both coenzyme A (CoA) and ATP. Esterified fatty acids may undergo oxidation or incorporation into triglycerides.

Activated fatty acids in the cytosol cannot be oxidized directly. They are first transported across the mitochondrial membrane by acyl CoA carnitine transferases specific for chain length and intimately associated with mitochondrial membranes. Carnitine-dependent translocation facilitates ingress of acyl CoA into the mitochondrial matrix where beta-oxidation occurs. Acyl CoA is oxidized to produce acetyl CoA which is oxidized via the Krebs cycle with liberation of CO_2 and synthesis of intracellular ATP. The knowledge of altered fatty acid metabolism in myocardial ischemia stimulated labeling procedures with FFA for the detection of CAD.

Metabolism and pharmacokinetic behaviour of labeled FFA

The first efforts with radiolabeled FFA were mainly pointed at the search for myocardial imaging agents. It was only recently that the noninvasive study of regional metabolic turnover rates in the myocardium has become a potential issue. For quantification of metabolic rates, the pharmacokinetics of these tracers in the myocardium in terms of uptake and clearance and their relationship to the biochemical process must be known.

Previous experimental studies [1,2] have revealed a similar type of pharmacokinetics in the heart both for C-11-palmitic acid and for iodinated fatty acids (Figure 3). The kinetics exhibit a fast uptake which represents the extraction from blood (phase I). This first phase simply reflects perfusion as has been demonstrated by studies [3] comparing labeled ammonia (N-13-H3) and C-11-palmitic acid. Then, two elimination phases follow, a fast and a slow one. The fast elimination phase (phase II) is considered to represent beta-oxidation and is clinically the most relevant phase. The third phase can be attributed to release of fatty acids which has been stored before as triglycerides and phospholipids. Turnover rates of the labeled FFA can be expressed in terms of half-time values (minutes) calculated from the best-fit mono- or biexponential function of the different phases of the time-activity curve. For I-123 terminally labeled to heptadecanoic acid, the fast elimination phase has a half-time of about 25 min in man. Regarding C-11-palmitate, about similar half-time values have been clinically demonstrated [4]. The slow elimination (phase III) can hardly be seen in man and imaging is generally stopped 30 to 60 min after injection because the activity levels become too low for appropriate measurements.

The resemblance of the clearance curves of I-123-FFA and of C-11-palmitate suggests that clearance of I-123 reflects natural metabolism of FFA. Small differences in clearance pattern may still be expected since the C-11 label is removed from the fatty acid in the first step of beta-oxidation with subsequent degrading in the Krebs cycle and exhalation as C-11-02, while the radioiodine label at the terminal carbon atom is probably removed in the last step of beta-oxidation and released in to the circulation before or in the Krebs cycle.

Accordingly, the kinetics of I-123-FFA may parallel metabolism of FFA in uptake of FFA and beta-oxidation pathway. Therefore, clearance of I-123-FFA has been regarded to reflect metabolic turnover of FFA in the myocardium. This view is partly supported by Dudczak et al. [5] and Comet et al. [6], who experimentally demonstrated that halothane anesthesia and cardiac drugs, such as verapamil and propranolol, considerably influenced the clearance rates. In contrast, doxorubicin did not change the elimination rates of I-123-HDA, obtained from dog hearts. As a result, considerable debate has arisen about the proper explanation for the elimination half-time in the second phase. It has been postulated that the measured half-times of iodinated FFA do not correlate with beta-oxidation but are due to the rate of diffusion of free iodide from the mitochondria into the coronary circulation [8]. Such nonspecific deiodination would limit the use of iodinated FFA to evaluate oxidative FFA metabolism based on analysis of myocardial clearance curves.

On the other hand, with respect to C-11-palmitate, it remains to be proven that clearance of tracer is really due to oxidative metabolism with resultant formation of C-11-02 and not to washout of oxidation products, such as short-chain intermediates via the coronary circulation [9]. In experiments with C-14 palmitate in rabbit hearts [23] it was observed that at 5 min almost 40% of extracted myocardial activity was already in the aqueous phase, indicating the early presence of products of palmitate catabolism. These factors become of crucial importance during reduced oxidative metabolism induced either by the decreased coronary flow (ischemia) or diminished oxygen delivery (hypoxia).

Lerch et al. [10] demonstrated that clearance of C-11-palmitate was constantly depressed in regions with restricted oxygen supply regardless of concomitant reduction of flow, and they concluded that metabolism itself is the major determinant of reduced regional clearance. Schelbert et al. [11] suggested that results would be distorted because of altered residence time (i.e. duration of myocardial exposure to labeled substrates) or that altered washout would mask detection of impaired metabolism caused by ischemia or hypoxia. Later studies by his group indicated that measuring FFA oxidation rates is till possible in ischemia but probably with a lower accuracy than in normal myocardium [12].

The exact mechanism can only be clarified by experimentally studying the content of free I-123 or free C-11-02 per unit myocardial weight or from coronary venous blood when measured acutely after injection and under different pathophysiological circumstances.

Recent results obtained from canine studies by our group [13] and Kloster et al. [14], in which a rather high percentage of free iodide (40-60%) was found a few minutes after injection of I-123-heptadecanoic acid (I-123-HDA), suggest that the diffusion of iodide from the cell to the circulation is an important step in the description of myocardial clearance rates.

Fox et al. (66) reported that under normal conditions about 45% of C-11-palmitate has metabolized while 6% showed back-diffusion in unaltered form. In contrast, with ischemia 17% was metabolized to C-11-O2, while 16% (i.e. half of the amount cleared) evolved as C-11-palmitate. It was concluded that effects of nonmetabolized FFA must be taken into account when analyzing clearance curves.

Further studies are therefore needed to unravel the intimate relationship between uptake and clearance of labeled FFA, and to prove whether they really represent oxidative myocardial FFA metabolism.

Experimental and clinical results

C-11-palmitate

C-11 provides a particularly suitable label for FFA imaging because of its property as a positron emitting radionuclide. C-11 labeled to palmitate was first used for the visualization of the myocardium by PET in 1976 [2]. C-11-palmitate was found to accumulate substantially in isolated perfused hearts under aerobic conditions, and since reduction of coronary flow is accompanied by decreased FFA extraction, C-11-palmitate was utilized to image normal, transiently ischemic, and irreversibly injured myocardium in intact dogs.

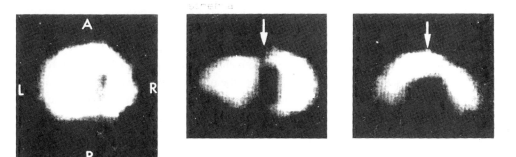

Figure 4

Positron-emission transaxial tomography after induction of transient myocardial ischemia by constriction of an exteriorized coronary artery occlusive cuff in an intact dog. Each image represents a reconstructed cross-sectional slice through the heart at the ventricular level. Anterior, posterior, left and right are indicated by the letters A, P, L, and R, respectively. In the top panel homogeneous accumulation of C-11-palmitate acid is evident in the normal left ventricular myocardium. The tomogram was obtained during a 20-min interval after intravenous injection of tracer. In the center panel, a transmural defect representing failure of accumulation (arrow) of C-11-palmitate is present anteriorly in an image obtained after 30 min of myocardial ischemia. The image shown in the lower panel was obtained during the 20-min interval immediately following release of the coronary artery occlusive cuff after an interval of ischemia of 30 min, hence insufficient to produce extensive infarction. As can be seen, after reperfusion, myocardial metabolic integrity is demonstrable in the area of the previous defect (arrow) and, in fact, the accumulation of tracer in this region exceeds that adjacent and presumably normal myocardium. (From E.S.Weiss et al., Circ Res 39:24-32, 1976. By permission of the American Heart Association Inc.)

In later studies, Weiss et al. [16] determined the distribution of the tracer in the dog heart by positron emission tomography (PET) and demonstrated that significant reversal of depressed C-11-palmitate accumulation in the ischemic zone occurred when coronary artery occlusion was maintained for less than 20 min, but that an irreversibly reduced uptake pattern was observed when reperfusion was delayed for 60 min or more (Figure 4). In a clinical study, Sobel et al. [17] demonstrated with PET that the distribution of C-11-palmitate in patients with remote myocardial infarction was analogous to the distribution observed in animals with experimentally-induced infarction. Subsequent studies in man have shown that infarct size determined by PET correlated with infarct size assessed by creatine kinase (MB) blood curves [18]. Geltman et al. [19] showed in 46 patients that both transmural and nontransmural infarctions could be detected with PET. All 22 patients with transmural infarctions had decreased C-11-palmitate uptake in the infarcted regions while in 23 out of 24 patients with nontransmural infarctions the area of diminished C-11-palmitate uptake was often nontransmural and a thin area of normal C-11 uptake was present. Moreover, a heterogeneous uptake pattern was observed in the adjacent myocardium, suggesting an admixture of normal cells in the surrounding area.

Regarding kinetics of C-11-palmitate Schön et al. [20] showed that labeled palmitate cleared from the myocardium in a biexponential fashion, indicating tracer distribution between at least two pools with different turnover rates. This clearance pattern reflects the distribution of FFA between immediate oxidation (the rapid turnover phase) and the intermediate storage in the endogeneous lipid pool (the slow turnover phase).

Al these studies indicate a promising and practical application for C-11-palmitate, especially since the evaluation of the effectiveness of therapeutic intervention for the protection of ischemic myocardium requires the quantitative assessment of the distribution and extent of jeopardized and irreversibly injured myocardium. Bergmann et al. [22] experimentally demonstrated in 1982 (by measuring uptake of C-11-palmitate) that successful streptokinase treatment, when initiated within 4 h after occlusion, showed preservation of cardiac metabolism while later treatment did not result in significant salutary metabolic effects. Also Ludbrook et al. [22] studied 17 patients with C-11-palmitate after therapy with intracoronary streptokinase and demonstrated in the 8 patients with successful thrombolysis increased uptake of C-11-palmitate in the affected areas indicating improvement of regional metabolism and salvage of jeopardized myocardial tissue. Recently reported studies [4, 9, 10, 20, 23] by the groups of Schelbert and Sobel have delineated the myocardial kinetics under normal and ischemic conditions, and the rate of clearance of C-11 activity from the myocardium was considered as an index of the oxidation rate of C-11-palmitate. It was shown in dogs and also in patients with exercise-induced ischemia that clearance of C-11-palmitate from ischemic regions was decreased compared to normal regions. Henze et al. [4] demonstrated in patients with pacemaker-induced ischemia that clearance from the ischemic regions was substantially decreased compared to normal myocardial regions.

On the other hand, increases in cardiac work and myocardial oxygen consumption raise the fraction of tracer entering the rapid turnover pool and accelerate the clearance rate of C-11 activity from myocardial tissue, which reflects enhanced FFA oxidation as a response to higher energy demands (Figure 5).

Table 2 shows the clearance rates of the most currently used labeled FFA expressed in minutes half-time.

Table 2
Metabolic clearance rates of various labeled FFA from normal and ischemic myocardial regions (in minutes).

FFA	Species	Clearance rates (Phase II) in minutes half time		Reference number
		normal	ischemia(I)[f]	
C-11 palmitate	dog	8.8 ± 3.5	14.9 ± 7.0	[62]
	dog	11.6	>12[g]	[9]
	man	22.6 ± 5.6	>23[g]	[4]
I-131-HA[a]	dog	20.0 ± 2.3	[h]	[2]
	dog	14.2 ± 1.4	22.6 ± 1.8	[36]
I-123-HA[b]	dog	14.0 ± 6.7	[h]	[6]
	man	25	>48[g]	[29]
	man	[h]	(18.5 ± 2.5, AMI)[e]	[33]
I-123-HDA[c]	man	25.0 ± 5.0	31.8 ± 19.6[i]	[30]
	man	24	46	[34]
	man	20-30	35-50	[63]
	man	27.5 ± 3.0	46 ± 7.1	[33,35]
			(16.8 ± 3.5, AMI)[e]	
I-1233-PPA[d]	dog	42	202, AMI[e]	[50]
	man	50-60	80-150	[53]
	man	46	61	[48]
	man	>60[g]	[h]	[51]

[a] I-131-hexadecenoic acid

[b] I-123-hexadecenoic acid

[c] I-123-heptadecanoic acid

[d] I-123-phenyl-pentadecanoic acid.

[e] Acute myocardial infarction.

[f] Transient ischemia, unless otherwise noted.

[g] No exact values mentioned.

[h] Not studied

[i] Obtained from the entire myocardium.

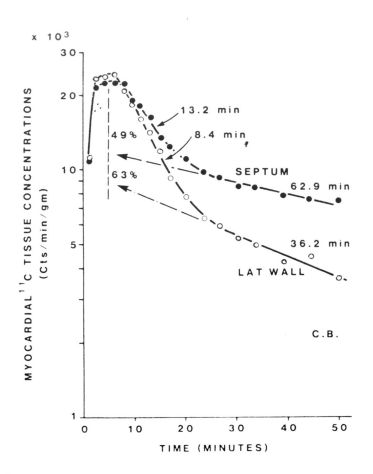

Figure 5

Time activity curves obtained during pacing-induced ischemia, derived from a region of interest over the nonischemic spectrum and the ischemia lateral wall. C-11 activity increases in both normal (open circles) and ischemic (closed circles) myocardium. Subsequent clearance of C-11 activity from ischemic and normal myocardium is biexponential. By back-extrapolation of the slow clearance phase, the relative sizes of the early rapid components can be estimated. In ischemic compared with normal myocardium, the relative size of the early curve component is smaller (49% vs 63%), and the half-time of the early clearance phase is slower (8.4 min vs 13 min). (From M. Grover and H.R. Schelbert, Positron emission computed tomography. In: Digital Cardiac Imaging, Eds. A.J. Buda and E.J. Delp, 1985, Martinus Nijhoff Publishers, with permission).

Radioiodinated FFA

One of the earliest attempts at cardiac imaging was performed with FFA labeled with iodine-131 (I-131, half-life 8.06 days). In 1965, Evans et al. [24] iodinated oleic acid across the double bond and demonstrated that this could be used to visualize the myocardium and to detect myocardial infarction. This substance never became clinically useful because of its low specific activity, poor imaging quality and limitations in administered activity, dictated by radiation dosimetry. Moreover, iodination of FFA at the double bond strongly influenced extraction and elimination of the labeled compound.

In 1975, Robinson et al. [25] made considerable progress by introducing radiation into the terminal (omega) position of a fatty acid (hexadecanoic acid) without altering its extraction efficiency compared to the naturally occurring compound. Poe et al. [26] postulated that the iodine atom in the terminal position maintains a configuration similar to a methyl group (both with an atomic radius of 2 Angstrom) and that the resultant molecule behaves as though it possesses an extra carbon atom.

In this context 16-iodo-hexadecanoic acid (HA) would behave like heptadecanoic acid (HDA). Furthermore, it was shown that a chain length of 15 to 21 carbon atoms had the most optimal myocardial extraction [27], indicating that for metabolic studies a chain length of 16 or 17 carbon atoms appears to be very suitable.

Terminally labeled hexadecanoic acid demonstrated an initial myocardial distribution proportional to blood flow and, when labeled with I-123, its myocardial extraction of 78% and blood clearance half-time of 1.7 min closely resembled K-43 and Tl-201 distribution [2, 28]). From these studies it was inferred that I-123-FFA are distributed according to myocardial blood flow and subsequently metabolized by known metabolic pathways. Compared to I-123, Tl-201 has a low photon-energy of 80 keV resulting in important tissue absorption, and moreover a rather long physical (72 h) and myocardial half-life (7 h) which gives a total body exposure of 210 mrads/mCi and precludes rapid sequential imaging. I-123 is a gamma-emitter with suitable photon-energy (159 keV) for the currently available gamma cameras, it has a favourable physical half-life of 13.3 h and offers a relatively low whole body radiation dose to the patient (30 mrads/mCi). Table 3 shows the most important radiophysical properties of Tl-201 and I-123-FFA.

In 1977, Poe et al. [29] injected 5 mCi I-123-HA intravenously in patients with CAD and images containing about one million net counts from the total myocardium could be obtained with 10 min. In 1978, Machulla et al. [1] experimentally used various radiolabeled FFA and showed that terminally labeled I-123-HDA had a myocardial uptake and elimination almost the same as that of C-11-palmitate. This study has been clinically extended in 1980 by the group of Feinendegen et al. [30] and demonstrated reduced tracer uptake in ischemic myocardial zones using I-123-HDA. Not only high quality images were obtained, but also elimination of I-123 from the myocardium could be followed by calculating clearance half-times of I-123-HDA from distinct myocardial regions. All these investigative studies emphasized the potential value of I-123-FFA (hexadecanoic and heptadecanoic acid) for myocardial scintigraphy not only for myocardial imaging purposes, but also to evaluate myocardial metabolism in patients with CAD.

Table 3
Radiophysical properties of TI-201 and of I-123-FFA

	T1-201	I-123-FFA
Gamma camera detection efficiency (keV)	80	159
Myocardial extraction (%)	87	78
Physical half-life (hours)	72	13
Biological half-life (hours)	7	0,5
Body exposure (mrads/mCi)	210	30

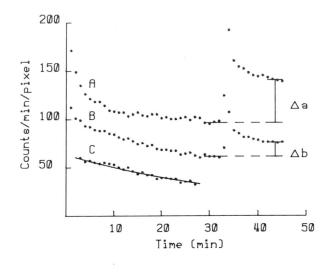

Figure 6
Schematic illustration of the correction method.

Regions of interest (ROI) are made over lung tissue and a distinct part of the myocardium, resulting in curve A, resp. B. After administration of 123-I-iodide, 30 min after injection of 123-I-FFA, in both regions an increase is found proportional to the amount of circulating blood in the ROI (△a, resp. △b).

Consequently the count-rate (CR) in lung tissue is proportional to the concentration of circulating in the blood i.e. CR (I-total, A) = CR(I⁻,A). Furthermore the CR in the myocardium will be proportional to the amount of circulating blood iodide plus the amount of "bound" fatty accid, CR(I-FFA,B). Therefore the following equation is valid:

$$CR \text{ (I-FFA, B} = CR \text{ (I-total, B)} - \frac{\triangle b}{\triangle a}. CR \text{ (I-total, A)}$$

If CR (I-FFA, B) is plotted versus time, the blood background corrected curve is found, which represents the net turnover of 123-I-FFA in the myocardium. So for every point (t)* in the corrected curve C holds:

$$C \text{ (t)} = b \text{ (t)} - \frac{\triangle b}{\triangle a}. A \text{ (t)}. \qquad * \text{ (every fifth point plotted)}$$

So far, clinical studies have been hampered by restricted commercial supply and the technical problem of a rapidly increasing background radioactivity due to release of free radioiodide into circulation after administration of I-123-FFA. It has been shown that within 15 min after intravenous administration of I-123-HDA, about 50% of the radioactivity in the blood consists of free iodide, which implies that only within this time-limit (preferably within 10 min after administration) good analogue images can be obtained [31]. Roesler et al. [32] studied patients with CAD, using a 7-pinhole collimator and compared the imaging quality of I-123-HDA with that of Tl-201. Similar images were observed and I-123-HDA proved to have no advantages over Tl-201 with respect to imaging quality.

The background problem has been met by a specially designed computer-aided correction procedure, described by Van der Wall et al. [33]. The correction method must be used to correct the serial images for background activity from the I-123 in the blood pool i.e. for iodide not bound to the myocardial cells. The procedure is based on the quantitative evaluation of the contribution of inorganic I-123 to the image. Its principle is schematically presented in Figure 6.

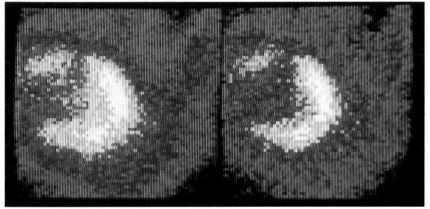

Figure 7
Myocardial I-123-heptadecanoic acid scintigram before (left) and after correction in a patient with antero-septal infarction.

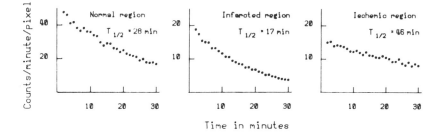

Figure 8
Time-activity curves derived from normal, ischemic and infarcted myocardial region.

The correction procedure results in good quality scintigrams which provide a better contrast between myocardial and surrounding tissue (Figure 7), and this procedure enables the calculation of time-activity curves which may serve as a parameter for the metabolic turnover of FFA in the myocardium. A drawback of turnover rate measurements is the long imaging period of 45 min and the acquisition of one single view per study which may underdiagnose the presence of CAD. The single view problem can of course be obviated by employment of a biplanar collimator [34].

We studied the kinetics of I-123-FFA in patients with stable and unstable angina pectoris, and patients with acute myocardial infarction (AMI) and we observed different turnover rates of normally perfused, transient ischemic and acutely infarcted areas [33,35]. With reference to half-time values measured in apparently normal regions (20-30 min), we demonstrated increased values in ischemic zones (> 40 min) and decreased values (< 20 min) in infarcted zones, suggesting a slow and a fast metabolic turnover of I-123-FFA respectively. Figure 8 gives schematically the observed turnover rates from different myocardial regions. Based on our results, it was postulated that I-123-FFA offer the diagnostic potential to distinguish reversible from irreversible ischemia. Although clinically interesting, and supported by animal experiments [36] and other clinical studies [37], these findings have to be confirmed by studies in much larger populations. Another application of I-123-HDA is its use in patients after successful thrombolysis. Two clinical studies [38, 39] reported the value of I-123-HDA in assessing the metabolic integrity of reperfused myocardium within 1 week after AMI, based on the reduction of defect size and normalization of half-time values. Also in patients with congestive cardiomyopathy (COCM), it has been shown that the determination of clearance rates could be of significant value [40]. All patients with COCM showed inhomogeneous tracer distribution and low clearance rates of I-123-HDA, suggesting altered FFA metabolism in diseases myocardial regions. In a recent study by Rabinowitz et al. [41] it was reported that scintigraphy with I-123-HDA should be of interest as a screening test for carnitine deficiency in patients with a variety of cardiomyopathies (see chapter 12).

Classification of primary cardiomyopathies is currently based on anatomic and functional abnormalities regardless of the underlying etiology. Biochemical studies will not only enhance our understanding of these disorders as well as their detection and characterization but will also aid in the development of effective treatment [65].

Also results of venous bypass surgery and the effect of cardiac rehabilitation have been assessed with I-123-HDA by the measurement of myocardial clearance rates [42, 43].

Future prospects

New biochemical concepts have been proposed to avoid the high background activity in imaging studies of the myocardium [44]. Attaching the iodine label to a benzene ring located in the terminal position of a fatty acid (I-123-phenyl-pentadecanoic acid; I-123-PPA) results in a radiopharmaceutical which shows essentially no release of

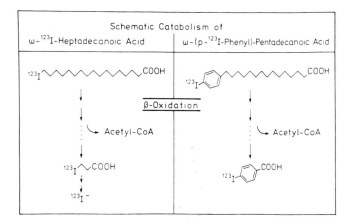

Figure 9

Final products from I-123-heptadecanoic acid (free radioiodide) and from I-123-phenyl-pentadecanoic acid (benzoic acid). Reproduced from Machulla, with permission [44].

free radioiodide into the circulation (Figure 9). The final catabolite of I-123-PPA consists of benzoic acid, which is fastly detoxificated and so obviates background problems.

Uptake of I-123-PPA parallels regional myocardial flow in both normal and ischemic myocardium [45], and I-123-PPA can therefore be employed for imaging purposes [46]. Since the breakdown products of phenyl-fatty acids will reside much longer in the cells, myocardial clearance will be considerably delayed and makes proper metabolic studies very complicated [47], although recent papers have reported the value of clearance rates of I-123-PPA for the detection of CAD and the evaluation of cardiomyopathies [48-51]. Reske et al. [52] compared quantitatively the uptake and metabolism of I-PPA with C-14-palmitate in rats, and observed a very similar pattern for both tracers. Moreover they showed in canine studies that initial uptake of I-PPA was related to myocardial uptake both under control conditions and in ischemia. In clinical studies, patients with significant CAD and with myocardial infarction were accurately detected and localized with I-123-PPA. In our institution, elimination half-times of much more than 60 min from normal human hearts have been calculated [51], which probably excludes measurement of oxidative metabolism and will only reflect turnover of triglycerides [53]. However, I-123-PPA has been shown a valuable metabolic tracer in many clinical studies.

A next labeled fatty acid that recently [54] has been proposed is tellurium-123m-9-telluraheptadecanoic acid (Te-123m-THDA). This radiopharmaceutical gives a reasonable imaging quality in dog hearts. However, the physical and myocardial biological half-lives of Te-123m are respectively 120 and 7 days, which precludes metabolic clearance studies. In addition, and apart from high radiation doses, experimental studies [55] showed toxic effects in rats, and further toxicity studies are necessary before considering Te-123m-THDA as a myocardial imaging agent in man.

Another new metabolic tracer is C-11-beta-methyl-heptadecanoic acid (C-11-BMHDA) [56]. This compound is obtained by inserting a methyl radical in the beta-position and so inhibits beta-oxidation. It is therefore trapped in the myocardium and can not further be metabolized (nearly constant level of activity in the dog myocardium for 60 min). Therefore, the beta-methyl branched FFA are very suitable for studies of regional distribution and can be used to study myocardial perfusion, but more importantly, can be used to study aberrations in FFA metabolism under normal flow conditions where regional FFA uptake may be correlated with several aspects of regional metabolism. In a recent study [57] by our group, we evaluated the uptake and kinetics of 15-p-(I-125)-iodophenyl-3-beta-methyl-pentadecanoic acid (I-125-BMPPA) in diabetic rats. It was shown that myocardial uptake in diabetic rats was higher than in normal rats despite increased plasma FFA. Furthermore, washout over 60 min was slower in the diabetic hearts compared to the normal hearts.

It was concluded that radiolabeled I-BMPPA handling is different in diabetic myocardium compared to nondiabetic myocardium, which may have important implications for myocardial imaging. Newer developments concern with different biochemical steps in the metabolism of FFA such as studies with C-11 labeled acetate and pyruvate. These labeled metabolic products may provide insight into the overall metabolism of the heart under various conditions. Moreover, enzyme deficiencies (for instance lack of carnitine) can be detected with these labeled metabolic products and the therapeutic effectiveness can be evaluated.

Conclusion

Cardiac disease, in particular CAD, is at present most frequently diagnosed and treated in its final stage, after structural or anatomic derangements are already present. However, disease begins at the biochemical level and therapies are designed to halt or reverse abnormal biochemical processes, restore delivery of biochemical nutrients, or supplement depleted ones. Any technique that provides biochemically specific information about the myocardium could play a vital role in the early diagnosis and effective management of human cardiac disease [65].

Until now, clinical studies have been scarce mainly due to restricted availability of radiopharmaceuticals and to limited equipment facilities. Chapter 10 adresses the most relevant clinical applications of metabolic tracers.

Positron emission tomography

The PET technique potentially provides a unique tool to investigate regional myocardial metabolism noninvasively, although the initial as well as the operational costs of positron emission tomography have been major limitations for widespread application and the number of positron cameras throughout the world is still very small. In addition, one might legitimately question the usefulness of an imaging technique limited to the small number of positron-emitting radionuclides as compared to the considerably greater number of gamma-emitters, particularly in light of the fact that positron emission tomographs are expensive and complex devices which cannot be used for the imaging of the more common gamma-ray emitters. However, dedicated and reliable medical minicyclotrons with less technical requirements and lower costs are currently developed, combined with automated synthesis techniques. A substantial problem is the proper interpretation of clearance curves because of back-diffusion of nonmetabolized substrates.

At present, clinical studies with C-11-palmitate are limited and its interest remains of investigational value. In a recent experimental study by Schwaiger et al. [58], it was reported that C-11-palmitate in conjunction with PET may be helpful to identify reversibly injured myocardium. This finding stimulates continuation of metabolic studies with C-11-palmitate. Further studies will be needed to demonstrate the clinical utility of the PET technique for detection of cardiac disease prior to irreversible damage and to design therapeutic regimens more precisely.

Radioiodinated FFA

Radioiodinated FFA have become commercially available and can therefore be used on a routine basis in clinical practice [56-61, 67].

Regarding clinical use, we think it wise to make a clear distinction between studies for imaging purposes and for metabolic investigations. As for imaging in patients with CAD, excellent images can be obtained. Similar to C-11-palmitate, however, the value of the kinetics remain to be established. The study of myocardial FFA metabolism by the noninvasive measurement of turnover rates is still in the experimental phase and its understanding needs the combined efforts of both nuclear medicine and myocardial biochemistry. Adequate application of I-FFA will give more information of cardiac function than just the scintigraphic pictures do. Valid questions with respect to analysis of metabolic clearance rates are

1) how long after injection should we measure,

2) is the correction method really necessary,

3) which part of the curve has to be considered,

4) do we have to apply a mono- or biexponential curve fitting, and lastly

5) do we really measure FFA degradation or are other mechanisms responsible for the observed phenomenon.

Still controversies exist, whether deiodination of I-123-FFA is a nonspecific process or is related to oxidative FFA metabolism. An urgent problem that has to be solved is the understanding of the coupling of flow and metabolism i.e. the relation between uptake and elimination of metabolic tracers especially under conditions of myocardial exercise and ischemia. Unless the exact mechanism of the metabolic kinetics has been elucidated, the clinical value of labeled FFA as metabolic tracers will be limited. Well-controlled experimental studies have to be carried out to make the labeled FFA clinically useful and 'this general class' of studies will represent the next stratum of nuclear cardiology investigations.

41

References

1. Machulla HJ, Stöcklin G, Kupfernagel C, et al. (1978) Comparative evaluation of fatty acids labeled with C-11, Cl-34m, Br-77 and I-123 for metabolic studies of the myocardium: concise communication. J Nucl Med 19: 298 - 302.
2. Poe ND, Robinson jr GD, Graham LS, MacDonald NS (1976) Experimental basis for myocardial imaging with I-123-labeled hexadecenoic acid. J Nucl Med 17: 1077 - 82.
3. Schelbert HR, Henze E, Huang SC, Phelps ME (1981) Relationship between myocardial blood flow and uptake and utilization of free fatty acids (FFA) J Nucl Med (abstract) 22: P10.
4. Henze E, Guzy P, Schelbert HR (1983) Metabolic effects of cardiac work on normal and ischemic myocardum in man measured noninvasively with C-11-palmitate and positron emission tomography (PET). Eur Soc Cardiol Working Group on Use of Isotopes in Cardiol, Rotterdam (abstract).
5. Dudczak R, Kletter K, Frischauf H, Losert U, Angelberger P, Schmoliner R (1984) The use of I-123-labeled heptadecanoic acid (HDA) as metabolic tracer: Preliminary report. Eur J Nucl Med 9: 81 - 5.
6. Comet M, Wolf JE, Pilichowski P, et al. (1982) Influence du propranolol sur l'active myocardique apres injection i.v. d'acide 16 I(123) hexadecène-9-oique. In: Faivre G, Bertrand A, Cherrier F, Amor M, Neimann JL (eds) Noninvasive methods in ischemic heart disease. Nancy, Specia, pp 295 - 99.
7. Styles CB, Noujaim A A, Jugdutt BI, et al. (1983) Effect of doxorubicin on (omega-I-131) heptadecanoic acid myocardial scintigraphy and echocardiography in dogs. J Nucl Med 24: 1012 - 8.
8. Stöcklin G (1981) Evaluation of radiohalogen labelled fatty acids for heart studies. Nuklearmedizin (Suppl) 19: 1-6.
9. Lerch RA, Ambos HD, Bergmann SR, Welch MJ, Ter-Pogossian MM, Sobel BE (1981) Localization of viable, ischemic myocardium by positron-emission tomography with C-11-palmitate. Circulation 64: 689 - 99.
10. Lerch RA, Bergmann SR, Ambos HD, Welch MJ, Ter-Pogossian MM, Sobel BE (1982) Effect of flow-independent reduction of metabolism on regional myocardial of C-11-palmitate. Circulation 65: 731 - 8.
11. Schelbert HR, Phelps ME, Hoffman E, Huang SC, Kuhl DE (1980) Regional myocardial blood flow, metabolism and function assessed noninvasively with positron emission tomography. Am J Cardiol 46: 1269 - 77.
12. Schön HR, Schelbert HR, Najafi A, et al. (1982) C-11 labeled palmitic acid for the noninvasive evaluation of regional myocardial fatty acid metabolism with positron-computed tomography. II. Kinetics of C-11-palmitic acid in acutely ischemic myocardium. Am Heart J 103: 548 - 61.
13. Visser FC, Westera G, Eenige van MJ, van der Wall EE, den Hollander W, Roos JP (1985) The myocardial elimination rate of radioiodinated heptadecanoic acid. Eur J Nucl Med 10: 118 - 22.
14. Kloster G, Stöcklin G, Smith EF, Schrör K (1984) Omega-halofatty acids: A probe for mitochondrial membrane integrity. In vitro investigations in normal and ischaemic myocardium. Eur J Nucl Med 9: 305 - 11.
15. Weiss ES, Hoffman EJ, Phelps ME, et al. (1976) External detection and visualization of myocardial ischemia with C-11-substrates in vitro and in vivo. Circ Res 39: 24 - 32.
16. Weiss ES, Ahmed SA, Welch MJ, Williamson JR, Ter-Pogossian MM, Sobel BE (1977) Quantification of infarction in cross sections of canine myocardium in vivo with positron emission transaxial tomography and C-11-palmitate. Circulation 55: 66 - 73.
17. Sobel BE, Weiss ES, Welch MJ, Siegel BA, Ter-Pogossian MM (1977) Detection of remote myocardial infarction in patients with positron emission transaxial tomography and intravenous C-11-palmitate. Circulation 55: 853 - 57.
18. Ter-Pogossian MM, Klein MS, Markham J, Roberts R, Sobel BE (1980) Regional assessment of myocardial metabolic integrity in vivo by positron-emission tomography with C-11-labeled palmitate. Circulation 61: 242 - 55.
19. Geltman EM, Biello D, Welch MJ, Ter-Pogossian MM, Roberts R, Sobel BE (1982) Characterization of nontransmural myocardial infarction by positron-emission tomography. Circulation 65: 747 - 55.
20. Schön HR, Schelbert HR, Robinson G, Najafi A, Huang SC, Hansen H (1982). C-11-labeled palmitate acid for the noninvasive evaluation of regional myocardial fatty acid metabolism with positron-computed tomography. I. Kinetics of C-11-palmitic acid in normal myocardium. Am Heart J 103: 532 - 47.
21. Bergmann SR, Lerch RA, Fox KAA, et al. (1982) Temporal dependence of beneficial effects of coronary thrombolysis characterized by positron tomography. Am J Med 73: 573 - 81.
22. Ludbrook PA, Geltman EM, Tiefenbrunn AJ, Jaffe AS, Sobel BE (1983) Restoration of regional myocardial metabolism by coronary thrombolysis in patients. Circulation (abstract) (Suppl. III):325.

42

23. Goldstein RA, Klein MS, Welch MJ, Sobel BE (1980) External assessment of myocardial metabolism with C-11-palmitate in vivo. J Nucl Med 21: 342 - 8.

24. Evans JR, Phil D, Gunton RW, Baker RG, Spears JC, Beanlands DS (1965) Use of radioiodinated fatty acid for photoscans of the heart. Circ Res 16: 1 - 10.

25. Robinson jr GD, Lee AW (1975) Radioiodinated fatty acids for heart imaging: iodine monochloride addition compared with iodide replacement labeling. J Nucl Med 16: 17 - 21.

26. Poe ND, Robinson jr GD, MacDonald NS (1975) Myocardial extraction of labeled long-chain fatty acid analogs. Proc Soc Exp Biol Med 148: 215 - 8.

27. Otto CA, Brown LE, Wieland DM, Beierwaltes WH (1981) Radioiodinated fatty acid for myocardial imaging: Effects of chain length. J Nucl Med 22: 613 - 8.

28. Westera G, van der Wall EE, Heidendal GAK, van den Bos GC (1980) A comparison between terminally radioiodinated hexadecenoic acid (I-HA) and Tl-201-thallium chloride in the dog heart. Implications for the use of I-HA for myocardial imaging. Eur J Nucl Med 5: 339 - 43.

29. Poe ND, Robinson jr GD, Zielinski FW, Cabeen jr WR, Smith JW, Gomes AS (1977) Myocardial imaging with I-123-hexadecenoic acid. Radiology 124: 419 - 24.

30. Freundlieb C, Höck A, Vyska K, Feinendegen LE, Machulla HJ, Stöcklin G (1980) Myocardial imaging and metabolic studies with (17-I-123)iodoheptadecanoic acid. J Nucl Med 21: 1043 - 50.

31. Van der Wall EE, Heidendal GAK, den Hollander W, Westera G, Roos JP (1980) I-123 labeled hexadecenoic acid in comparison with thallium-201 for myocardial imaging in coronary heart disease. A preliminary study. Eur J Nucl Med 5: 401 - 5.

32. Rösler H, Hess T, Weiss M. et al. (1983) Tomoscintigraphic assessment of myocardial metabolic heterogeneity. J Nucl Med 24: 285 - 96.

33. Van der Wall EE, den Hollander W, Heidendal GAK, Westera G, Majid PA, Roos JP (1981) Dynamic myocardial scintigraphy with I-123 labeled free fatty acids in patients with myocardial infarction. Eur J Nucl Med 6: 383 - 9.

34. Aurich D, Reske SN, Biersack HJ, et al. (1982) Biplanar sequential scintigraphy of the myocardium by means of 123-I-heptadecanoic acid. In: Raynaud C (ed) Nucl Med Biol, Proc third World Congr Nucl Med Biol Paris II Pergamon Press, pp 1389 - 91.

35. Van der Wall EE, Heidendal GAK, den Hollander W, Westera G, Roos JP (1981) Metabolic myocardial imaging with I-123 labeled heptadecanoic acid in patients with angina pectoris. Eur J Nucl Med 6: 391 - 6.

36. Van der Wall EE, Westera G, den Hollander W, Roos JP, Visser FC (1981) External detection of regional myocardial metabolism with radioiodinated hexadecenoic acid in the dog heart. Eur J Nucl Med 6: 147 - 51.

37. Huckell VF, Lyster DM, Morrison RT (1980) The potential role of 123 iodine-hexadecenoic acid in assessing normal and abnormal myocardial metabolism. J Nucl Med (abstract) 21: P57.

38. Pachinger O, Sochor H, Ogris E, Probst P, Klicpera M, Kaindl F (1982) Salvage of ischemic myocardium by intracoronary streptokinase therapy? In: Faivre G, Bertrand A, Cherrier F, Amor M, Neimann J L (eds) Noninvasive methods in ischemic heart disease. Nancy, Specia, pp 410 - 4.

39. Visser F C, Westera G, van der Wall EE, Roos JP (1985) Dynamic free fatty acid scintigraphy in patients with successful thrombolysis after acute myocardial infarction. Clin Nucl Med 10: 35 - 9.

40. Höck A, Freundlieb C, Vyska K, Lösse B, Erbel R, Feinendegen LE (1983) Myocardial imaging and metabolic studies with (17-I-123)iodoheptadecanoic acid in patients with idiopathic congestive cardiomyopathy. J Nucl Med 24: 22 - 8.

41. Rabinovitch MA, Kalff V, Allen R, et al. (1985) 123-I-Hexadecanoic acid metabolic probe of cardiomyopathy. Eur J Nucl Med 10: 222 - 7.

42. Freundlieb C, Höck A, Vyska K, Erbel R, Feinendegen LE (1982) Fatty acid uptake and turnover rate in the ischemic heart before and after bypass surgery. In: Raynaud (ed) Nucl Med Biol, Proc third World Congr Nucl Med Biol Paris II Pergamon Press pp 1392 - 5.

43. Höck A, Freundlieb C, Vyska K, et al. (1982) The influence of rehabilitation training on fatty acid metabolism in patients with myocardial infarction. In: Faivre G, Bertrand A, Cherrier F, Amor M, Niemann JL (eds) Non invasive methods in ischemic heart disease. Nancy, Specia, pp 300 - 3.

44. Machulla HJ, Marsmann M, Dutschka K (1980) Biochemical concept and synthesis of a radioiodinated phenylfatty acid for in vivo metabolic studies of the myocardium. Eur J Nucl Med 5: 171 - 3.

45. Reske SN, Schön S, Knust EJ, et al. (1984) Relation of myocardial blood flow and initial cardiac uptake of 15-(p-I-123-phenyl)-pentadecanoic acid in the canine heart. Nucl Med 23: 83 - 5.

46. Sun QX, Zhang J, Ji QM, et al. (1984) Pharmacology of radioiodinated hexadecenoic acid. A myocardial imaging agent. Nucl Med 23: 73 - 4.

47. Coenen HH, Harmand MF, Kloster G, Stöcklin G (1981) 15-(p-(Br-75)bromophenyl)-pentadecanoic acid: Pharmacokinetics and potential as heart agent. J Nucl Med 22: 891 - 6.

48. Dudczak R, Schmoliner R, Kletter K, Frischauf H, Angelberger P (1983) Clinical evaluation of I-123-labeled p-phenylpentadecanoic acid (p-IPPA) for myocardial scintigraphy. J Nucl Med All Sci 27: 267 - 9.

49. Rellas JS, Corbett JR, Kulkarni P, et al. (1983) Iodine-123 -phenylpentadecanoic acid: Detection of acute myocardial infarction and injury in dogs using an iodinated fatty acid and single-photon emission tomography. Am J Cardiol 52: 1326 - 32.

50. Reske SN, Biersack HJ, Lackner K, et al. (1982) Assessment of regional myocardial uptake and metabolism of omega-(p-I-123-phenyl)-pentadecanoic acid with serial single-photon emission tomography. Nucl Med 21: 249 - 53.

51. Visser FC, van der Wall EE, Eenige van MJ. Elimination rates of I-123-labeled phenylpentadecanoic acid in patients after acute myocardial infarction. Preliminary results.

52. Reske SN (1985) 123-I-Phenylpentadecanoic acid as a tracer of cardiac free fatty acid metabolism. Experimental and clinical results. Eur Heart J (suppl B) 6: 39 - 47.

53. Reske SN, Machulla HJ, Biersack HJ, Simon H, Knopp R, Winkler C (1982) Metabolic turnover of P-I-123-phenylpentadecanoic acid in the myocardium. In: Raynaud C (ed) Nucl Med Biol, Proc third World Congr Nucl Med Biol Paris III Pergamon Press, pp 2522 - 5.

54. Okada RD, Knapp jr FF, Elmaleh DR, Yasuda T, Boucher CA, Strauss HW (1982) Tellurium-123m-labeled-9-telluraheptadecanoic acid: A possible cardiac imaging agent. Circulation 65: 305 - 10.

55. Elmaleh D , Knapp jr FF, Yasuda T, et al. (1981) Myocardial imaging with 9-(Te-123m)telluraheptade-canoic acid. J Nucl Med 22: 994 - 9.

56. Livni E, Elmaleh DR, Levy S, Brownell GL, Strauss H W (1982) Beta-methyl(1-C-11)heptadecanoic acid: A new myocardial metabolic tracer for positron emission tomography. J Nucl Med 23: 169 - 75.

57. van der Wall EE, Barrett E, Strauss HW, et al. (1985) Altered uptake and kinetics of radioiodinated 15-P-(I-125)-iodophenyl-3-methylpentadecanoic acid in diabetic myocardium. Circulation (abstract) 72 (suppl III): 424.

58. Schwaiger M, Schelbert HR, Keen R, et al. (1985) Retention and clearance of C-11-palmitic acid in ischemic and reperfused canine myocardium. J Am Coll Cardiol 6: 311 - 20.

59. Machulla HJ, Knust EJ (1984) Recent developments in the field of I-123-radiopharmaceuticals. Nucl Med 23: 111 - 8.

60. van der Wall EE (1984) Myocardial imaging with radiolabeled free fatty acids. In: Simoons M L, Reiber J H C (eds) Nuclear imaging in clinical cardiology. The Hague: Martinus Nijhoff, pp 83 -102.

61. van der Wall EE (1985) Myocardial imaging with radiolabeled free fatty acids: A critical review. Eur Heart J (suppl B) 6: 29 - 38.

62. Schelbert HR, Henze E, Keen R, Huang H, Barrio J, Phelps M (1982) Regional fatty acid metabolism in acute myocardial ischemia demonstrated noninvasively by C-11-palmitate (CPA) and positron tomography (PET). Circulation (abstract) 66 (suppl II): 126.

63. Vyska K, Höck A, Freundlieb C, et al. (1979) Myocardial imaging and measurement of myocardial fatty acid metabolism using omega-I-123-heptadecanoic acid. J Nucl Med (abstract) 20: 650.

64. Grover M, Schelbert HR (1985) Assessment of regional myocardial substrate metabolism with positron emission tomography. In: G Pohost (Ed) New concepts in cardiac imaging 1985 Boston. Hall Medical Publishers.

65. Schelbert HR, Phelps ME, Shine K I (1983) Imaging metabolism and biochemistry: a new look at the heart. Am Heart J 105: 552 - 26.

66. Fox KAA, Abendschein DR, Ambos HD, Sobel BE, Bergmann SR (1985) Efflux of metabolized and nonmetabolized fatty acid from canine myocardium tomographically. Circ Res 57: 232 - 43.

67. van der Wall EE (1986) Myocardial imaging with radiolabeled free fatty acids: Applications and limitations. Eur J Nucl Med 12: S11 - S15.

3.
Function:
Assessment of cardiac function by radionuclide angiography

Introduction

Radionuclide angiography techniques have been used for the noninvasive evaluation of ventricular performance since the late seventies. These techniques require peripheral intravenous injection of radioactive tracers remaining within the intravascular space during the period of study, a scintillation camera or probe, and a computer for data processing.

Radionuclide angiography studies are safe, repeatable during various interventions (exercise, drugs) and the injected radionuclides do not induce measurable hemodynamic alterations. These techniques are used for the evaluation of regional ventricular performance, measurement of various global ventricular performance indices such as right and left ventricular ejection fraction, quantitation of intracardiac shunts, valvular regurgitation, ventricular volumes, and diastolic filling rates.

Two techniques can be used for the assessment of cardiac function;
(1) first-pass radionuclide angiography, and
(2) multiple gated blood pool scintigraphy.

Usually for both methods technetium-99m (Tc-99m) is used as the imaging agent. The physical half-life of Tc-99m is 6 hours and its gamma energy 140 keV, ideally suited to current gamma cameras.

First-pass radionuclide angiography

With the first-pass technique, 15 mCi (550 MBq) Tc-99m pertechnetate is rapidly injected in an antecubital vein as a compact bolus. The scintillation data of the first pass through the central circulation are accumulated by a multicrystal or single crystal camera. Complete mixing of the bolus is assumed to have occurred by the time the radionuclide enters the left ventricle. As a result, changes in radioactivity during the ejection phase reflect proportional changes in chamber volume and are free of geometric assumptions. The efficacy of the first-pass method is dependent upon obtaining sufficiently high count rates to assume statistical accuracy. The multicrystal camera provides a much higher count rate capacity than the currently available singlecrystal gamma cameras (maximal 500.000 versus maximal 90.000

counts per second respectively). A time-activity curve is generated over an area of interest over the ventricle. A typical left ventricular time-activity curve in characterized by cyclical fluctuations (peaks and valleys) in count rate (Fig 1).

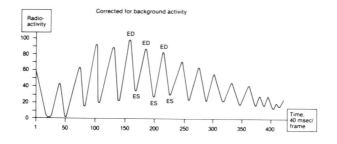

Figure 1
The time-activity curve of the first transit of the radioactive bolus through the left ventricle is shown. The peaks of the curve correspond to end-diastole (ED) and the valleys to end-systole (ES). Based on the mean ED and ES values of e.g. 3 consecutive beats, left ventricular ejection fraction (LVEF) can be calculated:

$LVEF = \dfrac{ED-ES}{ED}$. Since these results are based on counts, LVEF is not geometry dependent.

Each peak, or maximal ventricular activity, corresponds to end-diastole (ED) whereas each valley, or minimal activity, reflects end-systole (ES). These time-activity curves have to be corrected for non-cardiac background activity, which can be determined by different empirically found methods.

The left ventricular ejection fraction is calculated by the summation of 3-4 cycles: LVEF= ED-ES/ED. By choosing a region of interest over the right ventricle, the right ventricular ejection fraction can also reliably be determined by this technique. Qualitative information can be obtained by visual assessment of regional wall abnormalities of the right and left ventricle.

Multiple gated blood pool imaging

With the gated blood pool or equilibrium technique, the cardiac blood pool is imaged after injection of a radionuclide which remains entirely in the intravascular space. This can be achieved by two methods: Tc-99m tagged to human serum albumin or directly to the erythrocytes of the patient (Fig. 2). At present, it is generally agreed that labeling of the erythrocytes provides a more stable tag, which is important when serial studies are desired. Imaging is mostly performed in the 45-degree left anterior oblique position for optimal separation of the right and left ventricle. With the use of a gamma camera and a computer system, scintillation data are recorded continuously in synchrony with the R-wave of the electrocardiogram (Fig. 3). Data are recorded throughout the cardiac cycle and stored separately, depending on the relationship to each R-wave. The RR-interval is usually divided into 16 to 24 frames. Imaging is continued until 150.000-250.000 counts per frame are accumulated, which takes about 6 minutes. From these data, a time-activity curve can be generated over a region of interest over the left ventricle, which shows the activity accumulated over several hundred (300-500) cardiac cyles.

The time-activity curve has to be corrected for background activity and left ventricularejection fraction is then calculated by conventional equation:

(A)
$$LVEF = \frac{EDC - BC}{EDC - BC}$$

where LVEF = left ventricular ejection fraction, ED = end-diastole, ES = end-systole, B = background and C = counts (Fig. 4).

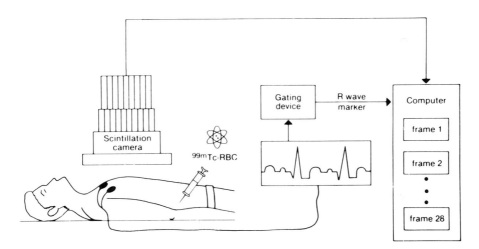

Figure 2
Equilibrium radionuclide angiocardiography or multiple gated cardiac blood pool imaging provides a means of assessing cardiac performance by synchronizing collection of scintillation data with electrocardiographic events (i.e. gating). Presently, the in-vivo labeling method is widely employed. First, the patient's own red blood cells (RBC) are "primed" with 5-15 mg of unlabeled stannous-pyrophosphate. Subsequently, after 15 minutes 20 mCi technetium-99m pertechnetate is administered, which then labels the red cells with high efficiency. The intravascular blood pool can now be visualized.

The radionuclide left ventricular ejection fraction compares well with the ejection fraction obtained from contrast left ventriculography. Similar to the first-pass technique, visual inspection allows the assessment of regional wall motion abnormalities. However, the spatial resolution of conventional systems is not much less than 1 cm.

When the first-pass technique is compared with the gated bloodpool scintigraphy, both techniques provide accurate data on cardiac function. Which technique to prefer depends on the expertise in the laboratory, the type of camera and specific clinical needs. An advantage of the gated blood pool technique is the possibility of data collection for several hours (4-6 hours) after tracer injection; serial measurements can be made after physiologic or pharmacologic intervention.

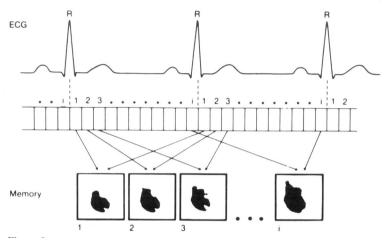

Figure 3

Schematic diagram of the technique of equilibrium radionuclide angiocardiography. The RR-interval is subdivided into 16-28 frames of 30-50 msec duration. Each frame has a fixed relationship to the preceding R wave and the acquired image is stored in the computer. Usually 300 to 500 cardiac cycles are needed to sample sufficient counts for reliable analysis of LVEF. After summation of all acquired data, a single representative cardiac cyle is generated with can be displayed as an "endless loop" movie. The cine display permits accurate assessment of relative chamber size and global and regional wall motion. (From Schelbert and Wisenberg, Current Problems in Cardiology, Yearbook Medical Publishers, 1979 with permission).

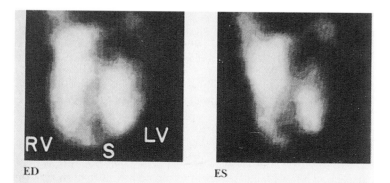

Figure 4A

Radionuclide angiograms in left anterior oblique view during end-diastole (ED) and end-systole (ES) obtained from a normal subject. The left (LV) and right ventricle (RV) show normal size and there is excellent inward systolic motion of all LV regions. S=septum.

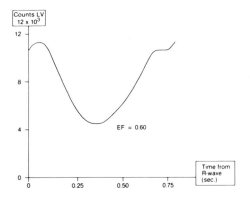

Figure 4B

Analysis of counts in the left ventricular regions of interest as a function of time relative to the R wave or the electrocardiogram results in a left ventricular time-activity curve. LVEF can be calculated from this curve. Good correlation with contrast ventriculography has been reported (r=0.95). Automated edge-detection programs have been developed, wich greatly enhance the reproducibility of calculation of LVEF.

TABLE I

Functional parameters measured in gated cardiac blood pool scanning

1. Wall motion assessment	Global (LV and RV)
	Regional (LV)
2. Ejection fraction	LV and RV
3. Regional ejection fraction	LV
4. End-diastolic and end-systolic volume	LV and RV
5. Stroke volume and cardiac output	LV and RV
6. Regurgitation fraction	LV
7. Systolic emptying and diastolic filling rate	LV
8. Time to peak systolic emptying and diastolic filling	LV

LV = left ventricle, RV = right ventricle

The assessment of left ventricular ejection fraction during rest and exercise is probably the most widely used clinical application of the above-described techniques. Both the first-pass technique and the gated blood pool study are used to evaluate

49

patients with suspected cardiac disease, although the gated blood pool study has shown to be more feasible. Supine exercise gated blood pool scintigraphy can be carried out with the patient exercising on a special 'bicycle stress' table under the camera. A resting study is performed with the patient in the same position as will be used later during exercise. This is usually the 45-degree left anterior oblique projection, so that the right and left ventricles can be viewed seperately, and with the patient supine or 45 degrees upright. The 45-degree upright position increases the likelihood that the patient will achieve an adequate exercise level but requires an appropriately designed table and camera mount. A high-sensitivity collimator is used because the acquisition time is short. A restraining harness is used to minimize patient motion under the camera during exercise. The imaging table should be secure, with minimal motion. Exercise loads are increased stepwise by 25-watt increments at 3-minute intervals until the patient experiences symptoms of angina, dyspnea, or fatigue of sufficient severity to limit further exercise or until the patient develops hypertension, severe arrhythmias, or marked ST-segment changes.

Electrocardiographic leads are recorded and monitored continuously throughout the study. At each level of the work load, data are acquired by the computer during a 2-minute period. In a normal subject, left ventricular ejection fraction will increase during exercise by at least 5%. In contrast, patients with significant coronary artery disease demonstrate generally an abnormal response on exercise: left ventricular ejection fraction fails to increase or falls even to lower values, while very often regional wall abnormalities develop. However, one must realize that only regional wall abnormalities are specific for coronary artery disease, since a decrease in global left ventricular ejection fraction can also occur in patients with valvular lesions and cardiomyopathies.

Non-imaging radionuclide angiography (Nuclear probe)

This is a modification of the radionuclide angiography technique involving the use of a specially collimated, high sensitivity, relatively small, and easily movable nuclear probe and dedicated microprocessor instead of the larger conventional scintillation gamma camera and computer. The data can be obtained, displayed, and analyzed on a beat-to-beat basis or added over 15-90 seconds to generate and electrocardiogram-gated relative volume curve. This technique allows rapid assessment of various indices of systolic and diastolic left ventricular performance without providing images or regional analysis. Left ventricular ejection fraction can be determined with similar accuracy as with the conventional gamma camera.

Right ventricular ejection fraction

Although equilibrium (electrocardiogram-gated) radionuclide ventriculography can

be used for the sequential assessment of global and regional left ventricular performance, there are anatomical differences between the left and right sides of the heart
that make assessment of right ventricular ejection fraction using count-rate
techniques and the equilibrium radionuclide angiocardiogram more difficult. The
right atrium lies behind the right ventricle to a greater extent than the left atrium
overlies the left ventricle. This interference is solved in first-pass radionuclide angiocardiography by imaging in the right anterior oblique projection, thus spatially separating the right atrium from the right ventricle. This cannot be done easily using equilibrium radionuclide ventriculography because the right ventricle is superimposed on
the left ventricle in that projection. Thus, initial attempts at measuring right ventricular ejection raction by equilibrium methods have necessitated the use of either
multiple regions of interest in an effort to define the right ventricular perimeter
throughout the cardiac cycle or a background region of interest extending into the
right atrium and pulmonary outflow tract.

Alternatively, right ventricular ejection fraction can be determined by using a slant-
hole collimator which provides a 30-degree caudal tilt that more effectively separates
the right atrium and the right ventricle. By using similar background correction
procedures as for left ventricular ejection fraction measurement, right ventricular
ejection fraction is calculated according the standard equation (A). The correlation
between right ventricular ejection fraction by both first-pass and equilibrium studies
is excellent.

Valvular regurgitation

The severity of aortic and mitral regurgitation can be measured from the radionuclide
angiocardiogram. While first-pass techniques have been described for assessing left-
sided regurgitation, the greatest experience has been derived from equilibrium
studies. Regions of interest are drawn over the left and right ventricles by visual
inspection, taking care to include the entire right ventricular or left ventricular area,
while excluding as much of the atria, pulmonary artery, and aorta as possible.
Changes in the counts in each ventricular area between systole and diastole are then
determined. Since the same regions of interest are used for both sytole and diastole,
and since only the absolute change in counts is recorded, background activity is not
subtracted. The results are expressed as a ratio of the change in counts in the left
ventricular area over the change in counts in the right ventricular area (LV/RV
stroke-index ratio). A regurgitation index can be calculated according to the
following equation:

$$\text{Regurgitation index} \quad = \quad \frac{\text{LVEDC - LVESC} = \text{LVSC}}{\text{RVEDC - RVESC} = \text{RVSC}}$$

(ED = end-diastole, ES = end-systole, LV = left ventricle, RV = right ventricle,
S = stroke, C = counts)

In patients without aortic or mitral regurgitation, the left-to-right ventricular stroke-index is 1.15±0.15. The ratio is greater than one in normal patients because the right ventricular stroke volume is underestimated owing to overlapping of the right atrium on the right ventricle. In patients with mitral or aortic regurgitation, the ratio is greater than 1.35. There is good agreement between the stroke-volume index and qualitative angiographic estimates or regurgitation.

The limitations of applying the regurgitation index are that (1) right-sided regurgitation should not be present, (2) global left ventricular ejection fraction should be greater than 30%, and (3) there should be good separation of the right atrium from the right ventricle (1,2). There is always some overlap of the right atrium on the right ventricle and this problem may be more severe with significant right atrial enlargement.

Range of normal values

Global ejection fraction
In order to reach a world-wide consensus on the normal range of left and right ventricular ejection fraction at rest and during exercise, pooled data of 1200 normal subjects from 28 leading centres in the field of nuclear cardiology was analysed (3).

Weighted mean normal values for left ventricular ejection fraction at rest were $62.3 \pm 6.1\%$ ($\pm$ 1SD) with a lower limit for normal of 50% and for right ventricular ejection fraction $52.3 \pm 6.2\%$ with a lower limit of normal of 40%. During exercise, left ventricular ejection fraction increased in 475 subjects by a mean of 8.0 ejection fraction% (range 3-15%), a normal increase being accepted to be >5% over a normal resting value for both left and right ventricular ejection fraction. Subgroup analysis of results at rest revealed no significant differences regarding selection of normal subjects (based on normal catheterization findings versus normal volunteers with low probability of disease), age or sex. Data on reproducibility and variability showed that radionuclide angiocardiography can be considered to be a reliable method today. These normal values may serve as general guidelines for future applications of the radionuclide angiography techniques (4) (See Chapter 16, Guidelines in Nuclear Cardiology).

Regional ejection Fraction
Although no world-wide consensus has been obtained for measurements of regional left ventricular ejection fraction, yet several methods have been applied for measuring regional ejection fraction. Basically, one method divides the ventricle into radial sectors while the other divides it into rectangular segments bordering the major and minor axes of the left ventricle. Background is substracted regionally, using areas adjacent to the various regions. Regional ejection fraction is then calculated from the count-rate changes in each segment using the standard equation (A) of left ventricular ejection fraction measurement.

Both methods yield similar results. With the rectangular method, normal regional ejection fraction is 0.66 ± 0.13 in the anteroseptum, 0.85 ± 0.12 in the apex, and 0.74 ± 0.16 in the inferoposterior segment.

Regional ejection fraction measurements are reproducible and useful in studies that require quantitative measures of wall motion, such as before and during drug therapy.

Clinical applications

Detection and evaluation of coronary artery disease

In patients with coronary artery disease who have not yet sustained an acute myocardial infarction, resting ventricular performance is usually normal because the myocardium is not ischemic. When these patients are stressed, an imbalance between oxygen supply and demand develops, resulting in ischemia. This, in turn, causes a fall in global left ventricular ejection fraction and the development of regional wall motion abnormalities. When radionuclide angiocardiography is applied during exercise in normal patients, left ventricular ejection fraction rises significantly compared to levels at rest, with no left ventricular wall motion abnormalities (Fig. 5). In patients with coronary artery disease and angina, left ventricular ejection fraction falls during exercise and new regional wall motion abnormalities may develop (Fig. 6).

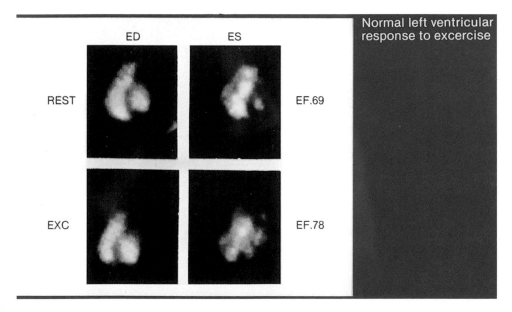

Figure 5
This figure shows a normal subject in left anterior oblique projection during end-diastole (ED) and end-systole (ES). LVEF increased from 69% at rest to 78% at peak exercise. This is a normal exercise response.

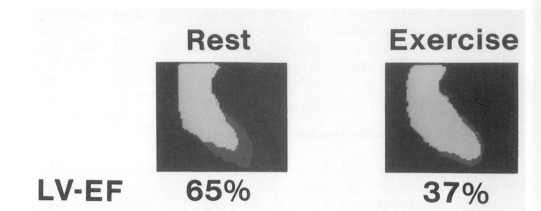

Figure 6
LVEF response during exercise in a patient with coronary artery disease and angina pectoris during exercise. It can be observed that LVEF decreases during exercise from 65% to 37%. (From Iskandrian, Nuclear Cardiac Imaging, F.A. Davis Company, 1987, with permission).

The normal increase in ejection fraction with exercise is due primarily to a decrease in end-systolic volume, while the exercise-induced decrease increase in ejection fraction in patients with angina is due to an increase in end-systolic volume. In patients with coronary artery disease without angina there is usually no change in ejection fraction during exercise, since there is no significant change in end-systolic volume (Fig. 7).

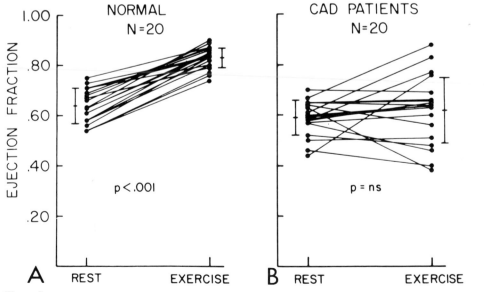

Figure 7
LVEF response in twenty normal subjects and in twenty CAD patients without angina during exercise. LVEF increases in normal subjects but shows no significant change in the asymptomatic patients.(From DS Berman and DT Mason, Clinical Nuclear Cardiology, Grune & Stratton, 1982, with permission).

54

At first glance, this technique would seem to be particularly accurate for the diagnosis of coronary artery disease. Reviewing the data in the literature from 1978 to 1987 it was found that the sensitivity for detection of regional wall motion abnormalities (the percentage of coronary artery disease patients with this finding) was 73%, while the specificity (the percentage of normal subjects without regional asynergy) was 100%. There was considerable variability in the sensitivity rates from study to study, however, with a range of less than 50% to 100%. It would seem that the sensitivity for detecting wall motion abnormalities should not be high with this method, since only one projection is obtained during exercise and the image has poor resolution because of the short acquisition time. However, the sensitivity of this method for detecting an abnormal left ventricular ejection fraction response in patients with coronary artery disease was as high as 87% with a specificity of 93%, when regional wall motion was included (Table II).

TABLE 2

Comparison of exercise electrocardiography and radionuclide angiography for the detection of coronary artery disease

	Sensitivity (%)	Specificity (%)
Electrocardiogram	65	92
Regional wall motion	73	100
LVEF	88	76
LVEF + regional wall motion	87	93

Data based on studies in 771 patients from 12 centers
LVEF = left ventricular ejection fraction

Other factors will play a major role in determining left ventricular response with exercise. For example, inadequate stress due to peripheral vascular disease or the concurrent administration of beta-adrenergic blocking drugs or calcium-antagonists may result in normal responses in spite of coronary artery disease. The ejection fraction response is greater with upright exercise than with supine exercise.

In fact, an abnormal ejection fraction response to exercise is expected in any condition in which there is reduced left ventricular reserve, such as volume- or pressure-overload states and states of decreased left ventricular compliance. As a result, abnormal responses have been reported in patients with valvular abnormalities and cardiomyopathies. Therefore, regional wall motion analyses should be included (Fig. 8).

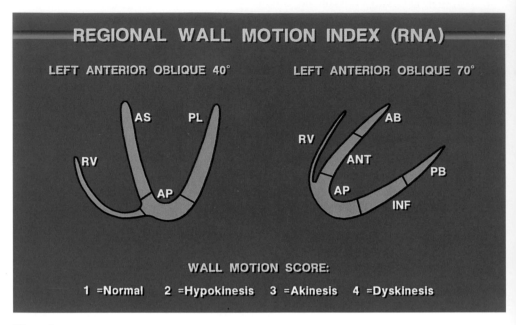

Figure 8

Evaluation of regional wall motion by radionuclide angiography. The radionuclide angiograms are evaluated in at least two different views; in our institution the left anterior oblique views 40° and 70° are used. The left ventricle is divided into 7 segments which are each visually scored from normal=1 to dyskinesis=4. Based on this scoring system a regional wall motion index is obtained. The presence of a regional wall motion abnormality is highly specific for coronary artery disease.

When interpreting the exercise radionuclide angiocardiogram, it is clear that additional information should be incorporated into the decision-making process. For example, almost 75% of patients suspected of having coronary artery disease with a low pretest probability of the disease (i.e. no previous infarction or no typical angina) can be diagnosed with an 85% certainty by combining the results of exercise radionuclide angiocardiography and clinical variables such as the presence of chest pain and ST-T segment changes with exercise. Thus, the radionuclide angiocardiogram is most useful in the noninvasive diagnosis of coronary artery disease when it is coupled with additional clinical information.

In the diagnostic evaluation of patients with suspected coronary artery disease, the exercise electrocardiogram may provide the necessary diagnostic information without resorting to additional noninvasive methods. If the exercise electrocardiogram is nondiagnostic, an exercise radionuclide study may be useful. At the present time, neither exercise radionuclide angiocardiography nor exercise myocardial perfusion scintigraphy clearly to be appears clearly to be the procedure of choice. Radionuclide angiocardiography provides higher sensitivity but poorer specificity in patients with valvular heart disease, primary myocardial disease, or severe lung disease.

56

Furthermore, particularly with supine bicycle ergometry, many patients may not achieve an adequate chronotropic response. The exercise radionuclide angiocardiogram does provide more complete information, particularly when imaging is performed at each stage of exercise, which allows cardiac performance to be assessed at various levels of submaximal exercise.

Unstable angina

Only a few studies have been performed in assessing radionuclide LVEF in the acute phase of unstable angina (5,6). These studies were performed as part of the Holland Interuniversity Nifedipine Trial (HINT). In these studies it was shown that left ventricular ejection fraction was abnormal in about 50% of patients who were studied within 12 hours after onset of symptoms. When patients were restudied after 48 hours, left ventricular ejection fraction was increased in particular in those patients on nifedipine.

Acute myocardial infarction

Left ventricular performance is an important factor in determining patient prognosis after acute myocardial infarction. Radionuclide angiography techniques provide information concerning global left ventricular function, the extent and location of regional abnormalities, and the presence and extent of right ventricular involvement. As a result, radionuclide angiography provides prognostic information, since left ventricular ejection fraction is a predictor of early mortality and the development of congestive failure or sudden death. In addition, approximately 50% of the patients with inferior infarction will have abnormalities in right ventricular performance.
Ventricular function can also be used to assess patient recovery. Global and regional ventricular performance will improve gradually over the first two weeks after infarction but will show a significant improvement by two to four months if uninterrupted by complications such as reinfarction. Also acute therapeutic interventions can followed over time. For instance, one of the mainstays of the Working Group on Thrombolytic Therapy under the auspices of the Netherlands Interuniversity Institute of Cardiology was the assessment of radionuclide left ventricular ejection fraction 2 days, 2 weeks and 3 months after acute thrombolytic therapy (7-9). Before the beneficial effects of recanalization on mortality were demonstrated in this study, a significant increase of left ventricular ejection fraction in the thrombolysis group compared to the conventionally treated control group was already apparent in the early period after the intervention, in particular in patients with an anterior infarction.

Risk stratification

Additional prognostic information may be gained from (sub)maximal exercise testing of patients prior to discharge from the hospital, since the ventricular response to exercise appears useful in selecting patients at high risk for subsequent complications.

Pryor et al. (10) determined which radionuclide variable obtained at rest and during exercise predicted subsequent survival or cardiac events defined as cardiovascular death or nonfatal acute myocardial infarction in 386 patients with stable angina pectoris who were followed for up to 4,5 years. There were a total of 27 cardiovascular deaths and 28 nonfatal acute myocardial infarctions. Univariate analysis revealed that the exercise left ventricular ejection fraction was the variable most closely associated with future events. The second best variable was the resting ejection fraction followed by wall motion abnormalities and then the exercise duration. The change in ejection fraction from rest to exercise was not a significant predictor. Multivariate analysis revealed that once the exercise ejection fraction was known, no other radionuclide variables contributed independent information about the likelihood of future events. Kaplan-Meier survival curves showed that patients with exercise ejection fraction of <35% has significantly more events during the follow-up period than patients with exercise ejection fraction of 35 to 49%, and those, in turn had more events than patients with exercise ejection fraction >50%.

Bonow et al. (11) found that among patients with three-vessel disease, minimal syptoms, and preserved resting left ventricular function, those who had both ST-segment depression and decreased ejection fraction during exercise in association with an exercise tolerance of 120 watts or less, the probability of survival is significantly lower than in patients who had no ischemia during exercise.

Studies by Morris et al. (12), Starling et al. (13), and Ong et al. (14) showed that rest and exercise radionuclide angiography after acute myocardial infarction provides significant information regarding specific events during follow-up independent of that provided by clinical assessment.

Iskandrian et al. (15) examined the value of rest and exercise radionuclide ventriculography in risk stratification in patients with known or suspected coronary artery disease. When these patients were divided into those who did not have previous coronary artery bypass grafting and those who did, the exercise left ventricular ejection fraction remained the most important predictor of death and total events. The risk of future events is significantly lower among patients with an exercise ejection fraction >50% than among those patients with an exercise ejection fraction of <50%, regardless of whether or not these patients had previous revascularization. Furthermore, the risk for future events increased in a stepwise fashion as the exercise ejection fraction decreased, patients with exercise ejection fraction >50% had higher survival rates than patients with exercise ejection fraction of 30-49% and those in turn had higher survival rates than patients with exercise ejection fraction <30%. These data again indicate that exercise left ventricular ejection fraction is a powerful prognostic indicator which identifies patients at risk for future cardiac events in patients with or without prior bypass surgery.

Clinical implications in patients with coronary artery disease

Based on the afore-mentioned results, several guidelines for patients after acute myocardial infarction have been advised to obtain an optimal dedicated post-infarction diagnostic strategy (16,17). The following approach can be recommended.

First, a symptom-limited exercise test should should be performed at discharge as a routine procedure. Second, in case of equivocal results, exercise radionuclide angiography will be performed within 1 week. Based on these results, patients with a resting left ventricular ejection fraction of <30% and patients with a resting ejection fraction between 30 and 70% with inadequate ejection fraction response during exercise will be considered for coronary arteriography since these patients have a high risk profile. Conversely, patients with a resting left ventricular ejection fraction between 30 and 70% with an adequate response during exercise, and patients with a resting ejection fraction of >50% can be considered as low risk patients and they will primarily be assigned to medical therapy.

Valvular heart disease

Radionuclide angiography provides the only readily available, noninvasive means for quantifying the degree of left-sided valvular regurgitation. While echocardiography offers excellent visualization of valve motion, assesses aortic dilatation, and measures the degree of mitral stenosis, the severity of regurgitation can be estimated only qualitatively, even with Doppler methods.

In addition to its ability to detect and measure left-sided regurgitation, radionuclide angiocardiography may play a role in the management of patients with aortic valve regurgitation. In these patients, the decision to intervene surgically depends on the degree of left ventricular dysfunction. The dysfunction may not be apparent at restand may show up only during exercise. It has been suggested that by the time symptoms develop in these patients, irreversible myocardial dysfunction has occurred and that functional abnormalities may appear during stress even in the asymptomatic patient. As a result, radionuclide assessment of left ventricular function during exercise has been suggested as a means of following patients with aortic regurgitation to determine the optimal time for valve replacement. However, the optimal management of patients with severe aortic insufficiency is still a matter of debate, in particular in asymptomatic patients. In most centers a left ventricular end-systolic dimension of 55 mm or more as determined by M-mode echocardiography has been accepted as the optimal moment for appropriate surgical intervention. However, this approach has been questioned by Fioretti et al. (18) who demonstrated that a preoperative left ventricular end-systolic dimension of 55 mm or more does not preclude successful aortic valve replacement. This might be due to the highly variable echocardiographic measurements of the left ventricular dimensions in severe aortic insufficiency with variations of as much as 20%. Moreover, in a recent article by Szlachcic et al. (19) it was found in 22 patients with significant but asymptomatic aortic insufficiency that a 9 mm increase in left ventricular systolic or diastolic dimension, as measured by M-mode echocardiography, is required to state with confidence that a change has occurred. In a subsequent editorial comment (20) it was therefore recommended to use the radionuclide left ventricular ejection fraction as the most reliable parameter for choosing the adequate moment for operation; surgery has to be considered if left ventricular ejection fraction is less than 50%, preceded by contrast angiography.

While this approach appears promising, further validation is required before it can be recommended for routine clinical use (21,22). In a superb review article, Iskandrian et al. (23) emphasized the need for patients with asymptomatic aortic insufficiency to undergo serial evaluation of the radionuclide angiography studies combined with exercise testing, although they state that an abnormal ejection fraction response to exercise should not be the only indication for valve replacement. Also other radionuclide-derived indices such as end-systolic volume and pressure/volume relationship at rest and during exercise should be taken into account.

A suggested guideline in these patients is the performance of a radionuclide angiography exercise study on a one-yearly basis; in case of a significant change to abnormal left ventricular ejection fraction values at rest or a fall to abnormal ejection fraction values during exercise surgery should be considered.

Cardiomyopathies

Radionuclide angiography techniques provide useful information in determining the diagnosis, prognosis and therapeutic responses in patients with any of the several forms of cardiomyopathy. Radionuclide angiography may allow the differential diagnosis between those forms of cardiomyopathy in which the diastolic dysfunction is the major problem and those forms in which the systolic function dominates. This is of particular interest in patients with hypertrophic cardiomyopathy, since it has been shown that patients with hypertrophic cardiomyopathy manifest abnormal diastolic function in terms of prolonged relaxation-time index, impaired diastolic filling and increased chamber stiffness. Bonow et al. (23) studied 40 patients with hypertrophic cardiomyopathy and used the radionuclide angiography technique for the evaluation of left ventricular systolic function and diastolic filling, and for the effects of oral verapamil (320-480 mg/day) on these parameters. All but one patient had normal or supernormal systolic function, but 28 patients (70%) showed evidence of diastolic dysfunction as indicated by a diminished peak filling rate and a prolonged time to peak filling rate. Verapamil did not change the systolic function parameters, but improved diastolic function in 18 patients (40%). This study, therefore, showed that diastolic filling is abnormal in a high number of patients with hypertrophic cardiomyopathy, and that verapamil normalizes or improves these abnormalities without altering systolic function. The exact indications for the use of nifedipine in hypertropic cardiomyopathy are not yet clear, although it may be more promising than verapamil because of its effects on improving ventricular filling. Also diltiazem improves left ventricular relaxation and diastolic filling in patients with hypertrophic cardiomyopathy without altering left ventricular systolic function (See Chapter 12 on Cardiomyopathies).

Assessment of ventricular dysfunction

Radionuclide angiocardiography is most useful in patients with symptoms suggesting ventricular dysfunction because it can 1) detect ventricular aneurysm, 2) distinguish regional from global dysfunction, 3) evaluate myocardial viability, 4) evaluate right en left ventricular function, and 5) evaluate the effectiveness of therapeutic interventions. It provides a noninvasive method for accurate quantitation of ventricular hemodynamics and regional wall motion in patients too ill to undergo invasive cardiac catheterization. In addition, the technique can be performed sequentially to evaluate the natural history of heart disease and the effectiveness of medical or surgical therapy.

The technique is comparable in sensitivity to contrast ventriculography in detecting and assessing aneurysm and in determining the location and extent of dyskinetic segments and the status of the remaining ventricular regions. These factors are particularly important in patients with coronary artery disease in whom aneurysmectomy is being considered. As a result, the radionuclide method can be used to screen patients to separate those with diffuse hypokinesis, who are poor candidates for surgery from those with localized akinesis or aneurysm, who may then undergo cardiac catheterization prior to surgery.

Regional wall motion abnormalities present at rest may be due to scar from previous myocardial infarction or to reversible ischemia of viable tissue. Since revascularization may improve regional function if the tissue is viable, it is important to differentiate between reversible ischemia and scar. Postextrasystolic potentiation and nitroglycerin have been used to help make this distinction, usually at the time of catheterization. The exercise radionuclide angiography study can be used to evaluate the change in regional wall motion after exercise. In most patients with surgically reversible regional abnormalities, left ventricular function in that region improves immediately after exercise compared to function at rest.

Radionuclide angiocardiography provides a noninvasive method for monitoring the acute and chronic effects on drugs on ventricular performance. A wide variety of drugs has been studied, including inotropic agents, afterload-reducing agents, bronchodilators, beta-adrenergic blockers, antiarrhythmics, and calcium-antagonists. For example, it was shown that the calcium-antagonist diltiazem, even in high doses (360 mg/day), did not produce any significant left ventricular dysfunction but actually increased left ventricular ejection fraction, both at rest and during exercise, probably as a result of reduction in aortic impedance to left ventricular emptying (24).

Ventricular performance is an important indicator of cardiotoxicity with drugs, such as doxorubicin, that have a potentially detrimental effect on the heart (25). By sequentially assessing patients who are receiving these agents, it might be possible to predict when irreversible cardiac failure might develop in an individual patient. As a result, medication can be continued as long as possible and stopped while cardiac failure is still reversible.

Conclusion

Radionuclide angiography studies have been shown safe and easily repeatable during various interventions (exercise, drugs). These techniques can usefully applied in patients with diverse manifestations of cardiac disease. Radionuclide angiography allows the evaluation of regional ventricular performance, measurement of various global ventricular performance indices such as right and left ventricular ejection fraction, quantitation of intracardiac shunts, valvular regurgitation, ventricular volumes, and diastolic filling rates. Currently, it is the most suited noninvasive technique to assess cardiac function during exercise.

References

1. Lam W, Pavel D, Byrom E, Sheikh A, Best D, Rosen K. Radionuclide regurgitant index: Value and limitations. Am J Cardiol 1981;47:292-8.
2. Ormerod OJM, Barber RW, Stone DL, Wraight EP, Petch MC. A comparison of radionuclide methods of evaluating aortic regurgitation with observations on the effect of exercise and symptoms. Eur J Nucl Med 1986;12:72-6.
3. Pfisterer ME, Battler A, Zaret BL. Range of normal values for left and right ventricular ejection fraction at rest and during exercise assessed by radionuclide angiography. Eur Heart J 1985;6:647-55.
4. Zaret BL, Battler A, Berger HJ, Bodenheimer MM, Borer JS, Brochier M, Hugenholtz PG, Neufeld HN, Pfisterer ME. Report of the Joint International Society and Federation of Cardiology/World Health Organization Task Force on Nuclear Cardiology. Circulation 1984;70:768A-781A.
5. Van der Wall EE, Kerkkamp HJJ, Lubsen J, Simoons ML, Van Rijk PP, Reiber JHC, Bom N, Roos JP, Lie KI. Left ventricular performance in unstable angina: assessment with radionuclide techniques. Int J Cardiol 1985;8:287-99.
6. Van der Wall EE, Kerkkamp HJJ, Simoons ML, Van Rijk PP, Reiber JHC, Bom N, Lubsen JC, Lie KI. Effects of nifedipine on left ventricular performance in unstable angina pectoris during a follow-up of 48 hours. Am J Cardiol 1986;57:1029-33.
7. Simoons ML, Scrruys PW, Van den Brand M, Res J, Verheugt FWA, Krauss XH, Remme WJ, Bär F, De Zwaan Ch, Van der Laarse A, Vermeer F, Lubsen J. Early trombolysis in acute myocardial infarction: limitation of infarct size and improved survival. J Am Coll Cardiol 1986;7:717-28.
8. Van der Wall EE, Res JCJ, Van Eenige MJ, Verheugt FWA, Wijns W, Braat S, De Zwaan Ch, Remme WJ, Vermeer F, Reiber JHC, Simoons Ml. Effects of intracoronary thrombolysis on global left ventricular function assessed by an automated edge detection technique. J Nucl Med 1986;27:478-83.
9. Res JCJ, Simoons ML, Van der Wall EE, Van Eenige MJ, Vermeer F, Verheugt FWA, Wijns W, Braat S, Remme WJ, Serruys PW, Roos JP. Long term improvement in global left ventricular function after early thrombolytic treatment in acute myocardial infarction. Br Heart J 1986;56:414-21.
10. Pryor DB, Harrell FE, Lee KL, Rosati RA, Coleman E, Cobb F, Califf RM, Jones RH. Prognostic indications from radionuclide angiography in medically treated patients with coronary artery disease. Am J Cardiol 1984;53:18-22.
11. Bonow RO, Kent KM, Rosing DR, Lan KKG, Lakatos E, Borer JS, Bacharach SL, Green MV, Epstein SE. Exercise-induced ischemia in mildly symptomatic patients with coronary artery disease and preserved left ventricular function: Identification of subgroups at high risk for death during medical therapy. N Engl J Med 1984;311:1339-45.
12. Morris KG, Palmeri ST, Califf RM, McKinnis RA, Higginbotham MB, Coleman E, Cobb FR. Value of radionuclide angiography for predicting specific cardiac events after acute myocardial infarction. Am J Cardiol 1985;55:318-24.
13. Starling MR, Crawford MH, Henry RL, Lembo NJ, Kennedy GT, O'Rourke RA. Prognostic value of electrocardiographic exercise testing and noninvasive assessment of left ventricular ejection fraction soon after acute myocardial infarction. Am J Cardiol 1986;57:532-7.
14. Ong L, Green S, Reiser P, Morrison J. Early prediction of mortality in patients with acute myocardial infarction: A prospective study of clinical and radionuclide risk factors. Am J Cardiol 1986;57:33-8.
15. Iskandrian AS, Hakki AH, Schwartz JS, Kay H, Mattleman S, Kane S. Prognostic implications of rest and exercise radionuclide ventriculography in patients with suspected or proven coronary heart disease. Int J Cardiol 1984;6:707-18.
16. Fioretti P, Brower RW, Simoons ML, Ten Katen H, Beelen A, Baardman T, Lubsen J, Hugenholtz PG. Relative value of clinical variable, bicycle ergometry, rest radionuclide ventriculography and 24 hour ambulatory electrocardiography monitoring at discharge to predict 1 year survival after myocardial infarction. J Am Coll Cardiol 1986;8:40-9.
17. Nienaber CA, Bleifeld W. Personal view: In-hospital patient management strategies after acute myocardial infarction. Eur Heart J 1985;6:640-6.
18. Fioretti P, Roelandt J, Bos RJ, Meltzer RS, Van Hoogenhuize D, Serruys PW, Nauta J, Hugenholtz PG. Echocardiography in chronic aortic insufficiency. Is valve replacement too late when left ventricular end-systolic dimension reaches 55 mm? Circulation 1983;67:216-21.

19. Szlachcic J, Massie BM, Greenberg B, Thomas D, Cheitlin M, Bristow JD. Interest variability of echo-cardiographic and chest X-ray measurements: implications for decision making in patients with aortic regurgitation. J Am Coll Cardiol 1986;7:1310-7.
20. Butman SM. When is a change in left ventricular function significant in the asymptomatic patient with aortic insufficiency. J Am Coll Cardiol 1986;7:1318-9.
21. Bonow RO, Rosing DR, McIntosh CL, Jones M, Maron BJ, Lan G, Lakatos E, Bacharach SL, Green MV, Epstein SE. The natural history of asymptomatic patients with aortic regurgitation and normal left ventricular function. Circulation 1983;68:509-17.
22. Iskandrian AS, Heo J. Radionuclide angiographic evaluation of left ventricular performance at rest and during exercise in patients with aortic regurgitation. Am Heart J 1986;111:1143-9.
23. Bonow RO, Rosing DR, Bacharach SL, Green MV, Kent KM, Lipson LC, Maron BJ, Leon MB, Epstein SE. Effects of verapamil on left ventricular systolic function and diastolic filling in patients with hypertrophic cardiomyopathy. Circulation 1981;64:787-96.
24. Hung J, Lamb IH, Connolly SJ, Jutzy KR, Goris ML, Schroeder JS. The effect of diltiazem and prop-ranolol, alone and in combination, on exercise performance and left ventricular function in patients with stable effort angina: a doubleblind, randomized, and placebo-controlled study. Circulation 1983;68:560-7.
25. Palmeri ST, Bonow RO, Myers CE, Seipp C, Jenkins J, Green MV, Bacharach SL, Rosenberg SA. Prospective evaluation of doxoribicin cardiotoxicity by rest and exercise radionuclide angiography. Am J Cardiol 1986;58:607-13.

4.
Planar Thallium-201 imaging:
Useful in clinical cardiology?

Summary

Thallium-201 (Tl-201) was first proposed and introduced for myocardial perfusion imaging in the mid-seventies(1). Tl-201 myocardial perfusion imaging since has evolved into an important diagnostic modality aiding significantly in the diagnosis and management of patients with coronary artery disease. Tl-201 exercise scintigraphy has been shown to increase the sensitivity and specifity for detection of coronary artery disease in comparison to the standard electrocardiographic stress test. In addition, Tl-201 imaging provides significant prognostic information in a variety of clinical situations. Depending on the specific clinical question addressed by the cardiologist, Tl-201 myocardial perfusion imaging is employed either in conjunction with exercise or at rest. Pharmacologic stress with dipyridamole in conjunction with Tl-201 imaging has become an useful alternative for patients who are unable to perform adequate physical exercise (See Chapter 11). For successful Tl-201 imaging, a thorough understanding of the technique of image acquisition and possible pitfalls associated with image interpretation is necessary. This chapter addresses the clinical value of planar Tl-201 imaging, in particular its diagnostic and prognostic value.
For a better interpretation of routine Tl-201 myocardial perfusion images, the biophysical profile and myocardial kinetics need to be clarified.

Biophysical characteristics

Unfavorable physical characteristics of several radioactive cations that accumulate in myocardial cells, such as potassium-43 (K-43) and rubidium-81 (Rb-81), limited their broad use for noninvasive measurement of myocardial blood flow. The physical properties of Tl-201 were more favorable and led to its widespread use for myocardial perfusion imaging. The main advantages of Tl-201 include a sufficiently long half-life of 73 hours for convenient delivery and a biological half-life in the myocardium of 7.5 hours permitting an adequate injected dose without excessive radiation exposure to the patient. A relative disadvantage of this radiopharmaceutical is the low photon energy emission of 80 keV, which results in significant tissue attenuation and scatter, degrading the images. The total myocardial accumulation of Tl-201 in humans is approximately 4% of the administered dose following intravenous injection. The largest radiation dose is absorbed by the kidneys. The renal dose ranges from 0.84-1.34 rad/mCi, and the whole body radiation is 0.21 rad/mCi.

Tl-201 myocardial kinetics at rest

Tl-201 is extracted very efficiently by normal myocardial cells. The cellular uptake is mediated by active and passive membrane transport, the former likely related to the $Na^+K^+ATPase$ pump. The mean myocardial extraction of Tl-201 after a bolus injection into the coronary circulation in experimental dog studies is almost 90% and remains relatively unaltered under varying physiologic and metabolic conditions.

In humans, following an intravenous injection at rest, rapid accumulation in normal myocardium occurs, reaching a peak activity at approximately 20 minutes. Within minutes, 80-90% uptake of the peak activity in normal myocardium is reached, followed by a near plateau phase of up to 60 minutes. This is the result of both physical decay and slow loss of Tl-201 from the myocardial cells into the capillary blood pool. Following a rest injection, accumulation is significantly slower, but adequate images can be obtained as early as 20 minutes after injection.

Abnormally decreased myocardial uptake following a rest injection may indicate several clinical conditions: 1) Acute myocardial infarction. Regional myocardial blood flow is severely reduces because of acute thrombosis in a major epicardial artery, usually at the site of severe stenosis. 2) Regional reduction of viable myocardial mass because of prior myocardial infarct and scar tissue. 3) Myocardial ischemia at rest (e.g., resting angina pectoris, unstable angina, or coronary artery spasm). Severely diminished resting blood flow will result in reduced initial myocardial Tl-201 uptake. Later, Tl-201 will distribute according to viability of the myocardial cells. 4) Noncoronary diseases, such as rheumatic connective tissue disorders, sarcoidosis or myocardial abscesses, may involve the myocardium and can produce perfusion defects.

Tl-201 myocardial kinetics at peak exercise

Patients with chronic stable coronary artery disease are frequently asymptomatic at rest. In contrast, during episodes of increased myocardial oxygen demand (e.g., physical exercise), an imbalance between the regional coronary oxygen delivery and local metabolic requirement exists in the perfusion territory of a coronary artery with a hemodynamically significant stenosis. The consequent regional myocardial ischemia is responsible for clinical sequele, such as angina pectoris, arrhythmias and, finally, myocardial infarction.

During exercise, under normal physiologic conditions an increase (up to 4 -5 times) of the coronary blood flow occurs to ensure adequate regional myocardial oxygen supply. Patients with a hemodynamically significant coronary artery stenosis demonstrate a locally reduced coronary flow reserve. During exercise myocardial blood flow cannot increase of the same extent as in the normal myocardium. Thus regional heterogeneity of myocardial blood flow is created. Following intravenous injection, Tl-201 distributes in the body proportional to cardiac output and within the myocardium relative to regional distribution of myocardial blood flow. As a result, imbalances between regional coronary flow can be visualized as regional differences in Tl-201 accumulation. Although the extraction of Tl-201 is rapid, an 'ischemic steady state' time window of approximately 1-2 minutes, during which the relative coronary blood flow does not change, is needed following intravenous injection at peak exercise in order to optimally visualize differences in regional Tl-201 distribution. The kinetics of Tl-201 uptake and washout from the myocardium can be evaluated using computer assisted quantitative image analysis. Tl-201 uptake and washout patterns are different in normal and ischemic myocardium.

In normal myocardium, uptake of Tl-201 injected at maximal exercise reaches an early peak after several minutes followed by a subsequent gradual decrease. The latter part of the myocardial uptake curve is referred to as washout of Tl-201 and gives additional useful clinical information.

Tl-201 uptake kinetics of ischemic myocardium are markedly different. The initial uptake in the hypoperfused myocardium is less and time to peak activity is delayed, resulting in continued myocardial uptake at a time that washout occurs from normal myocardial cells. Therefore, images obtained immediately after the exercise will demonstrate less accumulation of the radiopharmaceutical in the area of diminished blood flow, which improves on delayed imaged due to a relative or absolute increase of Tl-201 in the previously ischemic area compared to the normal myocardium.

Tl-201 washout is the net result of continued uptake from the residual Tl-201 in arterial-capillary blood and the ongoing loss of cellular Tl-201 to the capillary-venous circulation. Ischemic myocardium demonstrates either diminished Tl-201 washout, no net Tl-201 change, or even an absolute increase of Tl-201 myocardial activity.

Shortly after injection, a linear relationship exits between the regional Tl-201 myocardial uptake and the regional blood flow at reduced, normal and increased coronary flow levels. Under conditions of extremely high flow, such as in reactive hyperemia, Tl-201 myocardial uptake may underestimate coronary flow(2). Later, i.e. at least 2 hours after injection at peak exercise, the distribution of Tl-201 reflects the potassium pool or viable myocardial cells.

In order to evaluate these differences in Tl-201 kinetics for practical Tl-201 imaging, routinely a set of images is obtained shortly following termination of the exercise (starting within minutes) and a second set of images with identical acquisition parameters 2-4 or 24 hours later.

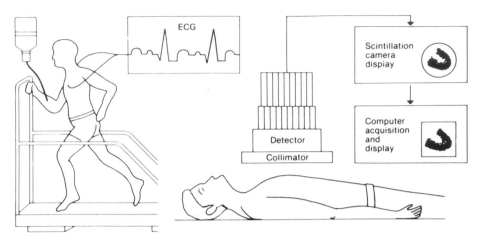

Figure 1

The drawbacks of exercise electrocardiography have prompted the development of radionuclide techniques for the detection of coronary artery disease in order to improve sensitivity, specificity and the predictive value. In particular, Tl-201 is employed as the radionuclide of choice for evaluating myocardial perfusion. Tl-201 exercise scintigraphy is nowadays widely used as a noninvasive test for the detection of coronary artery disease. The test is performed in conjunction with exercise electrocardiography. The patients are exercised on a motor driven treadmill or on a bicycle ergometer, untill the patient stops because of symptoms (chest pain, fatigue or hypotension). During the exercise test, a 12-lead electrocardiogram (ECG) should be obtained every 3 minutes. At peak exercise 75 MBq (2mCi) of Tl-201 is injected intravenously. Myocardial imaging is performed within 5 minutes after termination of the exercise in the following three projections: left anterior oblique (LAO), anterior (ANT), and left lateral (LL). Delayed or redistribution imaging is performed 2-4 hours later using identical timings and similar projections as for the initial imaging. For quantitative analysis of the Tl-201 imaging, it is essential that adequate count rates are obtained in the initial image: i.e. at least 400.000 counts in the whole field of view.

Protocol Tl-201 exercise scintigraphy

There is a general agreement on a standard protocol for myocardial perfusion scintigraphy with Tl-201. The patients are usually exercised on a treadmill or a bicycle ergometer with an intravenous line inserted into a dorsal hand vein (Fig. 1). Long-acting antianginal medication should be discontinued at least 48 hours before the test provided the condition of the patient allows such a regimen. Also food intake before the test should be kept to a minimum. A 12-lead electrocardiogram, modified according to Mason-Likar, is obtained every minute and patients exercise until the appearance of symptoms (angina or fatigue). Next criteria for discontinuation of the exercise are the occurrence of hypotension and/or the development of malignant arrhythmias. The patients are injected with a bolus of 55-75 MBq (1.5-2.0 mCi) Tl-201 intravenously at maximal exercise and asked to continue the exercise for 30 seconds during which time the Tl-201 is effectively taken up by the myocardium. Imaging starts preferably within 5 minutes after termination of the exercise with the use of a standard gamma camera interfaced with a nuclear medicine computer. A low-energy high-sensitivity collimator is employed with a 20% window around the 80 keV energy peak of Tl-201. Images of 6-8 minutes duration each are collected in three views: the anterior, 35° and 70° left anterior oblique positions (Fig. 2). Routinely, 500.000 counts per image are collected with a maximal acquisition time of 8 minutes per projection. The three projections are collected again 3-4 hours after the initial series of images without the need for an additional thallium injection. These late images are called delayed or redistribution images. Between the exercise and redistribution images the patient is asked to refrain from substantial meals and to preferably limit his intake to soft drinks.

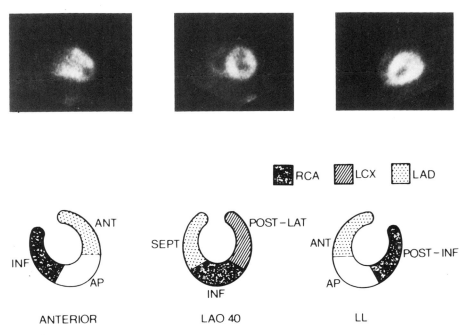

Figure 2
Scintigraphic and schematic representation of the location of the territories of the various coronary arteries on Tl-201 images: left anterior descending coronary artery (LAD), right coronary artery (RCA) and left circumflex coronary artery (LCX). LAO = left anterior oblique, LL = left lateral, ANT = anterior, AP = apical, INF = inferior, SEPT = anteroseptal, POST-LAT = posterolateral, POST-INF = postero-inferior

Reinjection of Tl-201
Recently, it has been demonstrated that reinjection of Tl-201 following the acquisition of the redistribution images may show additionally filling in of seemingly persistent defects. This finding indicates that some areas that were presumed to be necrotic still contain viable tissue. Since this may have important consequences for patient management, it is our policy to follow a standard reinjection procedure in all patients referred for Tl-201 exercise scintigraphy. The excess radiation dose (18 MBq, 0.5 mCi) is largely compensated by improved diagnosis and subsequent better management strategy for the patient.

Interpretation of Tl-201 images

The normal Tl-201 left ventricular image is horseshoe or doughnut shaped, with a central portion formed by the left ventricular cavity and thus having much less uptake. Areas of decreased tracer accumulation may also be seen normally at the apex, where the myocardial wall is thinner, and at the sites of insertion of the papillary muscles. Also the base of the heart has a reduced uptake of radioactivity because of attenuation by less vascular structures such as mitral and aortic valves. The right ventricular wall is also often seen on exercise studies. On stress images the myocardial-to-background activity ratio is about 2:1. This is higher than in rest images and possibly due to less splanchnic uptake.

To interpret the myocardial perfusion images visually or qualitatively, the intensity of Tl-201 uptake of the various regions of the myocardium is compared in various projections (usually: anterior, left anterior oblique 30° or 45° and left anterior oblique 70° or left lateral). The scintigram shows an abnormality when a region of the heart has a decreased radioactivity compared to another region in the same projection. Generally, there must be a 2:1 reduction in blood flow in a stenotic artery before a defect is apparent on the thallium scintigram. Abnormalities on thallium images may be caused by ischemia, infarction or both and are usually classified as "fixed" or "reversible". A fixed defect is one which is present on the rest or redistribution image and is attributes to the presence of myocardial fibrosis or scarring. A reversible defect is one which is seen on a stress study (directly post-exercise) but not on a redistribution image (after 4 hours) and generally indicates viable ischemic myocardium (Fig. 3). A partly reversible defect indicates that there is superimposed ischemia in an infarcted region.

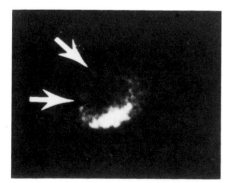 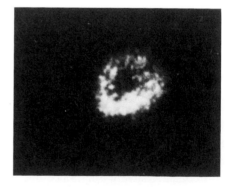

Figure 3A
Tl-201 exercise scintigraphy in a patient who developed an anteroseptal myocardial perfusion defect, observed on the anterior view (indicated by arrows). The defect fills in at the redistribution images, indicating exercise-induced transient myocardial ischemia.

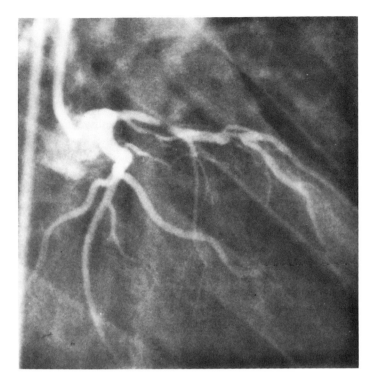

Figure 3B
Coronary arteriography revealed a 99% proximal narrowing of the left anterior descending coronary artery.

Tl-201 exercise scintigraphy may be of particular value in conditions when the exercise electrocardiogram is difficult to interpret, such as hyperventilation-induced abnormalities, left bundle branch block, left ventricular hypertrophy, old myocardial infarction, and nonspecific ST-T segment abnormalities at rest. Another group of patients in which Tl-201 imaging has been shown to be of value are those who have equivocal test results at exercise electrocardiography e.g. post myocardial infarction.

In most centers thallium myocardial images are analyzed visually. Various computer manipulations of the images are used to improve the quality of the images, including colour coding, contrast enhancement, smoothing and background subtraction. The effect of these manipulations is that any gain in sensitivity is counteracted by a loss of specificity. Visual interpretation is open to inter- and intraobserver variability. Also there is a limited sensitivity in the detection of individual coronary stenoses in patients with multivessel disease, especially if the degree of stenosis is not severe in proportion to the other stenoses vessels. It remains difficult to detect multivessel disease because of reduces spatial contrasting in so-called global myocardial hypo-perfusion. Also, visual analysis gives insufficient information about washout kinetics of Tl-201, and some possible temporal information remains unclear.

Visual versus quantitative thallium-201 scintigraphy

Because of the subjective nature of the visual analysis, quantitative (computerized) methods have been made to improve the accuracy of analysis (3). These methods typically use either a circumferential profile analysis of thallium distribution and washout or a horizontal profile or "slice" approach in which regional counts profiles are delineated in various myocardial regions (Fig. 4). Quantitation can be undertaken excellently both on spatial and temporal levels. There are several important advantages in quantifying myocardial uptake and washout of Tl-201. First, quantitative analysis permits less reliance on visual interpretation alone, and can be used to develop objective numerical standards, leading to more optimal reproducibility. Second, it is found by several groups that quantitative analysis enhances disease detection in individual coronary arteries and results in improved recognition of multivessel disease. Lastly, by measuring Tl-201 uptake in the initial uptake phase and characterizing washout from the redistribution images, quantitation offers a potential estimation of the amount of ischemic myocardium and distinguishing scar from hypoperfused but still viable segments.

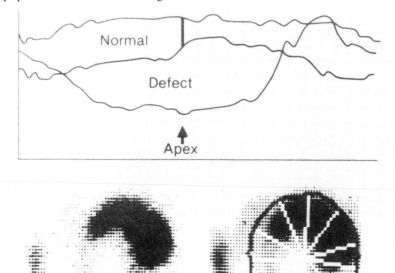

Figure 4
Although in general visual analysis of thallium-201 stress scintigraphy is highly specific for the overall detection of coronary artery disease, it has major limitations in sensitivity for detection of individual coronary artery stenoses, especially in patients with multivesssel disease. Therefore, quantitative analysis has been developed as a more reliable approach for interpretation of Tl-201 images. One method involves the construction of circumferential profiles using a minicomputer. In the example shown, such a profile is constructed from count values of 12 radii spaced at 30° intervals, plotted clockwise. (Currently, most circumferential profile methods employ 36 radii, spaced at 10° intervals). These profiles quantitate the

72

segmental Tl-201 activity as an angular function from the center of the left ventricular cavity. These profiles are then aligned by visually identifying the location of the scintigraphic apex on the stress and redistribution profiles. Fig. 4 shows an example of this analysis obtained from a patient with a large infero-septal perfusion defect. The two profiles connected by black bar represent the mean (± two standard deviations) distribution of Tl-201, derived from normal volunteers. The lower profile is a plot of the patient's myocardial distribution of Tl-201, showing reduced activity corresponding to the inferoseptal defect on the image shown at the bottem. (From Silverman et al. Circulation 1980;61:996, with permission)

It has to be stressed that sole reliance on the computer-derived quantitative scan interpretation may be hazardous. A great deal of experience is needed when dealing with the variability encountered in normal scan patterns. For example, breast attenu-ation, alterations in cardiac positions, such as counterclockwise or clockwise rotation can produce false positive defects if the reader is unfamiliar with the appearance of these variation (4). The outflow tracts which are photon deficient areas might also be misinterpreted as myocardial defects on automated, quantitative methods for scinti-graphic interpretation. Whichever scintigraphic technique is used, sufficient training and experience is necessary before optimal results of either approach are obtained. Quantitative analysis alone does not ensure improved sensitivity and specifity.

Limitations of exercise thallium-201 myocardial imaging

Thallium-201 scintigraphy is not a perfect test, and false negative and false positive results occur. Identifying situations in which such results might be expected could improve the clinical interpretation of a given test in an individual patient and could lead to bypassing this technique in favor of a more diagnostic tool (5).

False negative results

The cause of false negative test results of exercise thallium scintigraphy can be:
1) overestimation of the severity of coronary artery disease by angiography
   Perfusion abnormalities are more likely to be seen in the distribution of vessels with severe (>90%) stenoses than in vessels with moderate stenoses (50-70%). Overestimation of the severity of coronary angiography may be a cause of false negative thallium tests. Quantitative assessment of the degree of stenosis requires biplane studies and is only limited to a few centers but also has some technical limitations (because of overlap of secondary branches). It is also stated that the percentage of diameter of stenosis is a poor assessment of hemodynamic severity of coronary artery stenosis.
2) localization of coronary artery disease: circumflex artery, branch disease and peripheral vessel disease
   Detecting circumflex, marginal or diagonal branch vessel stenoses are more difficult than detecting left anterior descending or right coronary artery obstruc-tion. Perhaps, this is explained by the posterior location of the circumflex-

perfused myocardial regions being further away from the gamma camera. Small defects (<6 g) may be beyond the resolving power of the planar imaging method.

3) collaterals

The influence of the collateral flow on the sensitivity remains controversial. Collaterals develop in response to the presence of severe coronary artery stenosis. Angiographic appearance of collaterals may not correlate with their physiologic function and sometimes they may be present but angiographically invisible. It should be emphasized that the visibility of collaterals by angiography is determined by several (technical) factors. Such as, variation of force of injection into "collateral" vessels, duration of viewing during angiography. Some investigators have reported that collateral arteries are not protective in maintaining normal or increased perfusion during exercise evaluated by thallium scintigraphy. Another group has reported that perfusion abnormalities are more frequent in the distribution of occluded arteries not fed by collaterals compared with collateral emanated occluded vessels. It is also of great importance if the collaterals are "jeopardized" or not. However, it is possible that collaterals limit the area of ischemia rather than prevent it.

4) less stenosis severity

The sensitivity of the stress electrocardiogram is lower in single vessel disease than in multivessel disease. For detecting patients with one-, two-, and three-vessel disease some investigators have reported similar sensitivity, whereas others showed that the sensitivity decreased as the number of vessels involved decreased, especially when only visual analysis is used.

5) poor technical quality and improper interpretation of the images

6) diffuse ischemia

Approximately more than 50% of patients with three-vessel disease have multiple thallium defects in two or more vascular regions. As previously discussed quantitative analysis of thallium scintigrams increases the detection rate of multiple coronary stenoses. There is a group of patients that will demonstrate a diffuse slow washout pattern with no numerically significant defects or a maximum of one regional perfusion defect. So when only visual analysis is applied, some patients with diffuse ischemia could be missed.

7) inadequate level of exercise

The level of exercise achieved during stress testing is of greater influence to the exercise electrocardiogram than to the thallium scintigram. In patients achieving >85% of their predicted maximum heart rate the sensitivities of both tests are quite comparable, the thallium scan will have a greater frequency of being abnormal in the submaximal tests than the exercise electrocardiogram. This may be explained by the induction of heterogeneity of flow almost immediately on increasing myocardial oxygen demand with particular low levels of exercise. Whereas, it may take a significantly higher level of exercise to induce the myocardial cellular alternations that cause ST-segment changes.

False positive test results

The causes of false positive test results of exercise thallium scintigraphy can be:
1) underestimation of the severity of coronary artery disease on angiography
2) attenuation of thallium activity by breast tissue
   Specifity is considerably lower in women because of breast attenuation, particularly in the anterior and upper septal areas. Some investigators even found thallium scintigrams less sensitive for detecting coronary artery disease in women than in men, although this is not generally approved.
3) improper interpretation of the images
   The number of observers can both affect specifity and sensitivity. When averaging the multiple observer scores, both sensitivity and specificity can be maximized.
4) unrecognized excessive cardiac rotation
5) defect on the posterior wall due to attenuation from the diaphragm
6) other forms of heart disease, e.g. hypertrophic or idiopathic dilated cardiomyopathy, sarcoidosis, mitral valve prolapse, myocardial bridging, left bundle branch block, aortic valve disease, mitral valve prolapse, or myocardial tumors
7) marked obesity
8) right ventricular dilatation
9) exaggerated apical thinning

Detection of coronary artery disease

The traditional "gold standard" for the diagnosis of chronic coronary artery disease is angiography. This invasive technique relies solely on the presence of anatomical disease, and, although the only available comparative technique, may lack as a standard for the noninvasive physiologic information derived from the Tl-201 scintigraphy. The interpretation of quantitative analysis of Tl-201 stress studies should always be preceded by visual analysis of analogue or analogue equivalent digital images. A systematic approach of interpretation will minimize the effect of false negative and false positive results.

Many clinical studies have demonstrated the usefulness of planar Tl-201 stress scintigraphy in patients with chronic coronary artery disease. The overall sensitivity and specificity of Tl-201 stress imaging by visual analysis for the detection of coronary artery disease in a review study involving >2000 patients were 83% and 90% respectively (6). The standard electrocardiography stess test, compared in the same study, had a sensitivity of only 58% and a specificity of 82%.

Quantitative analysis of planar Tl-201 imaging increased the sensitivity and specificity for the detection of coronary artery disease. Visual Tl-201 stress imaging has a sensitivity and specificity of 65% and 100% respectively. The discrepancy with the reported values in the literature may reflect our conservative approach to image analysis. Quantitative analysis of the same studies increased the overall sensitivity for coronary artery disease detection to 89%. The same study revealed visual analysis to have a respective sensitivity of 55%, 79% and 80% for the detection of single-, double- and triple-vessel disease. The quantitative analysis added subsequent important clinical information and the overall sensitivity for single-, double- and triple-vessel disease increased to 84%, 94% and 100% respectively. The predicted accuracy for the presence of single-, double- and triple-vessel disease was still limited but improved over visual analysis (69%, 34% and 26% respectively). Other investigators have confirmed the substantial improvement of the detection of chronic coronary artery disease by Tl-201 stress imaging with quantitative analysis (7).

Prognostic implications of Tl-201 stress imaging

Regional myocardial ischemia detected by noninvasive Tl-201 stress imaging is an excellent predictor of the presence of anatomic coronary artery disease when compared to angiography. However, several studies demonstrated Tl-201 stress imaging to be a superior predictor of future cardiac events. In patients without prior myocardial infarction, the number of reversible Tl-201 defect was the most important predictor of future cardiac events (angina pectoris, infarction, cardiac death) (8). A similar study measuring the extent and severity also correlated with the occurrence of cardiac events (9) (Fig. 5). Patients studied with limited exercise protocol, involving quantitative Tl-201 stress scintigraphy following an uncomplicated myocardial infarction, had low subsequent event rate (6%) when only single fixed defects were present at discharge from the hospital. In contrast, patients with "high risk" findings (increased lung uptake, multipele perfusion abnormalities and reversible defects) had a 51% cardiac event rate (10).

Several studies have shown similar results in terms of prognostic value derived from Tl-201 stress imaging in patients following myocardial infarction. Another report showed early Tl-201 stress scintigraphy following percutaneous transluminal coronary angioplasty to be a better predictor (74%) of restenosis than the exercise electrocardiogram (54%).

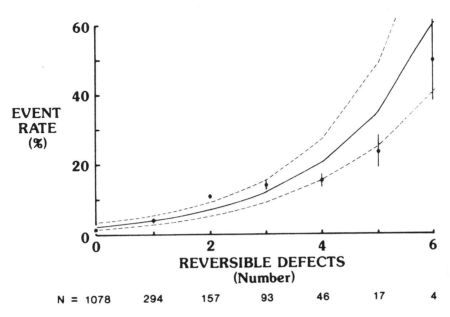

Figure 5

Relationship between the number of reversible defects (at redistribution) and subsequent cardiac event rate in 1078 patients undergoing Tl-201 exercise scintigraphy. Note the exponential increase in event rate corresponding to the increasing number of reversible perfusion defects. (From Ladenheim et al. (9), with permission)

Prognosis following a normal Tl-201 stress test

A normal Tl-201 stress imaging study had demonstrated to have be an excellent prognostic indicator. Even in the presence of angiographically demonstrated coronary artery disease, a normal Tl-201 stress test predicts a very low nonfatal infarction and mortality rate (0.6 and 0.5% respectively) (11-13). This is in sharp contrast to the above described negative prognostic outcome after an abnormal Tl-201 stress test. A similar study with a two-year follow-up involving 819 patients without previous myocardial infarction or coronary bypass grafting demonstrated a positive correlation between the magnitude of the perfusion defect and the frequency of subsequent cardiac events (14).

Conclusion

Thallium-201 is still the most frequently used radioisotope for myocardial perfusion imaging. Both for diagnostic and prognostic purposes, planar Tl-201 stress imaging (either visual or quantitative) has proved to provide unique information to the clinical cardiologist (15). Currently, the most important clinical applications of Tl-201 include: 1) detection of coronary artery disease, 2) risk stratification, 3) selection of patients for surgical or nonsurgical interventions, 4) follow-up of patients after interventions, and 5) assessment of myocardial viability. In particular, the viability issue has gained renewed interest after the reappraisal and large-scale application of the reinjection technique. Despite the development of new perfusion tracers, Tl-201 has obtained a fixed (no reversible) place in clinical cardiology.

References

1. Lebowitz E, Green MW, Fairchild R, et al. Thallium-201 for medical use. J Nucl Med 1975;16:151-60.
2. Strauss HW, Harison K, Lagan JK, et al. Thallium-201 for myocardial imaging: relation of thallium-201 to regional myocardial perfusion. Circulation 1975;51:641-5.
3. Wackers FJTh, Fetterman RC, Mattera JA, et al. Quantitative planar thallium-201 stress scintigraphy: a critical evaluation of the method. Semin Nucl Med 1985;15:46-66.
4. Dunn RF, Wolff L, Wagner S, et al. The inconsistent pattern of Tl-201 defects: a clue to the false positive perfusion scintigram. Am J Cardiol 1981;48:224-32.
5. Wackers JFTh. Thallium-201 myocardial imaging. In: Wackers FJ, editor. Thallium-201 and Technetium-99m Pyrophosphate myocardial imaging in the coronary care unit. The Hague: Martinus Nijhoff Publishers, 1980: 71-104.
6. Gibson RS, Beller GA. Should exercise electrocardiographic testing be replaced by radioisotope methods? In: Rahimtoola SH, Brest AN, editors - Controversies in Coronary Artery Disease. Philadelphia: FA Davies, 1981, 1-33.
7. Maddahi J, Garcia EV, Berman DS, et al. Improved noninvasive assessment of coronary artery disease by quantitative analysis of regional stress myocardial distribution and washout of thallium-201. Circulation 1981;64:924-35.
8. Brown KA, Boucher CA, Okada RD, et al. Prognostic value of exercise thallium-201 imaging in patients presenting for evaluation of chest pain. J Am Coll Cardiol 1983;1:994-1001.
9. Ladenheim ML, Pollock BH, Rozanski A, et al. Extent and severity of myocardial hypoperfusion as predictors of prognosis in patients with suspected coronary artery disease. J Am Coll Cardiol 1986;7:464-71.
10. Gibson RS, Watson DD, Craddock GB, et al. Prediction of cardiac events after uncomplicated myocardial infarction: prospective study comparing predischarge exercise thallium-201 scintigraphy and coronary angiography. Circulation 1983;68:321-36.
11. Wackers FJTh, Russo DJ, Russo D, et al. Prognostic significance of normal quantitative planar thallium-201 stress scintigraphy in patients with chest pain. J Am Coll Cardiol 1985;6:27-30.
12. Pamelia FX, Gibson RS, Watson DD, et al. Prognosis with chest pain and normal thallium-201 exercise scintigrams. Am J Cardiol 1985;55:920-6.
13. Wahl JM, Hakki AH, Iskandrian AS. Prognostic implications of normal exercise thallium-201 images. Arch Intern Med 1985;145:253-6.
14. Staniloff HM, Forrester JS, Berman DS, et al. Prediction of death, myocardial infarction and worsening of chest pain using thallium-201 scintigraphy and exercise electrocardiography. J Nucl Med 1986;27:1842-8.
15. Wackers FJTh. Myocardial perfusion imaging. In: Gottschalk A, Hoffer PB, Potchen EJ, editors. Diagnostic Nuclear Medicine. 2nd ed. Baltimore: Williams & Wilkins, 1988: 291-354.

5.
Cardiac single photon emission computed tomography:
SPECT, a new aspect in myocardial imaging?

Summary

The overlap of myocardial segments and the variable attenuation of radionuclide activity on routine planar thallium images may obscure accurate detection of perfusion defects and can also lead to errors in quantitative analysis. These major drawbacks can be overcome by employing tomographic techniques which improve the detection of ischemic myocardial regions and may even define zones with subendocardial ischemia. In particular, rotational tomography enhances the detection of regional perfusion abnormalities by providing a three-dimensional representation of myocardial thallium uptake.

Single photon emission computed tomography (SPECT) has now been used for several years in nuclear cardiology and recent studies have suggested that SPECT will become a more important clinical tool in clinical practice. Major advantages are the detection of mild coronary artery disease, the identification of multivessel disease, and the quantification of the area at risk after myocardial infarction. As a result, SPECT will become the preferred method for performing thallium myocardial perfusion scintigraphy.

Introduction

The noninvasive assessment of myocardial perfusion scintigraphy with thallium-201 has achieved wide acceptance as an important addition to the standard electrocardiographic exercise test (1). Thallium-201 imaging has become the technique of choice for assessing regional myocardial perfusion and has been shown to have a high sensitivity and specificity in identifying patients with coronary artery disease (CAD)(2). Although visual interpretation of planar thallium images has a sensitivity for detecting CAD in the range of 80 to 90% , it has significant inter- and intra-observer variability. Therefore, quantitative methods have been developed for a more objective analysis of thallium images resulting in increased sensitivity, particularly for detecting multivessel disease (3). However, quantitative planar thallium imaging fails to address the inherent limitations of two-dimensional planar scintigraphy that result from overlapping of myocardial segments and attenuation of radiation. The introduction of single photon emission computed tomography (SPECT) may overcome the limitations of planar imaging by providing a three-dimensional view of the myocardium which avoids superimposition of myocardial regions and enhances lesion contrast. As commercial SPECT camera computer systems are nowadays widely available, SPECT will become increasingly used in clinical cardiology. This chapter addresses the essential aspects of SPECT imaging and reviews current clinical applications.

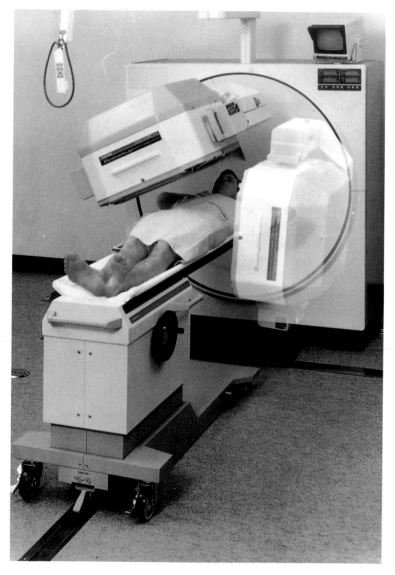

Figure 1
Tomographic system for SPECT imaging (Toshiba GCA 90B). The rectangular detector can move in two directions around the patient describing an arc of 360°. Two different detector positions are shown.

Methods

The two major categories of cardiac tomography are : 1) longitudinal tomography, and 2) transaxial tomography. With the longitudinal approach the image plane through the patient is parallel to the long axis of the body, while with the transaxial approach the image plane is transverse through the long axis of the body. Seven-pinhole tomography employs the longitudinal approach, whereas rotational tomography -including both SPECT and positron emission tomography (PET)- embodies the transaxial approach.

Seven-pinhole tomography

Although both tomographic modalities are quite capable to detect small perfusion abnormalities, the seven-pinhole approach may produce images with substantially reduced spatial resolution and diminished image contrast due to radioactivity from overlying and underlying structures. Data are collected over a limited angular range (26.5°) and result in image distortion. Therefore, the activity concentration in a perfusion defect is not accurately reconstructed and defects may be propagated longitudinally into adjacent reconstructed planes that are actually without defects. Since the results were shown to be not superior to planar thallium imaging, seven-pinhole tomography has been virtually abandoned in clinical practice and we will therefore focus on rotational tomography (SPECT).

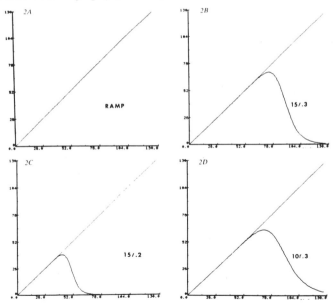

Figure 2

The pure ramp filter (upper left, 2A) attenuates the low frequencies and transmits more high frequencies, which mainly contain noise. By application of a window to the ramp filter the high frequency noise will be reduced. The other figures (upper right, 2B; lower left, 2C; and lower right, 2D) show different Butterworth filters with several orders (15, 15, and 10 respectively) and cutoff frequencies (0.3, 0.2, and 0.3 respectively).

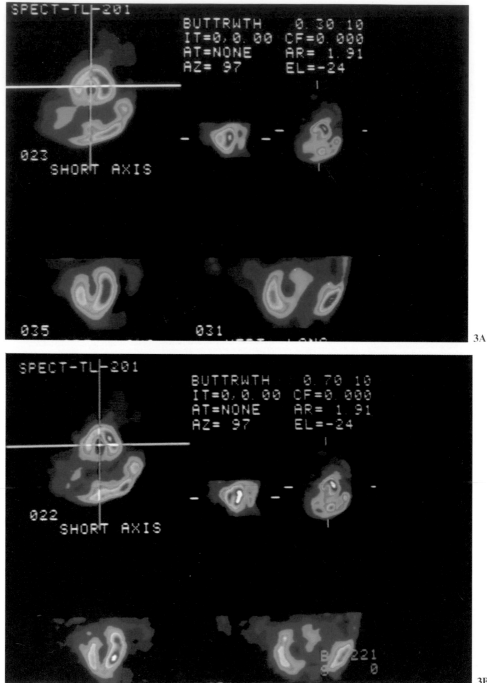

Figure 3
Reconstructed tomographic data by use of two different Butterworth (Buttrwth) filters. The low cutoff value (0.3) will produce oversmoothed images thereby disguising a lesion (upper image, 3A). A too high cutoff frequency (0.7) produces more noisy images, but will also show more details (lower image, 3B). The choice of the filter should reflect both the frequency context of the noise and the signal in the projection data.

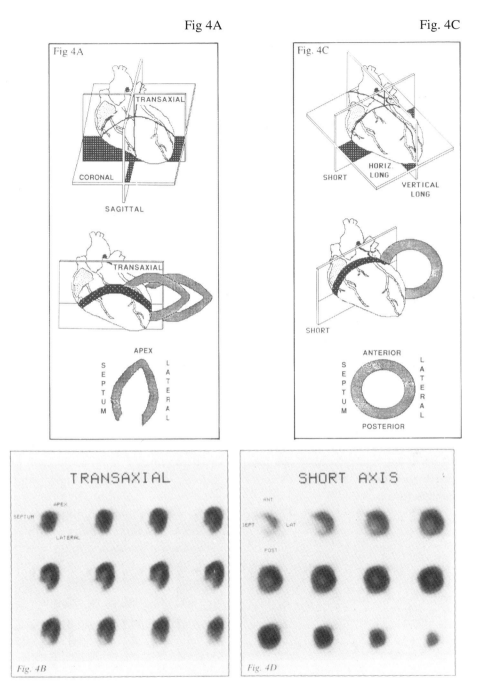

Fig 4A   Fig. 4C

Figure 4

Standard reconstruction (upper left, 4A) of the acquired data results in transaxial image slices (upper right, 4C). Coronal and sagittal tomographic planes can be obtained by reorganization of the transverse imaging data. Oblique images (short axis, horizontal and vertical long axis) which are parallel to the long axis (lower left, 4B) of the heart can be computed by using interpolation methods resulting in short axis images (lower right, 4D). ANT = anterior, LAT = lateral, POST = posterior, SEPT = septum

Rotational tomography

The general concept of SPECT imaging is circular angular sampling around the patient. The imaging instrument is a rotating Anger camera system that allows reconstruction of three-dimensional tomographic data. Images can be reconstructed in any plane. In our institution we use a large field of view digital gamma camera (Toshiba, GCA 90B), equipped with rectangular detector (50x30cm), and a low-energy, all purpose parallel-hole collimator centered on the 80 keV thallium x-ray peak (Fig. 1). The camera is interfaced to a dedicated computer and all projections are stored on a magnetic disk with a 128x128x12 bit matrix.

Imaging technique

The exact imaging technique varies slightly from laboratory to laboratory. Generally, a larger dose of thallium (100-150 MBq, 3.0-3.5 mCi) is recommended than usual (75 MBq, 2 mCi) since reliable reconstruction depends on an adequate number of myocardial counts. The acquisition arc may be 180° or 360°, but cardiac SPECT studies are generally acquired with 180° rotation from 45° right anterior oblique to the 45° left posterior oblique view. The 180° arc is preferred since this provides better image contrast and is less time-consuming than the 360°arc (4). The number of angular steps with our camera is 30 (6° per angle), each step being acquired for 60 seconds resulting in an imaging period of approximately 30 minutes. Approximately 100.000 counts per projection are obtained. The patient is positioned supine on the imaging table, and the left arm has to be placed above the head. To avoid image artifacts, patient motion should be kept to a minimum.

Recently it has been advocated that patients should be imaged in prone position to improve the specificity in the detection of inferior wall defects by suppressing attenuation artifacts (5).

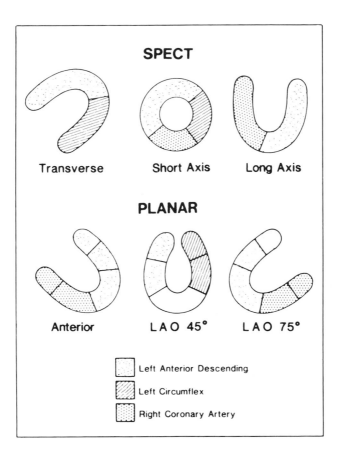

Figure 5
Comparison between tomographic and planar image interpretation. Upper panel: vascular territories in each tomographic image orientation (transverse, short axis, and long axis). SPECT = single photon emission computed tomography. Lower panel: vascular territories in each planar image orientation (anterior, 45° left anterior oblique (LAO), and 75° LAO). Reproduced by permission from Fintel et al. (14).

Imaging protocol

The imaging protocols at rest and during exercise are similar to those of planar thallium imaging. With thallium exercise SPECT, thallium is intravenously administered at peak exercise and the exercise is continued for an additional 60 seconds to allow adequate circulation of the radioisotope. Imaging is started within 5 minutes after exercise and repeated after 3-4 hours delay to obtain redistribution images. In patients who are unable to exercise dipyridamole perfusion scintigraphy with SPECT offers a valuable alternative pharmacologic stress method for detecting CAD. Patients receive dipyridamole either orally (300 mg) or by infusion (0.56 mg/kg) whereafter thallium is injected (40-50 minutes after oral medication or 2 minutes after intravenous injection).

Analysis of tomographic data

Image reconstruction

During the rotation of the camera around the long axis of the patient, information of all transaxial planes are simultaneously recorded. At reconstruction time only projection data corresponding with the slice to be constructed are taken into account. The simplest technique for reconstruction from projections is the back-projection algorithm. However, in this way the images become blurred. In general, an adapted algoritm called filtered back-projection is used for reconstruction of transaxial images. Different types of filters can be used to improve signal to noise ratio (Figs. 2 and 3). The filters may also influence the resolution of the imaging system. The standard reconstruction results in transaxial slices whereafter, by simple reorganization of the data, coronal and sagittal slices can be obtained. Since the heart is rotated in the thorax, oblique reconstruction has to be performed to provide short-axis, horizontal long-axis and vertical long-axis tomograms (Fig. 4).

Quantitative analysis

Visual interpretation of thallium SPECT images is often difficult and time-consuming particularly for the cardiologist accustomed to the conventional planar images. Typically, a myocardial SPECT study comprises about 10 short-axis slices, eight vertical long-axis slices, and eight horizontal long-axis slices. When both exercise and redistribution images are acquired, a total of 52 images must be reviewed which requires considerable interpretive expertise (Fig. 5). Therefore, a number of three-dimensional display formats has been developed to facilitate image interpretation. These quantitative methods are used to quantify and to display the data from an entire study in one single functional image. Circumferential profile analysis similar to that used with planar imaging has been applied to the short-axis SPECT data. Usually 10 slices are obtained from the normal-sized heart. The slices are divided into 40 sectors of 9° each and the maximum counts per pixel within each sector is determined (Fig. 6). The circumferential profiles of the short-axis slices are not displayed as curves but the curve values are color-coded and displayed as concentric circles. By superimposing each of the concentric circles -each representing one profile- a polar map called a bull's-eye plot is created with the apex at the center and the base of the heart at the periphery. The bull's-eye display allows the three-dimensional spatial distribution of thallium-201 to be reduced to a two-dimensional format that provides for better detection and localization of CAD both by visual and quantitative analysis (Figs. 7 and 8).

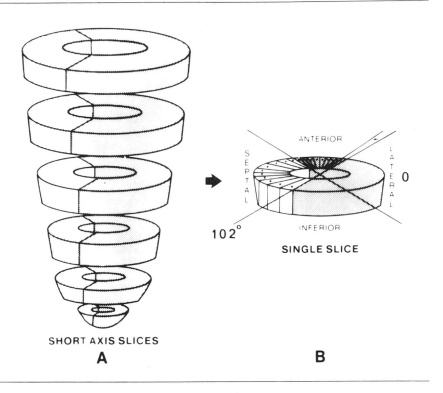

SHORT AXIS SLICES

A   **B**

Figure 6

Alternating short axis slices of the left ventricle (A) are displayed with the middle slice highlighted. A septal defect is present from base to apex. The highlighted slice (B) is divided into 40 sectors of 9 degrees each. The right ventricular junction (i.e. transit zone inferior and septal area) is always positioned at 102°. Adapted from DePasquale et al with permission. (22).

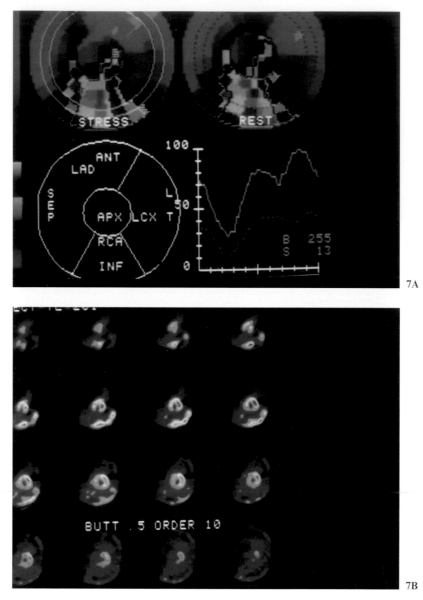

7A

7B

Figure 7
Polar plot map (bull's-eye view) showing the stress and delayed distribution of thallium (upper image, 7A). The center corresponds to the apex of the left ventricle, and the outer ring represents the most basal slice that was analyzed. The polar plot map is graphically divided into regions corresponding to the location of the major coronary arteries. The count profile plot represents the count distribution that extends clockwise from the left lateral wall, with the right ventricular junction always at 102° position. The exercise count profile is depicted by the dotted green line, and the resting count profile by the dotted blue line. A persistent defect is shown in the inferior region from a patient with sustained inferior infarction and is visible as a green-color enhanced area on both the stess and rest thallium image. The normally perfused areas are red-colored. On the lower image (7B) the short axis slices of this patient are shown. A Butterworth filter 0.5, order 10, was used. ANT = anterior, APX = apex, LT = lateral, INF = inferior.
LAD = left anterior descending coronary artery, LCX = left circumflex coronary artery, RCA = right coronary artery.

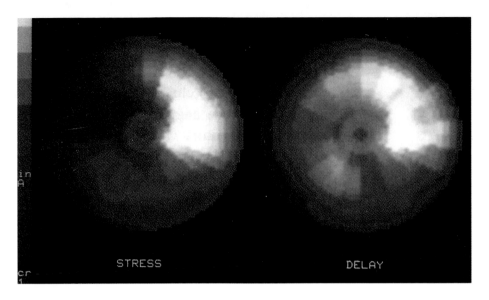

Figure 8
Bull's-eye views (stress and delay) from a patient with an 85% diameter stenosis of the left anterior descending coronary artery. Areas of maximal activity are displayed in yellow and red, whereas areas of diminished activity are shown in blue and green. There is a large anteroseptal defect during exercise (left), while the redistribution image (right) is normal indicating reversible ischemia in the anteroseptal region. Reproduced with permission from DePasquale et al. (22).

Another quantitative scheme is the three-dimensional reconstruction of the tomographic slices using surface mapping techniques (7). By geographical mapping both the extent, location and the severity of the perfusion abnormalities can be visualized in a three-dimensional display.

In summary, quantitative methods are preferred to visual analysis because they make interpretation more reproducible and less dependent on the skills of the observer.

Artifacts

Common potential difficulties in SPECT imaging include patient motion, inappropriate correction for center of rotation and camera nonuniformity. Each of these problems can create artifacts which, if not properly evaluated, will decrease the specificity of thallium SPECT imaging. In particular, upward motion of the heart during image acquisition ("upward creep") has been reported as a frequent cause of false positive studies. Patient motion can be minimized by comfortably keeping the arms of the patients outside the field of view and by carefully instructing the patients, while upward creep can be reduced by either delaying SPECT acquisition until 15 minutes postexercise (8) or by interposing a 5 minute anterior view planar acquisition between postexercise and the start of SPECT acquisition (9). Also following acquisition, SPECT is more subject to errors than planar imaging in selection of myocardial slices for visual display and quantitation. Therefore, SPECT requires greater attention to quality control than planar imaging for optimal image acquisition and analysis (10). Table I shows the advantages and disadvantages of thallium SPECT.

Table I
Advantages and disadvantages of SPECT compared to Planar thallium imaging

Advantages	Disadvantages
Improved image contrast	Prone to artifacts
Detection of extent of CAD	No better overall detection of CAD
Identification LCX lesions	More attention to quality control
Better infart sizing	Redistribution during acquisition of immediate postexercise images
Less inter- and intraobserver variability with quantitative analysis (bull's-eye view)	High costs of instrument

CAD = coronary artery disease, LCX = left circumflex coronary artery

Tomographic imaging versus planar imaging

In several studies planar thallium imaging has been compared with SPECT imaging. Most studies have indicated that SPECT is superior to planar thallium imaging both in patients with suspected CAD and in patients with acute or sustained myocardial infarction (11-19).

Exercise thallium SPECT

Table II shows the comparison between the results of exercise planar imaging and SPECT imaging. Exercise thallium SPECT, like planar thallium imaging, provides an excellent tool for the detection of patients with CAD but is generally superior in localizing disease in individual vessels.

The largest comprehensive comparison of SPECT and planar imaging has been reported by Fintel et al. (14), who studied 112 patients undergoing coronary arteriography and 23 normal volunteers by randomly sequenced exercise planar and tomographic imaging. The visual diagnostic performance of the two imaging techniques were compared using receiver operating characteristic (ROC) analysis. Thallium SPECT proved to be superior in identifying left anterior descending (LAD) and left circumflex disease (LCX), and also in detecting multivessel disease in patients with previous myocardial infarction.

Table II
Comparison between Planar and SPECT thallium exercise scintigraphy*

	Overall Detection	LAD	LCX	RCA
Sensitivity(%)				
Planar	90-91	58-73	36-39	55-85
SPECT	91-95	70-88	55-78	66-96
Specificity(%)				
Planar	83-100	89	100	87
SPECT	89-93	100	100	92

* Values are based on References 11-14
LAD = left anterior descending coronary artery
LCX = left circumflex coronary artery
RCA = right coronary artery.

Resting thallium SPECT

Resting thallium SPECT imaging has also been shown to be superior to planar imaging both in the detection of acute or sustained myocardial infarction and severe CAD. Tamaki et al. (15) measured perfusion defect size both by conventional thallium scintigraphy and by thallium SPECT in 18 patients with myocardial infarction. Creatine kinase MB release was compared with scintigraphic infarct size and showed a better correlation with SPECT (r=0.89) than with planar imaging (r=0.69). Maublant et al. (16) observed in 64 patients after myocardial infarction that the sensitivity of resting thallium SPECT was 98% in the detection of transmural infarction versus 93% with planar imaging. Specificities were 93% for both techniques. Ritchie et al. (17) found a sensitivity of 87% in detecting remote infarction in 38 patients using SPECT compared to 63% with planar imaging and was especially superior in patients with inferior infarcts. Similar to the findings of Maublant et al. (16), specificities were 93% for both imaging techniques. Tamaki et al. (18) showed a 96% overall sensitivity with SPECT and a 78% sensitivity with planar imaging in 160 patients with a first myocardial infarction. Kirsch et al. (19) reported a sensitivity of 93% for SPECT compared to 68% for planar imaging in 95 patients with severe CAD, of whom 45 with a prior myocardial infarction and 40 without a history of infarction.

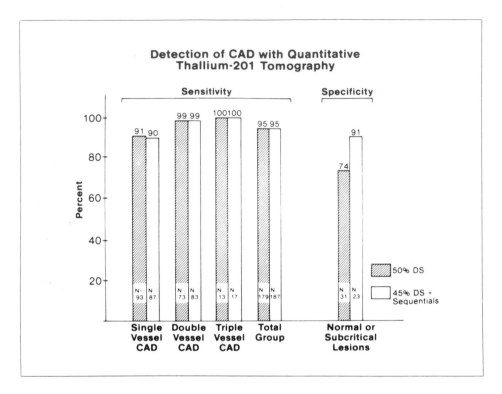

Figure 9
Comparison of the sensitivity and specificity of quantitative analysis for detection of coronary artery disease (CAD) when 50% diameter stenosis (DS) and 45% DS plus sequential lesions are used as the criteria for abnormality. The sensitivity in one-, two-, and three-vessel disease as well as the overall sensitivity and specificity are compared. Reproduced with persmission from DePasquale et al. (22).

Accordingly, the major improvements with thallium SPECT in patients with acute or previous myocardial infarction are the ability to localize inferior and posterior infarcts, to detect non-Q wave and small infarcts, and to quantify the extent of injured myocardial tissue.

Clinical applications of thallium SPECT imaging

A. Coronary artery disease

Visual analysis
Foster et al. (20) studied 37 patients with chest pain by exercise thallium SPECT and coronary arteriography. They observed by visual analysis a sensitivity of 97%, a specificity of 75%, and an overall accuracy of 95% for detecting CAD, indicating that thallium SPECT is an accurate noninvasive diagnostic test in patients with chest pain suggestive of angina.

Visual versus quantitative analysis

Tamaki et al. (21) found by visual analysis in 104 patients who underwent coronary arteriography a sensitivity of 93% for the overall detection of CAD, and sensitivities of 83%, 63%, and 88% for the detection of lesions in the LAD, LCX, and right coronary artery (RCA) respectively. When uptake and washout analysis were added, these values increased to 93% (overall detection CAD), 94% (LAD), 90% (LCX), and 88% (RCA), respectively. Depasquale et al. (22) studied 36 patients with a low probability of CAD to establish normal limits for the distribution of thallium, and 255 patients with angiographically documented CAD. Visual, quantitative, and combined visual and quantitative analysis were used for overall detection of CAD and the detection of individual vessel involvement. The overall sensitivities for detection of disease were 97%, 95%, and 95%; the specificities were 68%, 74%, and 71%, respectively. Regarding individual coronary artery lesions, the sensitivities for the LAD were 70%, 78%, and 75%; for the LCX 50%, 65%, and 55%; for the RCA 88%, 89%, and 87%, respectively.

These studies indicated that SPECT is a highly accurate technique for determining the presence and location of CAD. In addition, quantitative SPECT offered improvement over visual SPECT in the assessment of the extent of CAD and of subcritical stenoses (Fig. 9), and in particular in the detection of left circumflex artery disease and inferiorly localized segments.

Myocardium at risk

Prigent et al. (23) studied 22 patients with single-vessel coronary disease and demonstrated that SPECT was very useful to determine the extent of hypoperfused myocardium beyond the territory of the area supplied by the stenotic artery i.e. the myocardium at risk.

Silent ischemia

Hecht et al. (24) used exercise thallium SPECT in 112 patients with documented CAD of whom 84 patients had silent ischemia. It was observed that both patients with and without silent ischemia had perfusion abnormalities to a similar extent. The authors also suggested that future evaluation of silent ischemia by SPECT imaging may identify a greater number of patients with silent ischemia than previously suspected.

Dipyridamole thallium SPECT imaging

Borges-Neto et al. (25) studied 100 patients, of whom 84 with significant CAD, by thallium SPECT after a single oral dose of 300 mg dipyridamole and showed an overall sensitivity of 92% for detecting coronary artery disease. Dipyridamole thallium SPECT had a sensitivity of 80%, 51%, and 87% for localizing significant lesions in the LAD, LCX, and RCA, respectively. The corresponding specificities were 84%, 92%, and 92%. Severe multivessel disease (70% stenotic lesions) was identified with a sensitivity of 79% and a specificity of 87%. Huikuri et al. (26)

studied 73 patients with angina using a protocol of combining isometric handgrip exercise at the end of intravenous dipyridamole infusion and showed a sensitivity of 96% for detecting CAD. In addition, dipyridamole thallium SPECT proved to be superior to bicycle exercise thallium SPECT for the identification of multivessel disease.

Increased lung uptake
The additional value of increased lung uptake on thallium images, which is usually considered to reflect extensive coronary artery disease in planar thallium studies, proved to be at least questionable by SPECT imaging since this criterion did not provide supplementary information about the extent of disease on exercise SPECT images (27).

In summary, both visual and quantitative thallium SPECT -either by conventional exercise or after dipyridamole administration- have a high sensitivity and specificity for diagnosing CAD, ascertain the location of lesions in individual coronary arteries, and identify the presence of multivessel disease.

B. Interventions

Antianginal agents
Kugyama et al. (28) found that propranolol increased the thallium SPECT defect size in patients with variant angina while nifedipine decreased defect size. These changes were associated with concordant changes in symptoms and exercise tolerance. In patients with stable angina, however, Narahara et al. (29) demonstrated that beta-blocking agents significantly reduced exercise and redistribution thallium SPECT defect size and they concluded that thallium SPECT imaging is very useful in defining pharmacologically induced reduction of ischemia. Zannad et al. (30) showed that the calcium-antagonist diltiazem reduced ischemic injury after myocardial infarction in 34 patients who were serially studied by thallium SPECT before therapy (admission), after 48 hours, and 3 weeks later. The diltiazem group showed a significant decrease in perfusion defect scores and a better ejection fraction recovery.

Thrombolytic therapy
Several groups have used thallium SPECT in assessing infarct size after thrombolytic therapy. Kohn et al. (31) observed that infarct size determined by SPECT was significantly smaller in patients with successful thrombolysis after intravenous streptokinase than in conventionally treated patients.

Tamaki et al. (32) showed a better correlation between infarct size and enzyme levels (accumulated release of creatine kinase MB) in patients with unsuccessful than in patients with successful thrombolysis (r=0.91 vs r=0.80). The difference could be explained by changed kinetics in enzyme release, which shows a greater initial release in patients with reperfusion. Hashimoto et al. (33) examined by SPECT the significance of overlap between thallium-201 and technetium-99m pyrophosphate (i.e. a hot spot agent) as an indicator of early reperfusion. They studied 32 patients with acute myocardial infarction who received urokinase by infusion into the infarct-related artery. Myocardial imaging was performed at three days after infarction using simultaneous dual emission computed tomongraphy. The patients with unsuccessful reperfusion did not show any scintigraphic overlap, while the presence of overlap identified early reperfusion with a sensitivity of 80% and a specificity of 83%.

Maublant et al. (34) used thallium SPECT in 231 patients who were randomized to heparin or to APSAC (anisoylated plasminogen streptokinase activator complex) within 5 hours after acute myocardial infarction. Both radionuclide angiography and resting thallium SPECT were performed after 2-3 weeks and showed that both left ventricular function was improved and defect size was decreased by APSAC compared to heparin. The use of defect size assessment by SPECT proved to be as valuable for therapeutic evaluation as left ventricular function and wall motion analysis. Topol et al. (35) performed exercise thallium SPECT at 72 hours after acute myocardial infarction in 54 patients who received thrombolytic therapy and demonstrated that a positive thallium test result (i.e. reversible ischemia) was highly predictive for subsequent in-hospital cardiac events. In the patients with negative thallium results no cardiac events occurred. In addition, they showed that thallium exercise SPECT is already feasible at three days following myocardial infarction.

Percutaneous Transluminal Coronary Angioplasty
Cloninger et al. (36) performed quantitative thallium exercise SPECT scintigraphy in 141 patients before and after 160 percutaneous transluminal coronary angioplasty (PTCA) procedures. In the 123 patients without myocardial infarction, 67% had partial redistribution on delayed (4 hours) imaging. After PTCA, 76% showed improved thallium uptake in the areas with partial redistribution. In 40 patients with partial redistribution they also performed delayed imaging (8-24 hours) which demonstrated late redistribution in patients with and those without previous myocar-dial infarction. Therefore, additional imaging at 8-24 hours was recommended in patients with partial redistribution and no previous myocardial infarction, and in patients in whom the extent of myocardial scarring influences decisions regarding PTCA.

In a study by Jain et al. (37) in 53 patients to be treated by PTCA, thallium SPECT after dipyridamole (300 mg oral dose) allowed the assessment of the physiologic significance of both the coronary artery stenosis before angioplasty and of the residual stenosis after the intervention.

Coronary Artery Bypass Surgery
Fioretti et al. (38) studied 25 patients before and 2-3 months after coronary artery bypass surgery (CABG) by thallium exercise SPECT and showed that improvement of symptoms was accompanied by a marked improvement not only of transient, but also of persistent thallium defects. These findings indicated that seemingly persistent defects on pre-intervention tomograms are very well compatible with reversible

ischemic myocardial tissue post-intervention.

Kiat et al. (39) studied 21 patients by thallium exercise SPECT scintigraphy before and after CABG (15 patients) or PTCA (6 patients). Patients were imaged immediately after exercise, at 4 hours, and at 18-72 hours. The 4 hour redistribution images did not predict the postintervention scintigraphic improvement, while the 18-72 hour images were very useful in identifying viable tissue within the fixed defects at 4 hours: 95% of the late (18-72 hours) reversible segments improved after the intervention, whereas only 37% of the late nonreversible segments improved. They concluded that late redistribution images should be performed when nonreversible (fixed) defects are observed on 4 hour redistribution images.

C. Other cardiac diseases

Left bundle branch block
De Puey et al. (40) showed in 14 patients with left bundle branch block that thallium SPECT had a sensitivity of 75% but a specificity of only 10% for demonstrating coronary artery lesions in the LAD. The low specificity was due to the fact that 9 of 10 patients with a normal LAD showed septal perfusion defects, indicating that thallium SPECT is indeterminate for detecting lesions in the LAD in patients with left bundle branch block.

Cardiomyopathies
O. Gara et al. (41) studied 72 patients with hypertrophic cardiomypathy without objective signs of myocardial ischemia. Perfusion defects were identified in 41 patients (57%) of whom 17 patients had reversible defects and 24 patients irreversible thallium defects. The reversible defects occurred predominantly in patients with preserved systolic function, while the irreversible defects went along with depressed left ventricular function, suggesting that myocardial ischemia commonly occurs in patients with hypertrophic cardiomyopathy.

D. Other perfusion agents

Thallium-201 has a relatively long half-life (72 hours), and is a low-energy gamma-emmitter (80 keV) resulting in a substantial attenuation of gamma-rays. Moreover, evaluation of thallium exercise scintigrams relies on redistribution of thallium in the ischemic area, which may lower the sensitivity of tomographic imaging as redistribution could potentially occur during the 30 minutes between tracer injection and completion of the SPECT study. Therefore, alternative radiopharmaceuticals with shorter half-lives, higher gamma-energies, and without redistribution properties have been developed.

Technetium-99m isonitriles
One of such agents, technetium-99m labeled to isonitriles (MIBI), shows these

advantages: it has a 6-hour half-life, a gamma-emission of 140 keV, and when labeled to isonitriles it does not redistribute in ischemic myocardial areas. In particular, the absence of redistribution makes it ideal for longer imaging times required for SPECT. Therefore, technetium-99m MIBI is potentially more suitable than thallium for tomographic imaging. Iskandrian et al. (42) demonstrated in 39 patients, of whom 28 with CAD, that technetium-99m MIBI SPECT showed a similar sensitivity and specificity but a better image quality than thallium SPECT. Kahn et al. (43) used quantitative SPECT imaging with both technetium-99m MIBI and thallium-201 in 12 normal subjects and 38 patients with proven CAD. They observed that the image quality of technetium-99m MIBI was superior to thallium-201 and that reversible ischemic myocardial segments were better identified with technetium-99m MIBI. Similar findings were reported by Kiat et al. (44) who found that SPECT technetium MIBI was superior to planar technetium MIBI for the identification of individually diseased vessels. However, drawbacks of technetium-99m MIBI are the high liver uptake immediately following administration which postpones the image acquisition for at least one hour, and the separate injection of activity both at rest and during exercise needing a special imaging protocol. Furthermore, many more studies with technetium-99m MIBI have to be performed to establish its definite role in myocardial perfusion imaging. At present, thallium is still the most frequently employed radioisotope for myocardial perfusion imaging, both for planar and SPECT imaging.

Iodinated free fatty acids
Another alternative radiopharmaceutical with favourable imaging properties is iodine-123 (150 keV, half-life 13 hours) which, when labeled to free fatty acids, provides excellent insight in cardiac metabolism (45). Hansen et al. (46) used iodine-123 phenylpentadecanoic acid with exercise SPECT in 27 patients with CAD and showed that the metabolic compound was as sensitive as thallium for identification of myocardial ischemia.

Indium-111 antimyosin
SPECT imaging has also been applied for infarct-avid imaging using the hot spot agents technetium-99m pyrophosphate and the more recently developed indium-111 antimyosin. Radiolabeled antimyosin accumulates selectively in irreversibly damaged myocardial cells following acute myocardial infarction. Antunes et al. (47) studied 27 patients after acute transmural myocardial infarction by indium-111 antimyosin SPECT and showed that infarct size could be accurately measured between 1 and 4 days after the acute event.

Radionuclide angiography
Recent studies have demonstrated that radionuclide angiography by SPECT imaging allowed the automated identification of the left ventricular surface in gated tomographic radionulide ventriculograms. Global volumes computed from these surfaces

corresponded well with known volumes (48). Ohtake et al. (49) showed that the regurgitation fraction in patients with mitral and aortic insufficiency could be accurately measured by gated radionuclide angiography SPECT imaging.

SPECT versus PET

Positron emission tomography (PET) has theoretically several advantages over single photon techniques (50), including 1) the obtainment of both regional and absolute quantification of tracer distribution due to adequate correction for tissue attenuation, 2) improved spatial resolution and therefore high specificity for detecting CAD, 3) the rather short physical half-lives of positron emitters allowing the rest and exercise images to be acquired in rapid succession, and 4) assessment of myocardial viability by both perfusion agents and metabolic markers. Tamaki et al. (51) found in 28 patients with myocardial infarction that 38% of patients with fixed defects by exercise thallium SPECT had evidence of persistent metabolic activity by PET imaging when fluorine-18-deoxyglucose was used i.e they observed a mismatch between flow and metabolic activity. Also Brunken et al. (52) showed metabolic activity with glucose PET in almost half of the segments with fixed defects on thallium exercise SPECT images. These findings indicate remaining viability of apparently nonperfused myocardial areas and may be of clinical importance because myocardial areas with preserved glucose uptake can regain function after PTCA or revascularization. In another study, Tamaki et al. (53) compared exercise thallium SPECT with exercise PET using nitrogen-13-ammonia as a perfusion marker in 51 patients with CAD. They found no significant differences in sensitivity and specificity for overall CAD detection and identification of lesion in individual coronary arteries. Using a similar protocol, Tamaki et al. (54) showed in 31 patients following CABG that the preoperative prediction of reversible asynergy was only slightly better with ammonia PET compared to thallium SPECT. Thus, although the literature has been consistent with respect to advantages of PET, it has still to be settled whether PET is superior to SPECT in identifying patients with CAD. Table III shows a comparison between imaging characteristics of SPECT and PET.

Table III
Comparison between SPECT and PET imaging

	SPECT	PET
Spatial resolution (mm)	10-20	5-10
3D-reconstruction	Yes	Yes
Attenuation correction	limited	nearly exact
Quantitation of activity	limited	possible
Number of tracers	numerous	limited
Metabolic information	good	excellent
Acquisition time (min)	30	30
Interpretation	easy	needs expertise
Availability	increasing	still very limited
Costs of camera (Dfl)	2×10^6	6×10^6

SPECT, a new aspect and a new perspective?

Recent literature has convincingly shown that thallium SPECT imaging is superior to planar thallium imaging in patients with CAD. The most important advantages of SPECT over planar imaging are: 1) the three-dimensional presentation of the images, 2) improved contrast due to the lack of superimposition of normal and abnormal myocardial regions, 3) better assessment of the extent of CAD and recognition of individually diseased vessels, 4) increased detection of moderate or mild degrees of coronary artery stenoses, 5) improved quantitation of infarct size, and finally, 6) assessment of the myocardium at risk. Future SPECT studies are needed to demonstrate its prognostic power in risk stratification in addition to the prognostic information already established for planar thallium studies (55). With the development of the technetium-99m isonitriles, SPECT may become even more important for myocardial perfusion imaging. The recently demonstrated advantages of SPECT in cardiac patients put SPECT in a new perspective and advocate the use of SPECT imaging as the method of choice for myocardial perfusion scintigraphy.

References

1. Van der Wall EE, Braat S, Visser FC. Task Force Committee of The Netherlands Society of Cardiology. Guidelines for clinical use in nuclear cardiology. Neth J Cardiol 1988;1:45-52.
2. Okada RD, Boucher CA, Strauss HW, Pohost GM. Exercise radionuclide imaging approaches to coronary artery disease. Am J Cardiol 1980; 46:1188-204.
3. Wackers FJT, Fetterman RC, Mattera JA, Clements JP, Van der Wall EE. Kwantitatieve analyse van thallium-201 inspanningsscintigrafie. Hartbulletin 1986;17:4-20.
4. Knesaurek K, King MA, Glick SJ, Penney BC. Investigation of causes of geometric distortion in 180° and 360° angular sampling in SPECT. J Nucl Med 1989;30:1666-75.
5. Segall GM, Davis MJ. Prone versus supine thallium myocardial SPECT: a method to decrease artifactual inferior wall defects. J Nucl Med 1989;30:548-55.
6. Garcia EV, Van Train K, Maddahi J, et al. Quantification of rotational thallium-201 myocardial tomography. J Nucl Med 1985;26:17-26.
7. DePuey EG, Garcia EV, Ezquerra NF. Three-dimensional techniques and artificial intelligence in thallium-201 cardiac imaging. AJR 1989;152:1161-8.
8. Friedman J, Van Train K, Maddahi J, et al. "Upward Creep" of the heart: a frequent source of false-positive reversible defects during thallium-201 stress-redistribution SPECT. J Nucl Med 1989;30:1718-22.
9. Kiat H, Berman DS, Maddahi J. Comparison of planar and tomographic exercise thallium-201 imaging methods for the evaluation of coronary artery disease. J Am Coll Cardiol 1989;13:613-6.
10. DePuey EG, Garcia EV. Optimal specificity of thallium-201 SPECT through recognition of imaging artifacts. J Nucl Med 1989;30:441-49.
11. Tamaki N, Yonekura Y, Kukai T, et al. Segmental analysis of stress thallium myocardial emission tomography for localization of coronary artery disease. Eur J Nucl Med 1984;9:99-105.
12. Nohara R, Kambara H, Suzuki Y, et al. Stress scintigraphy using single-photon emission computed tomography in the evaluation of coronary artery disease. Am J Cardiol 1984;53:1250-4.
13. Port SC, Oshima M, Ray G, McNamee P, Schmidt DH. Assessment of single vessel coronary artery disease: results of exercise electrocardiography, thallium-201 myocardial perfusion imaging and radionuclide angiography. J Am Coll Cardiol 1985;1:75-83.
14. Fintel DJ, Links JM, Brinker JA, Frank RL, Parker M, Becker LC. Improved diagnostic performance of exercise thallium-201 single photon emission computed tomography over planar imaging in the diagnosis of coronary artery disease: a receiver operating characteristic analysis. J Am Coll Cardiol 1989;13:600-12.
15. Tamaki S, Nakajima H, Murakami T, et al. Estimation of infarct size by myocardial emission computed tomography with thallium-201 and its relation to creatine kinase-MB release after myocardial infarction in man. Circulation 1982;66:994-1001.
16. Maublant J, Gassagnes J, Le Jeune J, et al. A comparison between conventional scintigraphy and emission tomography with thallium-201 in the detection of myocardial infarction: concise communication. J Nucl Med 1982;23:204-8.
17. Ritchie JL, Williams DL, Harp G, Stratton JL, Caldwell JH. Transaxial tomographic with thallium-201 for detecting remote myocardial infarction. Am J Cardiol 1982;50:1236-41.
18. Tamaki S, Kambara H, Kadota K, et al. Improved detection of myocardial infarction by emission computed tomography with thallium-201. Relation to infarct size. Br Heart J 1984;52:621-7.
19. Kirsch C-M, Doliwa R, Buell U, Roedler D. Detection of severe coronary heart disease with Tl-201: comparison of resting single photon emission tomography with invasive arteriography. J Nucl Med 1983;24:761-7.
20. Foster CJ, Lawrence GP, Hastings DL, Prescott MG, Testa HJ. Evaluation of myocardial thallium tomography in patients with chest pain. Int J Cardiol 1989;22:203-11.
21. Tamaki N, Yonekura Y, Mukai T, et al. Stress thallium-201 transaxial emission computed tomography: quantitative versus qualitative analysis for evaluation of coronary artery disease. J Am Coll Cardiol 1984;6:1213-21.
22. DePasquale EE, Nody AC, DePuey G, et al. Quantitative rotational thallium-201 tomography for identifying and localizing coronary artery disease. Circulation 1988;77:316-27.

100

23. Prigent F, Maddahi J, Garcia E, Van Train K, Friedman J, Berman D. Noninvasive quantification of the extent of jeopardized myocardium in patients with single-vessel coronary disease by stress thallium-201 single-photon emission computerized rotational tomography. Am Heart J 1986;111:578-86.

24. Hecht H, Shwa RE, Bruce T, Myler RK. Silent ischemia: evaluation by exercise and redistribution tomographic thallium-201 myocardial imaging. J Am Coll Cardiol 1989;14:895-900.

25. Borges-Neto S, Mahmarian JJ, Jain A, Roberts R, Verani M. Quantitative thallium-201 single photon emission computed tomography after oral dipyridamole for assessing the presence, anatomic location and severity of coronary artery disease. J Am Coll Cardiol 1988;11:962-9.

26. Huikuri HV, Korhonen UR, Airaksinen KEJ, Ikä heimo MJ, Heikkilä J, Takkunen JT. Comparison of dipyridamole-handgrip test and bicycle exercise test for thallium tomographic imaging. Am J Cardiol 1988; 61:264-8.

27. Kahn JK, Carry MM, McGhie I, Pippin JJ, Akers MS, Corbett JR. Quantitation of postexercise lung thallium-201 uptake during single photon emission computed tomography. J Nucl Med 1989;30:288-94.

28. Kugiyama K, Yasue H, Horio Y, et al. Effects of propranolol and nifedipine on exercise-induced attack in patients with variant angina: Assessment by exercise thallium-201 myocardial scintigraphy with quantitative rotational tomography. Circulation 1986;74:374-80.

29. Narahara KA, Thompson CJ, Hazen JF, Brizendine M, Mena I. The effect of beta-blockade on single photon emission computed tomographic (SPECT) thallium-201 images in patients with coronary disease. Am Heart J 1989; 117:1030-5.

30. Zannad F, Amor M, Karcher G, et al. Effect of diltiazem on myocardial infarct size estimated by enzyme release, serial thallium-201 single-photon emission computed tomography and radionuclide angiography. Am J Cardiol 1988;61:1172-7.

31. Kohn H, Frohner K, Bialonezyk C, Unger G, Mostbeck A, Steinbach K. Intravenous streptokinase therapy in acute myocardial infarction: Assessment of therapy effect by quantitative thallium myocardial imaging (including SPECT) and radionuclide ventriculography. Eur J Nucl Med 1984;9:408-12.

32. Tamaki S, Murakami T, Kadota K, et al. Effects of coronary artery reperfusion on relation between creatine kinase-MB release and infarct size estimated by myocardial emission tomography with thallium-201 in man. J Am Coll Cardiol 1983;2:1031-38.

33. Hashimoto T, Kambara H, Fudo T, et al. Significance of technetium-99m/Thallium-201 overlap on simultaneous dual emission computed tomography in acute myocardial infarction. Am J Cardiol 1988;61:1181-6.

34. Maublant JC, Peycelon P, Cardiot JC, Verdent J, Fagret D, Comet M. Value of myocardial defect size measured by thallium-201 SPECT: results of a multicenter trial comparing heparin and a new fibrinolytic agent. J Nucl Med 1988;29:1486-91.

35. Topol EJ, Juni JE, O'Neil WW, et al. Exercise testing three days after onset of acute myocardial infarction. Am J Cardiol 1987;60:958-62.

36. Cloninger MG, DePuey G, Garcia EV, et al. Incomplete redistribution in delayed thallium-201 single photon emission computed tomographic (SPECT) images: an overestimation of myocardial scarring. J Am Coll Cardiol 1988;12:955-63.

37. Jain A, Mahmarian JJ, Borges-Neto S, et al. Clinical significance of perfusion defects by thallium-201 single photon emission tomography following oral dipyridamole early after coronary angioplasty. J Am Coll Cardiol 1988;11:970-6.

38. Fioretti P, Reijs AEM, Neumann D, et al. Improvement in transient and 'persistent' perfusion defects on early and late post-exercise thallium-201 tomograms after coronary artery bypass grafting. Eur Heart J 1988;9:1332-8.

39. Kiat H, Berman DS, Maddahi J, et al. Late reversibility of tomographic myocardial thallium-201 defects: an accurate marker of myocardial viability. J Am Coll Cardiol 1988;12:1456-63

40. DePuey EG, Guertler-Krawczynska E, Robbins WL. Thallium-201 SPECT in coronary artery disease patients with left bundle branch block. J Nucl Med 1988;29:1479-85.

41. O'Gara PT, Bonow RO, Maron BJ, et al. Myocardial perfusion abnormalities in patients with hypertrophic cardiomyopathy: assessment with thallium-201 emission computed tomography. Circulation 1987;76:1214-23.

42. Iskandrian AS, Heo J, Kong B, Lyons E, Marsch S. Use of technetium-99m isonitrile (RP-30A) in assessing left ventricular perfusion and function at rest and during exercise in coronary artery disease, and comparison with coronary arteriography and exercise thallium-201 SPECT imaging. Am J Cardiol 1989;64:270-5.

43. Kahn JK, McGhie I, Akers MS, et al. Quantitative rotational tomography with thallium-201 and technetium-99m methoxy-isobutyl-isonitrile. A direct comparison in normal individuals and patients with coronary artery disease. Circulation 1989;79:1282-93.

44. Kiat H, Maddahi J, Roy LT, et al. Comparison of technetium-99m methoxy isobutyl isonitrile and thallium-201 for evaluation of coronary artery disease by planar and tomographic methods. Am Heart J 1989;117:1-11.

45. Hansen CL, Corbett JR, Pippin JJ, et al. Iodine-123 phenylpentadecanoic acid and single photon emission computed tomography in identifying left ventricular regional metabolic abnormalities in patients with coronary artery disease:comparison with thallium-201 tomography. J Am Coll Cardiol 1988;12:78-87.

46. Van der Wall EE, Heidendal GAK, Den Hollander W, Westera G, Roos JP. Metabolic imaging with I-123 labeled heptadecanoic acid in patients with stable angina pectoris. Eur J Nucl Med 1981;6:391-6.

47. Antunes ML, Seldin DW, Wall RM, Johnson LL. Measurement of acute Q-wave myocardial infarct size with single photon emission computed tomography of indium-111 antimyosin. Am J Cardiol 1989;63:777-83.

48. Faber TL, Stokely EM, Templeton GH, Akers MS, Parkey RW, Corbett JR. Quantification of three-dimensional left ventricular segmental wall motion and volumes from gated tomographic radionuclide ventriculograms. J Nucl Med 1989;30:638-49.

49. Ohtake T, Nishikawa J, Machida K, et al. Evaluation of regurgitant fraction of the left ventricle by gated cardiac blood-pool scanning using SPECT. J Nucl Med 1987;28:19-24.

50. Van der Wall EE. Positron emission tomography in cardiology. From research device to clinical tool? Neth J Cardiol 1989;2:89-98.

51. Tamaki N, Yonekura Y, Yamashita K. et al. Relation of left ventricular perfusion and wall motion with metabolic activity in persistent defects on thallium-201 tomography in healed myocardial infarction. Am J Cardiol 1988;62:202-8.

52. Brunken RC, Kottou S, Nienaber CA, Schwaiger M, Ratib OM, Phelps ME, Schelbert HR. PET detection of viable tissue in myocardial segments with persistent defects at Tl-201 SPECT. Radiology 1989;172:65-73.

53. Tamaki N, Yonekura Y, Senda M, et al. Value and limitation of stress thallium-201 single photon emission computed tomography: comparison with nitrogen-13 ammonia positron tomography. J Nucl Med 1988;29:1181-88.

54. Tamaki N, Yonekura Y, Yamashita K, et al. Value of rest-stress myocardial positron tomography using nitrogen-13 ammonia for preoperative prediction of reversible asynergy. J Nucl Med 1989;30:1302-10.

55. Kaul S, Lilly DR, Gascho JA, et al. Prognostic utility of the exercise thallium-201 test in ambulatory patients with chest pain: comparison with cardiac catheterization. Circulation 1988;77:745-58.

6.
Positron emission tomography in cardiology: From research device to clinical tool?

Summary

Positron emission tomography is a rather new diagnostic modality for noninvasive studies of the heart using positron emitting tracers. Important advantages are the use of physiological substrates that can be labeled with positron tracers, the acquisition of accurate tomographic information, and the potential of quantitative measurements not obtainable with any other technique. Especially disorders in myocardial perfusion and metabolism can be studied in a very early stage of the disease process, which may result in application of more appropriate and earlier therapy. Major limitations are the expenses for the positron camera and, in particular, for a cyclotron. However, a positron tracer like rubidium-82 is generator-produced without the need for a cyclotron and provides accurate measurements of myocardial blood flow. Moreover, when effectively used, routine cardiac positron imaging may be cost-saving on the long run. At present, positron emission tomography has been evolved from a complex research device into routinely applicable clinical equipment. It will provide the basis for a specific therapeutic approach in patients with coronary artery disease, thereby justifying the routine, clinical and economic use of positron emission tomography in cardiology.

Introduction

Positron emission tomography (PET) is an advanced technique in nuclear medicine which permits accurate noninvasive quantification of cardiac perfusion, metabolism and function. Until now, PET has been widely considered as an expensive research tool rather than as a real clinical diagnostic modality. In addition, early PET investigations also required a fully equipped team of radiochemists, physicists and physicians to carry out appropriate research studies providing important basic scientific information, but limited in clinical application. However, tremendous progress in radiochemistry and technology have accounted for an important shift from experimental device to clinical equipment. The combination of automated synthesis techniques and clinically oriented positron cameras with dedicated software allows well-trained technicians or nurses to perform routine clinical PET studies under the supervision of a clinician. Although an on-site cyclotron is necessary for metabolic imaging, the development of generator-produced positron isotopes without a cyclotron, such as rubidium-82, permits routine clinical studies of cardiac perfusion and function. Since most positron-emitters have short half-lives ranging from a few seconds to several hours, their radiation exposure to the patient is minimal and they are very useful to study the physiological consequences of interventional procedures in cardiology. The effects of medical therapy, acute thrombolysis, percutaneous transluminal coronary angioplasty and coronary artery bypass grafting can be accurately assessed by the PET technique. The knowledge gained with PET may contribute to the development of alternative and less expensive diagnostic methods and to improvement in patient therapy.

So far, most experience has been obtained with the study of myocardial perfusion and metabolism (1,2). Future applications will pertain to the study of cardiac innervation by specific positron-labeled receptor ligands. This chapter will focus on cardiac positron instrumentation, the applied positron emitting radionuclides in cardiology, the main experimental and clinical applications, and the future role of positron emission tomography in cardiology.

Cardiac instrumentation

The current positron camera employs one or multiple rings arranged in opposing pairs around the patient. Only positron-emitting tracers can be detected on the basis of positron-electron annihilation. Positrons are positively charged electrons which travel only a very short distance (less than 1 mm) to encounter an electron. When the positron and the electron combine, both are annihilated and the energy of the two particles is converted to two high energy photons (511 keV) that are emitted 180° apart in opposite directions (Fig. 1). If two scintillation detectors are placed opposite one another, they will detect the annihilation photons simultaneously (coincidence detection). Scattered photons that reach only one of the detectors are rejected. The scintillation detectors provide multiple tomographic imaging planes of a three-dimensional reconstruction of activity in the field of view.

Major advantages of the PET approach include: 1) the incorporation of many positron tracers into naturally occurring substrates, 2) accurate tomographic localization of regional events in organs, and 3) adequate correction for photon attenuation and therefore better quantification of activity within the heart than is obtained with conventional gamma camera systems.

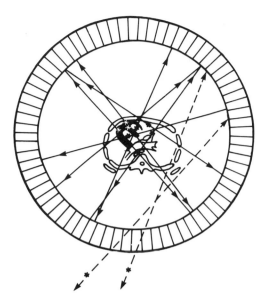

Figure 1

Schematic depiction of a ring of detectors from a positron emission tomographic system, including a cross section of the thorax and heart in the plane of the mitral valve apparatus. Positrons are emitted from the radiotracer within the heart, the blood pool and extracardiac structures. Annihilation of positrons results in emission of a pair of 511 keV photons at an angulation of 180°. Events which occur within the field of view activate a pair of opposing detectors if they arrive within a narrowly defined time interval (i.e. 500 picoseconds), thus providing electronic collimation by localizing the event along the line between that detector pair (solid lines). Extraneous activity is rejected because only a single detector is activated within the coincidence resolving time (broken lines). In practice, tomographs may be composed of multiple rings of adjacent detectors allowing visualization of a larger region axially and permitting reconstruction of images into transverse, sagittal, or coronal planes.*

Positron emitting radionuclides

Positron emitting radionuclides used for cardiac application are shown in Table 1. They can broadly be divided into those tracers that evaluate myocardial perfusion, those tracers that evaluate myocardial metabolism, and those that evaluate the myocardial nervous system.

Perfusion

The tracers for measurement of myocardial perfusion have to meet several require-ments: 1) they must remain in the heart for a sufficient time to acquire statistically adequate images, 2) the kinetics of the tracer should be known, and 3) the kinetics have to fit into kinetic models so that myocardial flow can be assessed from tracer distribution data. Positron-emitters used for evaluation of myocardial perfusion include isotopes of rubidium (^{82}Rb), nitrogen-13-labeled ammonia (employed in the form of $^{13}NH_4^+$), and labeled water ($H_2^{15}O$). The current positron instruments combine high sensitivity and high resolution for imaging myocardial perfusion. Recent studies by Gould et al. (3) indicate that reductions of luminal diameter of less than 50% can be detected when these radionuclides are administered in conjunction with dipyridamole vasodilatation. The regional distribution of both ^{13}N-ammonia and ^{82}Rb have excellent correlations with that of microspheres although they share the limitations of being diffusion-limited tracers. Extraction of ammonia and rubidium falls off at higher flows because shortened residence time in the capillary bed reduces uptake across capillary membranes.

Table 1.

Positron-emitting tracers for cardiac application

	Half-life	Intra-venous	Intra-coronary
A. Perfusion			
1. *monovalent cations*			
Rubidium-82 (^{82}Rb)	75 s	+	
Nitrogen-13-ammonia (^{13}NH$_4^+$)	10 min	+	
H$_2$^{15}O (labeled water)	2 min	+	
2. *Particulate agents*			
Carbon-11(11C)-microspheres	20 min		+
Gallium-68 (68Ga)-			
macroaggregates or albumin	68 min		+
B. Metabolism			
1. *Carbohydrates*			
2-fluorine-18-deoxyglucose (^{18}FDG)	108 min	+	
^{11}C-deoxy-D-glucose (^{11}CDG)	20 min	+	
^{11}C-pyruvate,^{11}C-lactate,^{11}C-acetate	20 min	+	
2. *Fatty acids*			
^{11}C-palmitate	20 min	+	
^{11}C-beta-methyl fatty acids	20 min	+	
3. *Amino acids*			
^{13}N-glutamate	10 min	+	
C. Nervous system			
^{11}C-labeled beta-adrenergic,	20 min	+	
muscarinic, and dopamine receptors			
6-(^{18}F)-fluorometaraminol	108 min	+	

Rubidium-82

Rubidium-82 (^{82}Rb, half-life 75 seconds) is a daughter of the cyclotron-produced strontium-82 (^{82}SR, half-life 25 days). The production of the parent strontium-82 requires a high-energy cyclotron, but ^{82}Rb can be produced from a Sr-Rb generator without the need for a cyclotron. Rubidium-82 (30-50 mCi) is eluted from the generator as a monovalent cation and, with a continuous supply from a bedside generator, an intravenous infusion results in an equilibrium in the arterial blood within four half-lives of ^{82}Rb. Myocardial imaging with ^{82}Rb requires fast acquisition of data. The images recorded during the first 1-2 minutes after intravenous administration depict the blood pool distribution of the radionuclide. If images are recorded with gating, also ejection fraction and regional wall motion can be determined, while images recorded after two minutes depict regional perfusion.

Rubidium-82 imaging provides a repeatable and noninvasive measure of regional myocardial perfusion since each patient can be used as his own control. This is a considerable advantage when evaluating the responses of the coronary circulation in various physiologic states. Several clinical studies have shown the value of ^{82}Rb for the detection of coronary artery disease by the measurement of coronary flow reserve after dipyridamole-induced vasodilation (3-5). In this way performed, clinical decisions are not only based on arteriographic data but mainly on functional degrees of coronary artery abnormality. The sensitivity of diagnosing coronary artery disease in comparison with coronary arteriography approximates 95% with an almost 100% specificity.

Relative disadvantages are 1) the remaining blood activity during the measurement after the infusion, 2) the inverse relation between flow and extraction, which may result in underestimation of increases in regional perfusion, and 3) the independent changes in rubidium uptake that can occur during metabolic abnormalities. However, all the experimental and clinical evidence to date indicates that regional decreases in coronary flow are reflected by changes in uptake of ^{82}Rb. For practical cardiology purposes, the application of ^{82}Rb is less expensive than the use of other positron tracers and yields important clinical information which cannot be obtained with any other technique.

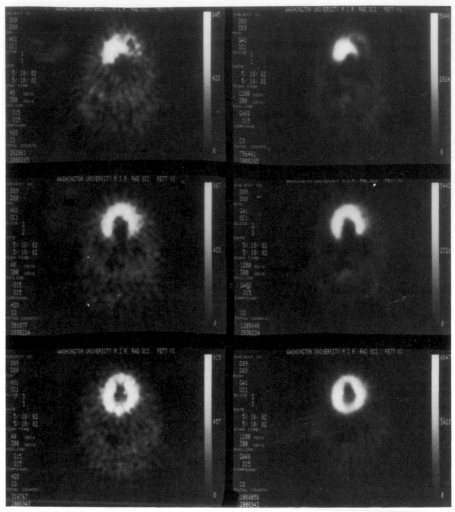

Figure 2

Tomograms from three adjacent planes through the ventricle of a normal dog. $H_2{}^{15}O$ distribution, corrected for vascular tracer with $C^{15}O$, is depicted on the left, and Gallium-68-microsphere distribution on the right. In each image, anterior myocardium is to the top, lateral wall to the left, and intraventricular septum to the right (i.e. as viewed from above). The much thinner right ventricle is not clearly defined (upper panels), and activity does not accumulate in the mitral valve region which is located posteriorly in the middle pair of images.*

Nitrogen-13 ammonia

Nitrogen-13 (^{13}N) labeled ammonia serves as a flow marker which concentrates in the myocardium with an extraction fraction of approximately 70%. Similar to ^{82}Rb, the net uptake of the tracer is related to blood flow in a curvilinear fashion. This means that the relation between blood flow and myocardial ^{13}N-ammonia is relatively linear over the physiological range of blood flow, but falls off at higher flows. Moreover, the uptake of ^{13}N-ammonia by the myocardium is also dependent on metabolic trapping catalysed by glutamine synthetase. However, changes in myocardial blood flow can adequately be recorded by PET, since ammonia activity concentrations measured by PET have been shown to correlate very well with the standard microsphere technique (6). Accurate quantitation of regional myocardial perfusion with ^{13}N-ammonia (and also with ^{82}Rb) has been difficult, although valuable clinical information has been obtained including determination of extraction of labeled metabolic substrates (labeled glucose) with reference to estimates of perfusion (See Section Labeled glucose).

In addition, like ^{82}Rb, alterations of perfusion and regional myocardial metabolism in response to pharmacological vasodilator stress may be used to assess severity of coronary artery disease. The relationship between abnormalities of ^{13}N-ammonia extraction and changes in accumulation of labeled glucose may provide a description of viable but transiently ischemic myocardium.

The detection of coronary artery disease by both ^{82}Rb and ^{13}N-ammonia during exercise or after dipyridamole administration has been improved compared to conventional planar thallium-201 scintigraphy; sensitivity as well as specificity approach 95%. To date, ^{13}N-ammonia has been used primarily as a qualitative index of the relative distribution of myocardial flow, although quantitative techniques to measure absolute blood flow are possible.

Radiolabeled water

A third short-lived, cyclotron-produced, positron emitting radionuclide, oxygen-15 (^{15}O), can be used for measurement of coronary blood flow. The tracer can be administered by inhalation of ^{15}O-labeled carbon dioxide, which results in the distribution of ^{15}O-labeled water. It has also been shown that labeled water can be administered as an intravenous bolus. The myocardial transit is recorded by PET, separate blood pool subtraction can be performed with ^{15}O-labeled carbon monoxide, and measurements can then be made of regional myocardial perfusion (Fig. 2). This provides another approach to the evaluation of coronary blood flow with negligible contribution from metabolic variables. The utility of this approach has been demonstrated in experimental canine preparations (7). In open chest dogs the single pass extraction of labeled water by the heart averaged 96 ± 5% and did not differ significantly over a wide range of flows (from 12 to 300 ml/100 g/min). Because the extraction fraction was high and consistent, the extraction of tracer appeared to be flow-limited rather than diffusion-limited over the ranges of flow studied. Thus, the tracer provided a good index of flow in vivo. The short physical half-life of ^{15}O (two minutes) allows sequential collection of the labeled water and labeled carbon monoxide images within approximately ten minutes. The radiolabeled water technique allows the study of the functional impact of subcritical coronary arterial stenoses on myocardial perfusion before and after pharmacologically induced vasodilatory stress (Fig. 3).

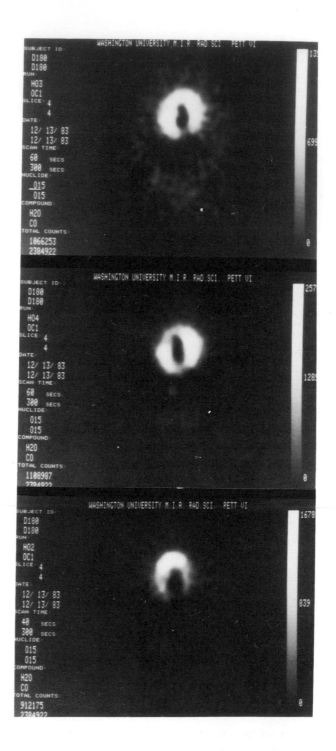

Figure 3

Midventricular tomograms from a single plane of a dog with a 70% diameter stenosis of the left anterior descending coronary artery. Images represent tissue $H_2{}^{15}O$ activity and are corrected for vascular tracer with the use of $C^{15}O$. The upper image was obtained under baseline conditions and reflects relatively homogeneous perfusion (mitral valve apparatus appears posteriorly in this plane). The middle image was obtained after administration of the coronary vasodilator dipyridamole. A relative defect in perfusion is apparent since the hyperemia in the normal region was much greater than in the anterior region supplied by the stenosed vessel. Actual blood flow was increased four-fold in the normal regions and two-fold in post-stenotic zones (confirmed with microspheres). The lower image was obtained immediately after occlusion and reperfusion of the stenotic artery and demonstrates hyperemia in the post-stenotic zone. This finding is consistent with the presence of a noncritical stenosis.*

Even when no perfusion defect is present at rest, the functional importance of a subcritical coronary stenosis is clearly visualized. A disadvantage of the labeled water technique is the high tracer activity in blood and lungs, which leads to activity cross-contamination. Nevertheless, it provides another approach for assessment of regional myocardial blood flow and represents therefore an interesting application of positron imaging.

Particulate agents

Microspheres labeled with ^{11}C or macroaggregates labeled with Gallium-68 have successfully been used to quantify regional myocardial blood flow in animals and in man. However, important limitations are the invasive nature of the technique, reason why the clinical utility of the particle technique is still no routine procedure in clinical practice.

Metabolism

The development of PET has been the greatest impetus to the study of regional myocardial metabolism. The regional, noninvasive assessment of myocardial functional integrity with the aim to distinguish normal from abnormal myocardial areas is highly desirable in patients with cardiac disease. Disease starts at the biochemical level and it is very likely that structural abnormalities are preceded by metabolic disorders of the myocardium. Therefore attempts have been made to determine the metabolic integrity of the myocardium quantitatively with radioactively labeled metabolic substrates. Since it became apparent that free fatty acids (FFA) are the primary substrates of the myocardium under normal physiological circumstances, much investigative work has been performed to label FFA with appropriate radionuclides and hence to study the metabolic processes of the normal and abnormal heart. Also glucose can be radioactively labeled to study the myocardial carbohydrate metabolism under different pathological conditions. Both FFA and glucose can be labeled with positron-emitting agents providing further important information of cardiac metabolism. In particular in patients with coronary artery disease, labeled metabolic substrates have been proven a valuable aid for the detection of ischemic myocardial areas. This has been achieved not only by visual inspection of the obtained images, but also by the measurement of metabolic turnover rates. Although metabolic imaging has as yet no worldwide application, its clinical relevance is growing and it will play a vital role in the early diagnosis and treatment of patients with cardiac disease (8).

Metabolic tracers

In general, metabolic isotope tracers should meet the following requirements; 1) they should be highly specific of a given metabolic pathway, 2) they must not change the physiological behaviour of the metabolic substrates, 3) they have to allow adequate external detection by currently available positron cameras, and 4) the metabolic tracers should have clinical application. These conditions are best fulfilled by radio-nuclides with chemical identities akin to those of physiological substrates such as carbon (^{11}C), nitrogen (^{13}N), and oxygen (^{15}O). At present, most clinical experience has been obtained with ^{11}C-palmitate and labeled glucose.

Carbon-11-palmitate

Under physiological circumstances FFA are the preferred substrates of myocardial metabolism. For PET studies the physiological positron-emitter ^{11}C has been shown to label adequately with palmitate.

^{11}C-palmitate follows the natural pathway of beta-oxidation and hence the rate of decrease in ^{11}C activity is proportional to the rate of FFA oxidation. An added advantage of ^{11}C is its short half-life of 20 minutes, allowing repeated measurements to be made at short intervals, which can be of great importance in intervention procedures. With respect to the kinetics of the labeled FFA, most studies have shown that they clear from the myocardium in a biexponential fashion, indicating tracer distribution between at least two different pools.

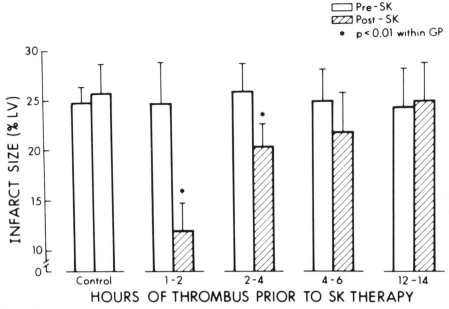

Figure 4

Histrogram of tomographically estimated infarct size for control animals with sustained coronary occlusion (n=6), and animals with 1-2, (n=4), 2-4 (n=6), 4-6 (n=4) and 12-14 hours of coronary occlusion prior to thrombolysis (n=3). Repeat tomography was performed 90 minutes after thrombolysis. Significant decreases of apparent infarct size (or increases in metabolic activity in jeopardized myocardium) occurred only in animals subjected to reperfusion within 4 hours of occlusion (values indicate means±SD) SK = streptokinase. The results illustrate the utility of PET for sequential characterization of myocardium before and after an intervention.*

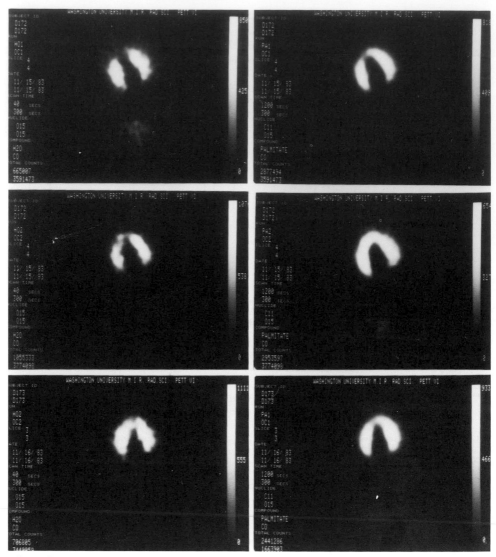

Figure 5

Tomographic reconstructions through a single midventricular plane of dog heart. All images have been corrected for activity in the vascular space with blood pool subtraction from an image obtained with $C^{15}O$. Perfusion images are on the left were obtained with $H_2^{15}O$. Images on the right depict the myocardial accumulation of ^{11}C-palmitate from 4 to 10 minutes after intravenous administration of that tracer. A defect is seen anteriorly (arrow) in perfusion and for ^{11}C-palmitate accumulation. In the plane illustrated the transverse section passes through the mitral valve apparatus posteriorly, consistent with the lack of activity in the inferior point of the images. The uppermost images were obtained during thrombotic occlusion of the proximal left anterior descending artery, induced with an intracoronary copper coil. Images in the center were obtained 1 hour after thrombolysis induced with intracoronary streptokinase. Incomplete restoration of perfusion and restoration of palmitate extraction are demonstrated. The lower images were obtained 24 hours following thrombolysis and show a further improvement in perfusion in the anterior zone but a decrease in palmitate accumulation.

The example illustrates differences in the time course of recovery of extraction of fatty acid with respect to perfusion after thrombolysis.

Alterations in the tissue distribution of fatty acid and the extent of oxidation may account for the differences in time course in metabolic images compared with perfusion images.*

114

This clearance pattern reflects the distribution of FFA between immediate beta-oxidation (rapid turnover phase) and the intermediate storage in the endogenous lipid pool (slow turnover phase). The rapid turnover phase is used for assessment of clearance rates and is commonly expressed in myocardial half-times. Normally functioning myocardial tissue shows homogeneous accumulation of ^{11}C-palmitate and the subsequent images show excellent imaging quality. At present, ^{11}C-palmitate has been mostly applied for the detection of coronary artery disease. Ischemic areas are characterized both by regionally diminished tracer accumulation and by the measurement of abnormal clearance rates in the affected areas. In myocardial ischemia FFA metabolism is decreased and glucose metabolism prevails. As a result, in ischemic myocardial regions decreased turnover of ^{11}C-palmitate is observed (prolonged myocardial half-times) indicating impaired myocardial FFA metabolism in ischemic areas.

Because of the very short half-life of ^{11}C-palmitate, also transient changes can be documented by repeated injections of the tracer. Transient ischemic regions will show augmented tracer accumulation after reperfusion, while zones of infarction show persistently diminished uptake. Bergmann et al. (9) experimentally demonstrated by measuring uptake of ^{11}C-palmitate that successful streptokinase treatment, when initiated within 4 hours after occlusion, showed preserved tracer accumulation while later treatment did not result in significant salutary metabolic effects (Fig. 4). Ludbrook et al. (10) studied 17 patients with ^{11}C-palmitate after treatment with streptokinase and demonstrated in the 8 patients with successful thrombolysis increased tracer uptake indicating improvement of regional myocardial metabolism and salvage of myocardial tissue. As a result, cardiac PET is particularly useful for characterizing the efficacy of interventions designed to salvage ischemic myocardium (Fig. 5).

Labeled glucose

Glucose analogues can be labeled either with ^{11}C or preferably with fluorine-18 (2-^{18}F-deoxyglucose). The residence time of 2-^{18}F-deoxyglucose in the myocardium is increased since this agent reaches a specific step in the catabolic process where it is recognized as different from the native substance. Therefore, it remains in the cell for a prolonged interval to over 100 minutes and the amount of 2-^{18}F-deoxyglucose taken up by the myocardium provides a measurement of exogenous glucose metabolism. The clinical value of 2-^{18}F-deoxyglucose is at the moment not very well

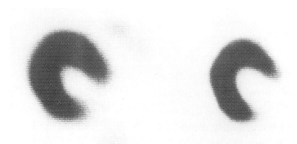

Figure 6A
Regional myocardial uptake of ^{13}N-ammonia (on the left) and 2-^{18}F-deoxyglucose (on the right) are displayed in a transverse slice of the left ventricle (normal young subject). From left to right, the free wall, the anterior wall and the septum show homogeneous and similar distribution of both tracers.**

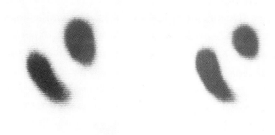

Figure 6B
Regional myocardial uptake of ^{13}N-ammonia and 2-^{18}F-deoxyglucose recorded in a patient who suffered an anterior myocardial infarction without thrombolytic therapy. Coronary angiography shows complete obstruction of the left anterior descending artery after the first diagonal branch. The uptake of both tracers is markedly decreased, in a similar proportion, in the anterior wall of the left ventricle.**

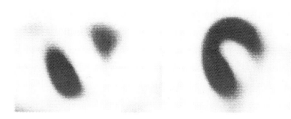

Figure 6C
Discordant uptake of ^{13}N-ammonia (left) and 2-^{18}F-deoxyglucose (right) in the anterior wall of a patient who suffered an anterior myocardial infarction treated by 1 million units of streptokinase intravenously administered 2.5 hours after the onset of pain. Coronary angiography performed after the thrombolysis reveals a 50% stenosis of the left anterior descending artery after the origin of the first diagonal branch. The corresponding affected area of the myocardium is akinetic and the global ejection fraction of the left ventricle is 25%.**

116

established, but it may have a supplementary role to perfusion markers for the detection of important coronary artery disease. It has been demonstrated that in injured but viable ischemic myocardium, myocardial perfusion determined by ^{13}N-ammonia may be markedly depressed while glucose uptake is increased, suggesting increased anaerobic metabolism of glucose in reversibly injured areas (11,12). With further injury resulting in cellular necrosis, both perfusion and uptake of glucose is depressed. As a result, in reversible ischemic myocardial regions a mismatch pattern can be observed i.e. the discrepancy between perfusion (cold spot) and glucose utilization (hot spot) in the same region. This phenomenon has become a hallmark of potentially reversible myocardial ischemia and denotes viability of myocardium recovering from ischemia (Fig. 6A,B,C). In this way used, 2-^{18}F-deoxyglucose could play an important role in predicting myocardial viability after administration of thrombolytic therapy.

Also ^{11}C-labeled pyruvate, lactate, and acetate may be useful markers to identify different steps in the pathways of myocardial oxidative carbohydrate metabolism. However, clinical experience at the moment is very limited.

Amino acids

Specific alterations of myocardial amino acid metabolism have been demonstrated in patients with coronary artery disease. A special metabolic function of glutamate has been suggested by the fact that glutamate is the only amino acid with a positive arteriovenous difference in the human coronary circulation. This difference is significantly greater in patients with coronary artery disease than in normal subjects, reason why labeled glutamate has been proposed for studying coronary artery disease. Glutamate labeled with ^{13}N has been shown to accumulate in human myocardium and preliminary reports have demonstrated apparent differences in myocardial distribution of ^{13}N-glutamate and thallium-201 (13). In reversible ischemic areas accumulation of ^{13}N-glutamate was observed, while thallium-201 uptake was decreased. This indicates the usefulness of a metabolic tracer in the differentiation between reversibly and irreversibly injured myocardium.

Nervous system

Apart from perfusion and metabolism, the future scope of PET cardiology studies will be directed to visualize different aspects of the myocardial nervous system. In particular, PET receptor ligand studies of the myocardium will become of main interest. Methods have already been reported for the measurement of beta-adrenergic receptors, muscarinic and dopamine receptors (14,15,16). For instance, practolol and pindolol can be labeled with ^{11}C and they have shown, after intravenous injection in humans, adequate cross-sectional images of the myocardium (17). Other studies with labeled guanethidine, that enters the adrenergic nerve endings, demonstrated in patients with a recent myocardial infarction that uptake of guanethidine was globally depressed but recovered at about two months (18). However, regional uptake persisted and corresponded to the site of the infarction. Recent studies with new a tracer, 6-^{18}F-metaraminol, a norepinephrine analogue, have shown neuronal dysfunction in acute myocardial ischemia (19). These preliminary results suggest that receptor ligand studies may be used for the noninvasive evaluation of structural and functional abnormalities of the myocardial nervous system (See Chapter 15)

CLINICAL APPLICATIONS

Coronary artery disease

Gould et al. (3) studied 50 patients with coronary artery disease using generator-produced rubidium before and after intravenous dipyridamole and the imaging results were compared with arteriographic data. Sensitivity for detecting coronary artery disease was 95% with a specificity of 100%. It was concluded that cardiac positron tomography of myocardial perfusion using rubidium provides sensitive and specific diagnosis of reduced coronary flow reserve due to coronary artery disease.

Tillisch et al. (20) studied 17 patients after myocardial infarction and observed that abnormal wall motion in regions with preserved 2-^{18}F-deoxyglucose uptake was highly predictive of reversible myocardial ischemia, while abnormal motion in regions with depressed glucose uptake was highly predictive of irreversible injury. The predictive accuracy for irreversibly damaged myocardium was 90% and it was postulated that the most important clinical application of 2-^{18}F-deoxyglucose is to predict viability of ischemic myocardium. Camici et al. (21) studied regional myocardial perfusion and metabolism with rubidium and 2-^{18}F-deoxyglucose at rest in 10 normal volunteers and in 12 patients with coronary artery disease and stable angina pectoris. Five volunteers and eight patients were also studied at maximal exercise. In patients at rest, the myocardial uptake of the two tracers did not differ significantly from that measured in normal subjects. All eight patients showed reduced segmental [82]Rb uptake during exercise, which returned to normal uptake values about 10 minutes after exercise. In seven of eight patients, it was observed that the regions with reduced [82]Rb uptake during exercise were characterized by increased uptake of 2-^{18}F-deoxyglucose in corresponding regions. The authors concluded that myocardial glucose transport and phosphorylation seem to be enhanced in the postischemic myocardium of patients with exercise-induced ischemia.

Schwaiger et al. (22) studied regional myocardial blood flow and glucose metabolism in 13 patients with acute myocardial infarction within 72 hours using the flow marker ^{13}N-ammonia and 2-^{18}F-deoxyglucose. Also two-dimensional echocardiography and radionuclide angiography were performed on the day of the tomographic study and 6 weeks later. Interestingly, they noticed that patients with persistent wall motion abnormalities had a concordant decrease in flow and glucose metabolism. In contrast, patients with improved wall motion over time showed the characteristic mismatch pattern i.e. diminished uptake of ^{13}N-ammonia but increased uptake of 2-^{18}F-deoxyglucose in similar regions. This study suggests therefore that the combined evaluation of blood flow and glucose utilization provides a noninvasive means to distinguish necrotic from potentially viable myocardial tissue in patients with acute myocardial infarction. However, the pathophysiologic mechanism of increased uptake of labeled glucose in ischemic mycardium remains to be elucidated.

Brunken et al. (23) studied 12 patients, who showed an exercise thallium-201 defect, with ^{13}N-ammonia and 2-^{18}F-deoxyglucose to assess perfusion and metabolism in 51 myocardial segments. All segments with a completely reversible thallium-201 defect were normal by PET, but in contrast in most of the fixed defects residual metabolic activity was observed. It was concluded that PET reveals evidence of persistent tissue metabolism in the majority of segments with a fixed defect, indicating that the use of perfusion markers alone may underestimate the extent of viable tissue.

Cardiomyopathies

In a report by Eisenberg et al. (24), 20 patients with dilated cardiomyopathy were studied with ^{11}C-palmitate in an attempt to differentiate nonischemic from ischemic cardiomyopathy. Regions of homogeneously severely depressed tracer accumulation were observed in eight of 10 patients with ischemic but in none of 10 patients with nonischemic cardiomyopathy. In addition, the patients with ischemic cardiomyopathy showed homogeneous tracer distribution, while in the nonischemic patients marked heterogeneity of ^{11}C-palmitate distribution was observed. These findings support the hypothesis that multiple myocardial infarctions underlie the process of dilated cardiomyopathy in patients with coronary artery disease. It was concluded that the use of ^{11}C-palmitate allows differentiation of ischemic from nonischemic cardiomyopathy.

Pharmacologic interventions

Few studies have reported on the evaluation of pharmacologic interventions by PET. Knabb et al. (25), in 16 dog hearts, examined the effects of intravenous diltiazem given 30 minutes before administration of streptokinase on myocardial blood flow (assessed by ^{15}O-labeled water) and salvage (assessed by ^{11}C-palmitate). Diltiazem had no additional effect on myocardial blood flow, but significantly improved uptake of ^{11}C-palmitate in the ischemic area (Fig. 7). Therefore, concomitant treatment of diltiazem enhances salvage of reperfused myocardium after coronary thrombolysis.

Future potential of PET

PET has been shown to be one of the most powerful research tools for noninvasively studying the heart. The early diagnosis of abnormalities in myocardial perfusion, metabolism or neuronal activity could lead to more effective, more specific, and

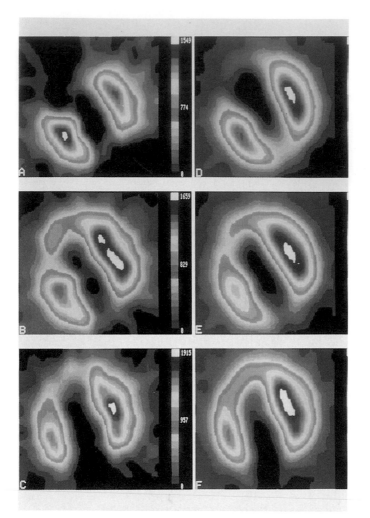

Figure 7

Transverse reconstructed tomograms from a dog given intravenous diltiazem before administration of streptokinase. Perfusion with ^{15}O-labeled water is depicted in A, B, and C. The distribution of ^{11}C-palmitate is shown in D, E, and F. Conditions were: A and D, occlusion; B and E, 1 hour after thrombolysis; C and F, 24 hours after reperfusion. Diltiazem had no effect on perfusion, but improved uptake of ^{11}C-palmitate compared with the restoration in dogs hearts given streptokinase alone, with substantial improvement evident at 24 hours. This finding indicates that administration of diltiazem before thrombolysis increases salvage of myocardium compared with salvage achieved by thrombolysis alone.

more economical treatment of the cardiac patient. Before PET will become a common diagnostic tool, its clinical utility has to be proven on a large scale. Major clinical applications have to be demonstrated to justify its existence in community hospitals. Factors limiting wider application of PET in the clinical environment are mainly the expenses for a positron camera and, in particular, for a cyclotron in case of metabolic imaging studies.

At present, a substantial capital investment of approximately Dfl 15.000.000,= is required for the combined purchase of a positron camera and a cyclotron (26). Fortunately, with the development of generator-produced positron isotopes, such as 82Rb, a cyclotron is no longer necessary to perform myocardial perfusion studies. In that case, the total estimated costs will be about Dfl 6.000.000,-- . In the Netherlands one PET centre has been established for multipurpose utilization. However, it would be very desirable to dispose in the Netherlands of several specially dedicated cardiac PET centers, since clinical applications of the PET technique are far most advanced in the field of cardiology.

The setting-up of a cardiac PET center entails three important issues. The first issue deals with the location of the PET facility. It is important that the PET centre has to be set up within a suitable infrastructure. First experience has to be gained in a university teaching hospital with excellently run departments of radiochemistry, nuclear medicine and clinical cardiology. The second issue regards the control of the PET facility, since PET requires multispecialty expertise from basic sciences to nuclear physics, and finally clinical cardiology. Therefore, the chief manager of a positron facility and its personnel has to dispose of technical, administrative, clinical, and social talents, and he should be able to integrate the various specialties, regardless of his own subspecialty. The third issue is to initiate the cardiac PET studies even if an on-site cyclotron is not immediately available. When a ^{82}Rb generator is present, one can already perform myocardial perfusion studies. At the same time, the PET research group can become familiar with the inherent problems of positron imaging including technical complications and appropriate patient management. The extension to a cyclotron facility may be then accomplished in a later phase.

Conclusion

Positron emission tomography in cardiology offers a new diagnostic tool for early noninvasive diagnosis and treatment of cardiac disease. Cardiac positron imaging can be used to assess the functional severity of coronary artery stenosis and to evaluate myocardial viability in patients with coronary artery disease. The use of generator-produced rubidium-82 makes this technique accessible to more cardiac centers. Rubidium-82 may also serve as a better alternative for the current standard perfusion agents. For larger number of cases, rubidium imaging is less expensive than thallium since a maximum of 6-7 thallium studies per day can be performed versus 15-20 rubidium studies. Moreover, it should also be realized that high technology in cardiology improves effective patient care and will be more cost-saving on the long run than "conservative" modalities relative to expenses, quality of life and lives saved (27).

Positron emission tomography represents one of the most advanced diagnostic modalities in cardiology and will provide the basis for specific therapeutic approaches in patients with cardiac disease, thereby justifying the routine, clinical, economic use of PET in cardiology.

References

1. Van der Wall EE. Noninvasive imaging of cardiac metabolism, 1987. Editor: van der Wall EE. Martinus Nijhoff Publishers, Dordrecht/ Boston/Lancaster.
2. Schelbert HR. Current status and prospects of new radionuclides and radiopharmaceuticals for cardio-vascular nuclear medicine. Seminucl Med 1987;17:145-81.
3. Gould KL, Goldstein RA, Mullani NA et al. Noninvasive assessment of coronary stenoses by myocar-dial perfusion imaging during pharmacologic coronary vasodilation. VIII. Clinical feasibility of positron cardiac imaging without a cyclotron using generator-produced rubidium-82. J Am Coll Cardiol 1986;4:775-89.
4. Goldstein RA, Mullani NA, Wong W-H et al. Positron imaging of myocardial infarction with rubidium-82. J Nucl Med 1986;27:1824-9.
5. Selwyn AP, Allan RM, L'Abbate AL et al. Relation between regional myocardial uptake of rubidium-82 and perfusion: Absolute reduction of cation uptake in ischemia. Am J Cardiol 1982;52:112-21.
6. Gould KL, Schelbert HR, Phelps ME, Hoffman EJ: Noninvasive assessment of coronary stenoses with myocardial perfusion imaging during pharmacologic coronary vasodilation. V. Detection of 47 percent diameter coronary stenosis with intravenous nitrogen-13 ammonia emisson-computed tomography in intact dogs. Am J Cardiol 1979;47:200-8.
7. Bergmann SR, Fox KAA, Rand AL et al. Quantification of regional myocardial blood flow in vivo with $H_2^{15}O$. Circulation 1984;70: 724-33.
8. Van der Wall EE. Metabolic imaging in cardiology. Current opinion in cardiology 1987;2:1051-57.
9. Bergmann SR, Lerch RA, Fox KAA et al. Temporal dependence of beneficial effects of coronary thrombolysis characterized by positron tomography. Am J Med 1982;73:573-81.
10. Ludbook PA, Geltman EM, Tiefenbrunn AJ, Jaffe AS, Sobel BE. Restoration of regional myocardial metabolism by coronary thrombolysis in patients. Circulation 1983;68:III,325 (abstract).
11. Marshall RC, Tillisch JH, Phelps ME et al. Identification and differentiation of resting myocardial ischemia and infarction in man with positron computed tomography, 18F-labeled fluorodeoxyglucose and N-13 ammonia. Circulation 1983;67:766-78.
12. De Landsheere C, Raets D, Piérard L et al. Residual metabolic abnormalities and regional viability after a myocardial infarction: a study using positron tomography, F-18 deoxyglucose and flow indica-tors. J Am Coll Cardiol 1985;5:451 (abstract).
13. Zimmermann R, Tillmanns H, Knapp WH et al. Regional myocardial nitrogen-13 glutamate uptake in patients with coronary artery disease: Inverse post-stress relation to thallium-201 uptake in ischemia. J Am Coll Cardiol 1988;11:549-56.
14. Seto M, Syrota A, Crouzel C et al. Beta adrenergic receptors in the dog heart characterized by 11C-CGP 12177 and PET. J Nucl Med 1986;27:P949 (abstract).
15. Syrota A, Comar D, Paillotin G et al. Muscarinic cholinergic receptor in the human heart evidenced under physiological conditions by positron emission tomography. Proc Natl Acad Sci US 1985;82:584-8.
16. Manger WM, Hoffmann BB. Heart imaging in the diagnosis of pheochromocytoma and assessment of catecholamine uptake: teaching editorial. J Nucl Med 1983;24:1194-96.
17. Syrota A, Dormont D, Berg J, et al. C-11 ligand binding to adrenergic and muscarinic receptors of the human heart studied in vitro by PET. J Nucl Med 1983;24:P20 (abstract).
18. Dae M, Herre J, Botvinick E et al. Scintigraphic assessment of adrenergic innervation after myocardial infarction. Circulation 1986;74:II-297 (abstract).
19. Guiborg H, Schwaiger M, Rosenspire KC et al. 6-(F18)Fluorometaraminol as marker for neuronal injury in "stunned" canine myocardium. J Nucl Med 1988;29:P938 (abstract).
20. Tillisch J, Brunken R, Schwaiger M et al. Reversibility of cardiac wall motion abnormalities predicted by positron emission tomography. N Engl J Med 1986;314:884-8.
21. Camici P, Araujo LI, Spinks T et al. Increased uptake of 18F-fluorodeoxyglucose in postischemic myocardium of patients with exercise-induced angina. Circulation 1986;74:81-8.
22. Schwaiger M, Brunken R, Grover-McKay M, et al. Regional myocardial metabolism in patients with acute myocardial infarction assessed by positron emission tomography. J Am Coll Cardiol 1986;8:800-8.

23. Brunken R, Schwaiger M, Grover-McKay M, Phelps ME, Tillisch J, Schelbert HR. Positron emission tomography detects tissue metabolic activity in myocardial segments with persistent thallium perfusion defects. J Am Coll Cardiol 1987;10:557-67.

24. Eisenberg JD, Sobel BE, Geltman EM. Differentiation of ischemic from nonischemic cardiomyopathy with positron emission tomography. Am J Cardiol 1987;59:1410-14.

25. Knabb RM, Rosamond TL, Fox KAA, Sobel BE, Bergmann SR. Enhancement of salvage of reperfused ischemic myocardium by diltiazem. J Am Coll Cardiol 1986;8:861-71.

26. Rapport van de Gezondheidsraad inzake advies Positron Emissie Tomografie, 1986.

27. Knoebel SB. Cardiology by the numbers and cost-containment. Am J Cardiol 1988;61:1112-5.

7.
Magnetic resonance imaging:
A new approach for evaluation coronary artery disease?

Summary

The cardiovascular applications of nuclear magnetic resonance imaging in coronary artery disease have considerably increased in recent years. Although many applications overlap those of other more cost-effective techniques, such as echocardiography, radionuclide angiography, and computed tomography, magnetic resonance imaging offers unique features not shared by the conventional techniques. Technical advantages are the excellent spatial resolution, the characterization of myocardial tissue, and the potential for three-dimensional imaging. This allows the accurate assessment of left ventricular mass and volume, the differentiation of infarcted tissue from normal myocardial tissue, and the determination of systolic wall thickening and regional wall motion abnormalities. Also inducible myocardial ischemia using pharmacologic stress (dipyridamole or dobutamine) may be assessed by magnetic resonance imaging. Future technical developments include real-time imaging and noninvasive visualization of the coronary arteries. These advances will have a major impact on the application of magnetic resonance imaging in coronary artery disease, potentially unsurpassed by other techniques and certainly justifying the expenses. Consequently, the clinical use of magnetic resonance imaging for the detection of coronary artery disease largely depends on the progress of technical developments.

Introduction

Nuclear magnetic resonance (NMR) imaging is a unique noninvasive method for visualization of the heart. Among other noninvasive imaging technologies NMR imaging offers the best anatomic resolution. The advantages of NMR in comparison with other imaging techniques are therefore the clear delineation of the subendocardial and subepicardial margins of the cardiac walls, the discrimination of intracardiac tumors and thrombi, and the direct visualization of pericardial structures. In particular the amount of cardiac mass can be accurately measured and diseases afflicting the cardiac walls are well defined by NMR imaging. Technical advantages are the potential for three-dimensional imaging, the free choice of tomographic planes and the lack of ionizing radiation. Disadvantages of NMR are (yet) the relatively long

125

imaging times and the lack of obtaining bedside information. Furthermore, it is difficult to study critically ill patients, although patients with acute myocardial infarction have been safely studied within 24 hours after the acute event. Real-time NMR imaging is not currently used, but the rapid development of ultrafast imaging techniques may permit soon the application of the 'echo-planar' techniques for routine clinical use.

Advantages of NMR imaging over echocardiography are that a complete study of the entire heart can be obtained without concern regarding acoustic window and transducer positioning. Unlike echocardiography, the image quality of NMR imaging is not operator-dependent and the NMR technique is not restricted in patients with thoracic deformities or emphysema. Technical difficulties in analyzing and reproducing echocardiographic endocardial tracings may substantially exaggerate the normal variability of left ventricular contraction. Three-dimensional reconstruction has made some progress in echocardiography, but this technique is still highly investigational and has presently no impact on clinical practice.

Radionuclide techniques employ radioactive materials and the images have a relatively low spatial resolution. In addition, most institutions use planar imaging techniques because tomographic radionuclide imaging is not universally applied on a routine basis. Cine computed X-ray tomography needs ionizing radiation and contrast material, and with the standard equipment the technique is restricted in the available imaging planes. The technique is not multislice and requires the patient to endure a large intravenous contrast load and to sustain prolonged breath holding.

Ultrafast computed tomography may circumvent some of these limitations but this technique has no wide application in clinical cardiology. Table I shows the various technical aspects of the currently used noninvasive imaging modalities.

Table 1 Comparison of technical aspects of noninvasive imaging methods

	Ionizing radiation required	Contrast media needed	Spatial resolution (mm)	Imaging time	Tomographic capability	Portability
Echocardiography	No	No	2-3	Real-time	Yes	Yes
Myocardial perfusion scintigraphy	Yes	No	10-15	Minutes	Yes	Yes
Radionuclide angiography	Yes	No	10-15	Minutes	No	Yes
Positron emission tomography	Yes	No	5-10	Minutes	Yes	No
Cine-computed tomography	Yes	Yes	~1	Seconds*	Yes	No
Magnetic resonance imaging	No	No	~1	Minutes*	Yes	No

* Real time approaches currently under development.

126

NMR imaging has opened new avenues for detecting cardiovascular abnormalities in an early stage of the disease process. This chapter describes the value of NMR imaging for detecting coronary artery disease. Although several other noninvasive imaging techniques like echocardiography and radionuclide imaging are very useful in the assessment of patients with coronary artery disease, NMR imaging may provide valuable information concerning the ischemic and infarcted heart which is not available from other diagnostic techniques. Before discussing the potential of NMR imaging to delineate and characterize myocardial ischemia and infarction, we will first address the most important physical principles and technical considerations of NMR imaging. Since NMR spectroscopy is a specialty of its own, this modality will not be described in this review article.

Physical principles, instrumentation, imaging techniques, technical and safety considerations.

Physical principles

Since NMR imaging is a rather new imaging modality, a brief outline of closely relevant physical principles is warranted. A more detailed description of the NMR physics has been described elsewhere (1,2).

NMR imaging is defined as a spatial two- or threedimensional map of nuclei which resonate at a characteristic frequency when placed in a magnetic field and when subjected to intermittently applied radiofrequency pulses. NMR imaging employs high strength static magnetic fields, low strength changing magnetic fields, and radiofrequency pulses to generate tomographic images of the body with high soft tissue contrast. Atomic nuclei with an odd number of protons or neutrons (e.g. hydrogen and phosphorus) have a magnetic moment which aligns along the direction of a magnetic field. Since hydrogen is by far the most commonly found nucleus in biologic systems, the discussion of NMR characteristics will refer to the hydrogen nucleus. Application of radiofrequency pulses of a specific frequency will partially align the magnetic moments of these atomic nuclei against the magnetic field and will induce resonance of these hydrogen nuclei. When the radiofrequency pulse ceases, the nuclei return to equilibrium and emit radiofrequency energy. The radio-frequency energy is transformed (Fourier transformation) by a computer allowing NMR images to be generated, whereby differences in signal intensity result in differences in greyscale. The signal intensity of the images is not only dependent on hydrogen density but also on the relaxation times T1 and T2 of the nuclei. Briefly, following application of radiofrequency pulses, T1 (longitudinal relaxation time) reflects the rate at which nuclei re-align with the external magnetic field and T2 (transverse relaxation time) reflects the rate at which nuclei lose coherence with each other. The relaxation times T1 and T2 are used to distinguish between different tissues and to characterize disease processes in myocardial tissue. In normal cardiac tissue, T2 is much shorter (±60 msec) than T1 (±500 msec) and differences in T1 and T2 relaxation times can be accentuated to produce contrast among various disease states. Generally, the NMR image contrast improves with increasing hydrogen density, shortening of T1, and lengthening of T2 relaxation time.

NMR system

Each NMR system consists of five major parts: the magnet, the transmitter, the antenna, the receiver, and the computer. NMR is best performed using a magnet with a high field strength to improve signal-to-noise ratio, with a very high field homogeneity, and with a large bore size to accomodate patients. Most modern NMR magnets are liquid-helium cooled, superconducting solenoids with a bore size varying from 1 meter (whole body magnets, field strength 0.1 to 2.0 Tesla) to a few centimeters (high resolution magnets, 2.0 to 14 Tesla). The transmitter is used for transmitting radiofrequency pulses to an antenna or coil, which in turn transmits the radiofrequency power to the patient and also receives the radiofrequency signal from the patient. The coil, made of wire or foil, usually surrounds the patient or may be directly put on the body of the patient (surface coils), depending on whether information is required from the whole body or from a selected organ of interest. Surface coils provide higher sensitivity and therefore excellent spatial localization of NMR signals for imaging studies, but have the disadvantage of an inhomogeneous radiofrequency field producing images of inhomogeneous signal intensity distribution. The receiver amplifies the signal picked up by the coil and the signal is processed by a computer, which is also needed to operate the entire NMR system.

Imaging techniques

Current NMR imaging exists in two basic forms; spin-echo imaging and gradient-echo imaging. With a spin-echo imaging sequence, images are produced after an initial 90° radiofrequency pulse (fixed pulse angle of 90°), followed by one or more 180° pulses. The gradient-echo technique allows a free choice of the angle of the initial radiofrequency pulse (pulse angle or flip angle between 0 and 90°, usually 30°). Spin-echo imaging provides high resolution images with clear anatomical definition of the intracardiac and intravascular structures in the presence of a low signal intensity of the blood pool. Currently, cardiac images are acquired using up to eight two-dimensional tomographic slices of 1 cm thickness or less. This procedure is called multislice imaging and takes about 7-10 minutes imaging time, depending on the desired image quality and the heart rate of the patient. To image the entire heart in various phases of the cycle, i.e. multislice-multiphase imaging, typically eight tomographic slices in eight different phases are obtained increasing the duration of the NMR procedure to approximately 30-35 minutes. In our institution we employ true orthogonal short-axis images to visualize the heart (Fig. 1).

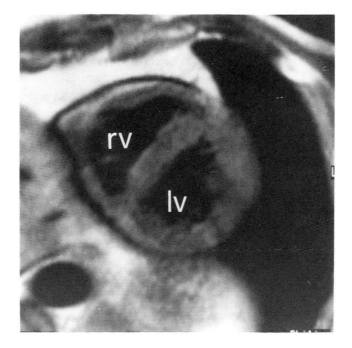

Figure 1
Orthogonal cardiac short-axis NMR image of a patient without cardiac disease. The myocardial walls of the left (lv) and right ventricle (rv) are clearly depicted.

Spin-echo imaging is the NMR technique of choice in assessing left ventricular mass by providing a three-dimensional direct visualization of the myocardium with excellent mural edge discrimination. Quantitation of left ventricular mass by NMR correlated closely with anatomical measurements in dog hearts (3-5). Using casts in dog hearts, NMR imaging allowed the accurate measurement of ventricular volumes independently from geometric assumptions (6). Cardiac and vascular anatomy have been examined in normal subjects and in patients with various forms of cardiovascular disease (7,8). Muscle mass and chamber dimensions correlated well with those obtained with echocardiography and contrast ventriculography (8-11). Left ventricular mass could be accurately measured in dog hearts before and after acute myocardial infarction, indicating that MRI is also reliable to calculate left ventricular mass in distorted ventricles (12). Left and right ventricular volumes, left ventricular ejection fractions, and regional left ventricular function can accurately be measured (13-20). NMR spin-echo imaging also allows the evaluation of changes in myocardial wall thickness during the cardiac cycle i.e. wall thickening or wall thinning. In normal hearts, systolic wall thickening is similar among different regional myocardial areas (21). Contrarily, ischemic and/or infarcted myocardial regions show absence of systolic wall thickening with increased wall thickening of adjacent normal myocardium (22,23). This indicates that NMR imaging is useful for detecting depressed function in ischemic and/or infarcted myocardium as well as increased function in regions of myocardium adjacent to injured myocardium.

Another unique feature of spin-echo imaging is the measurement of the myocardial relaxation times T1 and T2 in attempts to distinguish ischemic from normal myocardial tissue. Using pulse sequences with short echo-times (TE 30 msec, first spin-echo), predominantly T1 weighted images are obtained which are very useful for defining anatomic features. With TE of 60 msec (second spin-echo), relatively T2-weighted images are obtained which allow the evaluation of optimal contrast between different tissues i.e. the detection of cardiac masses and the distinction between myocardial scar, ischemic myocardium and normal myocardial tissue. On T2-weighted images the infarcted regions appear as regions with high signal intensity compared to normal myocardial regions (Fig. 2).

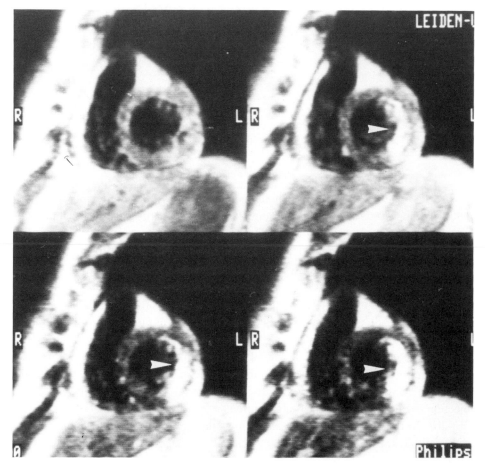

Figure 2
For T2-weighted NMR imaging a multi-echo study (TE 30-60-90-120 msec) was performed. This figure shows a short-axis NMR image of a patient with an inferoposterior wall infarction. Note the increased signal intensity (arrows) of the posterolateral wall on the images with (TE 60, 90 and 120 msec)

130

In our institution NMR imaging is performed with a 0.5 Tesla NMR instrument (Philips Gyroscan). Our procedure consists of applying the multislice technique using a TE of 30 msec and with a repetition time equal to the RR-interval of the electrocardiogram. After selecting the most suitable single slice, we employ the multi-echo technique using pulse sequences with TE of 30, 60, 90, and 120 msec.

Gradient-echo imaging employs the acquisition of 16 (or more) images of the cardiac cycle which can be played in a cine loop to show cardiac function (cine NMR imaging, four minutes imaging time). With cine NMR imaging the normal blood pool shows high signal intensity in all phases of the cardiac cycle which provides a constant contrast with the less intense myocardium, unlike conventional spin-echo imaging where intraluminal signal is usually low but may be variable and inseparable from adjacent myocardial tissue. Visual evaluation of global and regional myocardial dysfunction is facilitated by viewing the cinematic display of the NMR images. Cine NMR imaging appears to be the NMR technique of choice for assessing left ventricular function (24). Cardiac chamber volumes, ejection fraction, and regional wall motion and thickening can be reliably determined by cine NMR, and correlated well with two-dimensional echocardiography and contrast ventriculography (25,26). Buser et al. (27) studied 10 normal volunteers by cine NMR imaging and showed a mean endsystolic volume of 34 ± 4 ml, and a mean enddiastolic volume of 90 ± 7 ml. The correlation with two-dimensional echocardiography was excellent (r=0.91) and the plane of imaging was not critical for the quantitation of left ventricular volumes. Pflugfelder et al. (28) showed that the absence of systolic wall thickening proved to be a very specific marker of regional myocardial dysfunction. Basically, the cine NMR technique may be more accurate for defining regional myocardial dysfunction than cine angiography, since the latter depends upon the evaluation of wall motion only.

Volume or three-dimensional imaging of the heart has also been achieved using NMR imaging (29). Tomographic images of the heart can be acquired in any plane and at the same phase of the cardiac cycle. This permits the evaluation of many different parameters of cardiac funtion after three-dimensional reconstruction. For example, three-dimensional imaging shows less variability in normal wall thickening than planar imaging, and better discriminates ischemia from non-ischemia (30). However, at this moment the time cost of three-dimensional imaging is considerable.

The optimal approach for assessing global and regional ventricular function employs much faster scan methods than the spin-echo or the cine NMR technique. Therefore, 'instant' or echo-planar techniques have recently been developed which allow an image plane to be acquired in 30-50 msec (31). The technique uses oscillating field gradients (180° pulses could also be used) to refocus magnetization into spin-echo's, which can be collected and summed to markedly increase sensitivity per unit time. Cardiac function is observed by displaying multiple images acquired at different times in successive cardiac periods. As a result, a complete movie cycle can be obtained in real time. At present, echo-planar techniques can provide an image contrast similar to the conventional spin-echo imaging technique (32). The real-time approach will hopefully soon be implemented in NMR systems for routine clinical use.

Other recently developed methods for assessment of cardiac wall motion are myocardial tagging (33) and the so-called spatial modulation of magnetization (SPAMM)(34). With myocardial tagging the myocardial tissue is tagged with radiofrequency saturation before acquiring images. Specific myocardial regions can be tracked during contraction which enables the study of cardiac motion with the equivalent of multiple, noninvasively generated markers (33). SPAMM involves a pair of nonselective radiofrequency pulses separated by a magnetic field gradient pulse prior to imaging. The SPAMM technique produces images with a regular pattern of stripes that move with the cardiac wall. Using a two-dimensional grid of stripes in short-axis and long-axis views, it provides a unique method of analyzing regional ventricular strain and may offer the ability to accurately quantitate regional myocardial function (34).

Technical considerations

Several technical problems are encountered with NMR of the heart.

First, since the heart is in constant motion, the imaging process has to be gated to the cardiac cycle. Generally, triggering to the R-wave of the electrocardiogram provides the most reliable means of gating. Triggering may be complicated by magnetohydrodynamic effects and NMR-induced currents. These problems can be overcome by careful positioning of the electrocardiographic leads (R-wave larger than T-wave) and by electronic filtering of the signal. Furthermore, since multislice images are obtained at multiple time points in order to speed the imaging process, one obtains different slices at different phases during the cardiac cycle which limits the proper assessment of cardiac function. Therefore, time-consuming multislice-multiphase techniques have to be applied to obtain images of all the slices at the same phase of the cardiac cycle. The introduction of echo-planar techniques may overcome these limitations.

Second, an other problem is the variable orientation of the heart in the chest. The originally used standard imaging planes (transverse, sagittal, coronal) lead to varying obliquity of the cardiac slices, which may introduce partial volume effects. This may introduce anatomical artifacts such as abnormally increased wall thickness and improper volume calculations. As a consequence, the cardiac imaging planes have to be oriented corresponding to the functional axes of the heart to obtain valid information (35). A complete global and regional left ventricular function study has to include acquisition of serial true short-axis planes, preferably extended with the two true long-axis planes, which also permits appropriate comparison with other imaging techniques (36-38).

Third, the effects of flow have to be considered in the interpretation of the images. Flow may lead to signal loss (dark vessel lumen) or signal enhancement (bright intracardiac/intravascular signal) depending on the imaging technique used. However, with the even-echo rephasing phenomenon one can determine whether the signal intensity is due to slowly moving blood or to intravascular/intracardiac masses. Slowly moving blood can only be appreciated on second even-echo images (TE 60 msec), while thrombus is observed on both spin echo images (TE 30 and TE 60 msec).

Fourth, the presence of vascular clips, sternal wires, prosthetic valves and cardiac pacemakers may complicate NMR imaging. NMR should not be used in patients with vascular clips for cerebral aneurysm surgery. Patients with sternal wires after cardiac surgery are no major problem for low to midfield strength NMR instruments (less than 1.0 Tesla), because the presence of fibrosis around the wire will prevent NMR-induced motion. It is therefore generally recommended to postpone NMR studies for at least six weeks after cardiac surgery to allow fibrous tissue to surround mediastinal clips and to minimize clip motion.

Patients with prosthetic valves may only be imaged on the condition that no significant forces on the valve are generated. The latter information can be retrieved from data presented by Soulen et al. (39), who thoroughly examined the forces generated on different prosthetic heart valves at various magnetic fields. If no significant force is generated, the patient can be imaged by NMR. In general, nearly all patients with prosthetic valves can be safely imaged in NMR machines up to 1.5 Tesla field strength. The greatest valve deflection occurs with Starr-Edwards Pre-6000 valves which may angulate up to 27% when placed in a 2.35 Tesla NMR instrument. Randall et al. (40) showed a very little distortion of the NMR image outside the immediate area of the prosthetic valve and no symptoms of discomfort were mentioned by the patients studied. To summarize, NMR studies can be safely and reliably performed in patients with prosthetic heart valves, especially when problems as aortic dissection or perivalvular processes require evaluation.

The presence of a cardiac pacemaker remains an absolute contraindication for NMR imaging. In a NMR study of DDD pacemakers, most of them failed with total inhibition of atrial and ventricular output (41).

Safety considerations

A major concern regarding safety considerations has been the production of ventricular fibrillation through induction of a current into the patient by the rapidly changing magnetic field. In experimental studies in dogs the threshold rate of change of the magnetic field to produce ventricular fibrillation is approximately 500 Tesla/sec (42). The currently used clinical NMR instruments have a maximum rate of field change of about 3 Tesla/sec, indicating the enormous safety margin for the production of ventricular fibrillation in patients. Regarding imaging of patients with acute myocardial infarction, several patients within 24 hours after thrombolysis have been successfully studied (43). The emergency facilities for cardiovascular monitoring of these critically ill patients in the NMR machine have to be similar to those present in the coronary care unit. Constant infusion pumps can be safely applied in the NMR room without interfering with the magnetic field. A defibrillator is located in the NMR room, but adequate resuscitation needs to be performed in a nearby located room.

Finally, claustrophobia may impede NMR imaging in 2-5% of patients. This problem can be controlled by premedicating the patient with an anxiolytic agent.

Coronary artery disease

The use of NMR imaging in coronary artery disease falls into four main categories:
1. Evaluation of acute myocardial ischemia and infarction.
2. Assessment of the sequelae of myocardial infarction.
3. Evaluation of coronary artery bypass grafts, and
4. Visualization of the coronary arteries.

1. Acute myocardial ischemia and infarction
Experimental studies

The detection of acute myocardial ischemia and myocardial infarction is based on the alterations in tissue relaxation times T1 and T2 with resultant changes in image intensity. Early in vitro studies in dog hearts showed that the relaxation times T1 and in particular T2 are usually prolonged in disease states which are characterized by edematous changes that occur in regions with acute myocardial ischemia or infarction (44,45). Electrocardiographically gated NMR images of intact dog hearts also depicted regions of increased signal intensity at the site of the infarcted region (46,47). The magnitude of increase in T1 and T2 was proportional to the magnitude of changes in blood flow. Changes in T1 and T2 could be detected in vivo from 3 to 6 hours after infarction and maximal contrast between normal and infarcted myocardium was achieved at approximately 4 hours after occlusion. Serial imaging in dog hearts showed that signal intensity within the ischemic zone may remain elevated up to 20 days after coronary artery occlusion (48).

NMR imaging of dogs with reperfused myocardial infarctions showed a significant increase in signal intensity and T2 relaxation times already by 30 minutes after reperfusion (49-55). All these studies indicated that NMR imaging may detect ischemic myocardial areas soon after coronary occlusion and provides a method to discern reperfused myocardium acutely.

The use of relaxation times for detecting myocardial ischemia has been questioned (56). Only regions with moderate ischemia showed T1 and T2 prolongation, while in

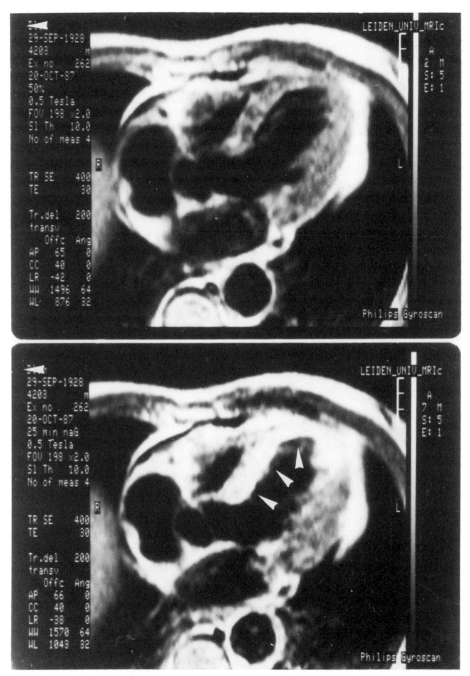

Figure 3

Transversal cardiac MRI scan of a patient with an anteroseptal wall infarction before (uppper image) and 20-25 minutes after administration of Gd-DTPA (lower image). Contrast enhancement is clearly visible in the anteroseptal areas with extension to the apex (arrows).

regions with severe ischemia no alterations in relaxation times were observed, sugge-sting that changes of T1 and T2 in ischemic myocardium are more complex than previously reported.

NMR imaging also allows the assessment of infarct size based on different T2-relaxation times between infarcted and normal tissue (57,58). However, infarct size may be slightly overestimated (59). Serial NMR studies in dogs after varying times of occlusion, either with or without reperfusion, showed that T1 and T2 abnormali-ties did not correlate well with the infarct zone prior to three weeks after occlusion implying that NMR imaging may not be suitable for early detection of infarct size (60). On the other hand, serial NMR imaging of left ventricular infarct size three and 21 days after coronary artery ligation using T2 measurements correlated well with histopathologically assessed infarct size (61). Based on these experimental findings, a T2 strategy has been advocated to evaluate healing patterns in patients following reperfusion after thrombolytic therapy (62).

Clinical studies

Clinical studies in patients with documented myocardial infarction have also shown T1 and T2 alterations in infarcted myocardium. McNamara et al. (63) studied nine patients with acute myocardial infarction 5-12 days after the acute onset and showed

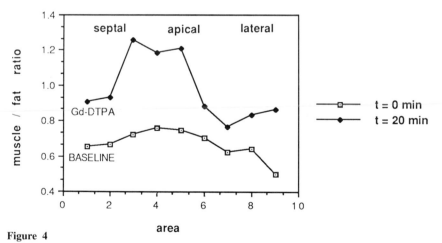

Figure 4

Computer-constructed signal intensity versus area curves from this patient (Fig. 3) both before (baseline) and after administration of Gd-DTPA obtained from 9 adjacent regions of interest (±1 cm3 per region). The antero-septal areas show the highest increase of signal intensity after Gd-DTPA. Also the non-infarcted areas show a slight, but definite increase of signal intensity. (Reproduced with permission, Van Dijkman et al. (112).

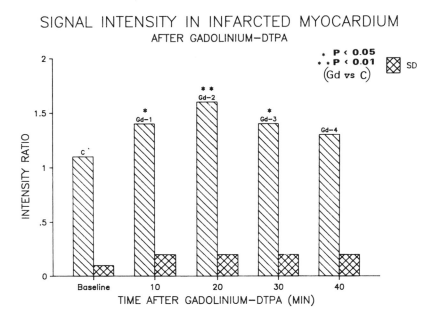

SIGNAL INTENSITY IN INFARCTED MYOCARDIUM
AFTER GADOLINIUM–DTPA

Figure 5
Overall results of the time course of mean signal intensity in 20 patients with acute myocardial infarction. Maximal contrast enhancement is observed 20 minutes after administration of Gd-DTPA. Gd = Gd-DTPA, C = baseline. (Reproduced with permission, Van Dijkman et al. (112))

that the infarcted areas were characterized by increased signal intensity of the infarcted region and prolonged T2 relaxation time. Distinction between normal and infarcted myocardium was sufficient to estimate infarct size. Johnston et al. (64) studied 34 patients 3-30 days after myocardial infarction and showed that regional increase of signal intensity was consistent with the electrocardiographic location of the infarction and with the presence of hypokinetic segments on the left ventriculogram. Fisher et al. (65) showed in 29 patients 3-17 days after myocardial infarction prolonged T2 relaxation times in infarcted myocardial regions. On the other hand, they observed that increased signal intensity on T2-weighted images may be very difficult to distinguish from slowly moving intraventricular blood flow. In addition, a recent study by Ahmad et al. (66) showed that T2 prolongation may be not a specific marker for acute myocardial infarction and can also be observed in abnormally perfused myocardial segments of patients with unstable angina. Been et al. (67) demonstrated in 10 of 13 patients with recent myocardial infarction a 40% increase of T1 values in the infarcted areas. In a subsequent study, Been et al. (68) showed in 41 patients with acute myocardial infarction that maximum T1 values were observed at two weeks after the acute onset, suggesting that the increase of T1 reflects cellular infiltration as much as or more than tissue edema. No differences in T1 values were observed between the patients with or without reperfusion, indicating that alterations

137

of T1 are complex and may bear no relationship with specific histological findings. In the absence of any histologic confirmation, these statements remain purely speculative. We showed in 20 patients with acute myocardial infarction, who underwent NMR studies with a mean of eight days after the acute event, that regional T2-abnormalities in 82% of patients correlated with the presence and location of thallium perfusion defects at rest emphasizing the value of NMR tissue characterization in flow-deprived injured myocardial tissue (69,70). In a subsequent study, Krauss et al. (71) showed in 20 patients 7-14 days after acute myocardial infarction that NMR imaging provided an accurate means of assessing infarct size based on calculation of T2 relaxation times. As the T1 and T2 relaxation times may be inaccurate as indices for tissue characterization in patients with myocardial infarction, other characteristics have to be taken into account. Infarcted myocardial areas may be seen by NMR imaging using morphological features like increased signal intensity, ventricular cavitary signal and regional wall thinning. Filipchuk et al. (72) showed increased myocardial signal intensity in 88%, cavitary signal in 74% and regional wall thinning in 67% of 27 patients with acute myocardial infarction. However, in 18 asymptomatic volunteers also increased myocardial signal intensity was observed in 83%, cavitary signal in 94%, and wall thinning in 11% of cases. These findings imply that increased signal both from myocardial tissue and from the cavity are sensitive but not specific at all for myocardial infarction. Of the three features therefore, wall thinning was the most predictive of and specific for acute myocardial infarction. White et al. (73) showed in 17 patients with a recent myocardial infarction a good comparison between NMR imaging and two-dimensional echocardiography for demonstrating regional wall motion abnormalities. They extended this study to 22 patients and observed that the extent of regional wall thinning by NMR imaging can be used to measure infarct size (74). Wisenberg et al. (75) showed in 66 patients three weeks after acute infarction that infarct size could very well be determined by NMR imaging based on signal intensity. They demonstrated that in the 41 patients who had reveived acute streptokinase therapy a significant reduction in NMR-measured infarct size was observed compared to the patients without thrombolytic therapy. Johns et al. (76) assessed NMR infarct size in 20 patients based on signal intensity at a mean of nine days after the acute onset of symptoms. NMR infarct size correlated very well with the extent of the region with severe hypokinesia visualized by left ventricular angiography.

All these clinical studies indicate that the use of relaxation times may be helpful for detection and characterization of infarcted areas but have to be analyzed concomitantly with other morphological NMR features.

Future directions for NMR research into recognition and sizing of acute myocardial infarction include the development of specific software programs and new pulse sequences that clearly define infarct borders and measure infarct mass, and the application of contrast agents to improve contrast between ischemic and normal myocardium.

138

Contrast agents

Despite the ability to generate images with varying image contrast, using the relaxation parameters T1 and T2, it is far from easy to detect abnormalities in tissue physiology in the early stage of myocardial ischemia. The detection of acute infarction with unenhanced NMR imaging does not occur until several hours after coronary occlusion. Moreover, the detection of myocardial infarction per se may be cumbersome, since prolongation of T1 and T2 in infarcted areas may not be sufficient to provide sufficient contrast to adequately visualize the infarcted area. As has been mentioned, normal subjects may also show myocardial regions with increased signal intensity comparable to those seen in patients with infarction. Furthermore, it is difficult to differentiate the wall signal from slowly moving blood in the ventricle, as well as artifactual variations in the myocardium due to respiratory or residual cardiac motion. In addition, the use of late echo's reduces the signal to noise ratio and leads to image degradation (78). Therefore, paramagnetic contrast agents have been developed to define functional and perfusion abnormalities in the setting of acute myocardial ischemia and infarction (79-89). In particular, Gadolinium-containing contrast agents (labeled with DTPA, DOTA, or albumin) have been shown to provide contrast on NMR images. Most clinical experience has been obtained with Gadolinium-DTPA, which can be safely used in patients with coronary artery disease.

Experimental studies

Gd-DTPA has been shown to improve contrast enhancement of ischemic and infarcted myocardium in dogs (90-94). Both T1 and T2 relaxation times are significantly shortened by Gd-DTPA in ischemic myocardial tissue after experimental coronary artery occlusion. The effect on T1 relaxation time is predominant and therefore T1-weighted images will show enhanced signal intensity in ischemic myocardium after administration of Gd-DTPA. The contrast enhancement at the ischemic area is probably caused by differences in wash-in and wash-out of Gd-DTPA from normal and ischemic myocardium. In acutely damaged myocardium, the increased accumulation of Gd-DTPA is dependent on blood flow, tissue blood volume, the size of the extracellular space, and the permeability of the capillaries, all of which causes slow wash-out from the infarcted zone. By 10 to 15 minutes after Gd-DTPA injection, it has largely washed out of the normal myocardium, while it remains in the infarcted zone suggesting that NMR imaging is preferably performed after 15-25 minutes. Gd-DTPA remains extracellular and is excreted by the glomerular filtration.

Gd-DTPA has been studied in several experimental models of myocardial ischemia that primarily differ from each other in the duration of coronary artery ligation, the time period between contrast administration and imaging, and the presence or absence of reperfusion (90-94). All these experimental studies using Gd-DTPA demonstrated that changes in relaxation times occur already very early (2 minutes) after coronary artery occlusion, implying that Gd-DTPA allows the detection of early myocardial ischemia even before the onset of myocardial edema formation or the development of irreversible damage. These studies also suggest that Gd-DTPA may be useful to outline distribution of regional myocardial blood flow. In a study by Miller et al. (95), NMR imaging was able to measure myocardial flow reserve during pharmacologic dilatation by dipyridamole. There was a significant correlation between changes in Gd-DTPA enhanced NMR signal and microsphere myocardial blood flow. Further experimental studies have shown that the use of Gd-DTPA may discriminate between occlusive and reperfused infarcts based on differences in signal intensities (96-99). Moreover, administration of Gd-DTPA early after reperfusion allowed the identification of the area at risk by selective concentration of Gd-DTPA in reperfused myocardium (100). In a recent experimental study, Nishimura et al. (101) measured infarct size both by NMR imaging using Gd-DTPA and indium-111 labeled antimyosin. Gd-DTPA showed significant contrast enhancement of the infarcted area and the extent of the contrast enhancement expressed infarct size precisely.

Other contrast agents

Apart from gadolinium-containing paramagnetic contrast agents, manganese-containing agents have been developed to detect acute regional perfusion abnormalities (102,103). These compounds concentrate in normal myocardium and distribute intracellularly in viable cells in proportion to organ blood flow. In contrast to the Gd-DTPA images, the manganese NMR images show increased signal intensity in the normally perfused myocardium (positive image) relative to ischemic myocardium. The manganese compounds are able to delineate the jeopardized area after acute myocardial ischemia (104), to discriminate between occlusive and reperfused infarcts (105), and to determine infarct size (106), all being studied in experimental settings. At present, the clinical use of manganese is limited by its short- and long-term effects (107). In the short-term, manganese behaves as a calcium-antagonist potentially leading to hypotension associated with decreased systemic vascular resistance. In the long-term, cerebral or hepatobiliary damage may occur. The results of clinical studies must be awaited.

Clinical studies with Gd-DTPA

Only few clinical studies with Gd-DTPA have been performed. Eichstaedt et al. (108) showed in 26 patients with acute myocardial infarction that the 11 patients who were studied with Gd-DTPA 5-10 days after the acute event had a 70% average increase of signal intensity within zones of infarcted myocardium, while only a 20% increase of signal intensity in normal myocardial tissue was observed. The other 15 patients were imaged later in the course of infarction and did not show differences in intensity ratio between infarcted and normal tissue. These findings were corroborated in a recent report by Nishimura et al. (109) who studied 17 infarct patients with NMR imaging and Gd-DTPA at an average of 5, 12, 30, and 90 days after the acute event. Increased signal intensity in the infarcted area was observed at 5 and 12 days, implying that only acute (or subacute) myocardial infarcts show significant accumulation of Gd-DTPA.

In an initial study from our institution by de Roos et al. (110), five patients underwent NMR imaging using Gd-DTPA 2-17 days after myocardial infarction. The signal intensity of infarcted versus normal myocardium was significantly greater after Gd-DTPA administration than before Gd-DTPA both by visual and computer-assessed analysis (Figs. 3 and 4). The use of Gd-DTPA improved infarct definition and obviated the need for multiecho imaging techniques. This study was extended to 20 patients with acute myocardial infarction and showed maximal contrast 20-25 minutes after administration of Gd-DTPA (Fig. 5)(111). Moreover, a good correlation between electrocardiographic infarct site and local increase of signal intensity based on region of interest analysis was observed. In 25 patients of whom 10 were studied within 72 hours after myocardial infarction, van Dijkman et al. (112, 113) showed that signal intensity of Gd-DTPA was significantly increased in the infarcted areas of the 15 patients who were studied more than 72 hours after the acute onset, indicating increased accumulation of Gd-DTPA in a more advanced stage of the disease process. These early encouraging results have led to initiation of a clinical study to determine whether the use of Gd-DTPA allows the discrimination of reperfused versus non-reperfused myocardial areas. Until now, two initial reports have shown that signal intensities do not differ between reperfused and non-reperfused myocardial areas (114,115). However, it was observed that the morphological appearance of contrast enhancement by Gd-DTPA may provide some clues as to the presence or absence of reperfusion; reperfusion goes along with a homogeneous aspect, while lack of reperfusion may be visualized as a heterogeneous enhancement of contrast (Fig. 11). These morphological characteristics had already been observed in experimental reperfusion studies (98). Further extension of these studies may provide the definite answers as to whether early reperfusion may be identified by Gd-DTPA enhanced NMR imaging.

In a recent study by de Roos et al. (116) in 20 acute infarct patients who received streptokinase, infarct size was determined by NMR imaging using Gd-DTPA. Nine slices (10 mm thick) perpendicular to the long axis of the left ventricle were obtained and for every slice the area with enhanced signal intensity (>mean normal intensity +2SD) was considered to be infarcted (Fig. 6). Following summation of these areas for all slices, infarct size proved to be significantly less in the patients who had reperfusion compared to the patients without reperfusion ($8\pm5\%$ versus $15\pm4\%$, $P<0.001$).

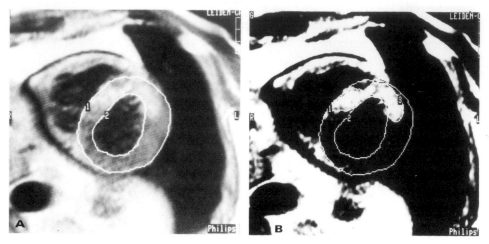

Figure 6

Computer-constructed contours of the subepicardial (1) and subendocardial (2) borders on the NMR image after Gd-DTPA administration in a patient with an anterior wall infarction. (**Fig. 6A, left**). After subtraction of the mean cardiac signal intensity + 2 standard deviations, the NMR image still shows marked contrast enhancement of Gd-DTPA in the anterior area (3), allowing the estimation of infarct size (**Fig. 6B, right**).

Cine NMR technique

The cine NMR technique can also be used for detection of myocardial ischemia and infarction. Myocardial infarction can be detected as an area of absolute decrease in signal intensity, presumably due to hemorrhage within the area of infarction and subsequent field inhomogeneity. Regional contractile abnormalities caused by ischemic heart disease are very well demonstrated by cine NMR. Both abnormal wall motion and more specifically abnormal wall thickening indicate diminished regional myocardial function. In particular decreased regional wall thickening is identified in patients with acute myocardial infarction (22). In a study by Pflugfelder et al. (29), 13 normal subjects and 15 patients with coronary artery disease were studied by cine NMR to document and quantitate regional left ventricular wall motion abnormalities. Abnormal wall motion was observed in 40 of 90 segments in patients with coronary artery disease, which correlated well with results of echocardiography or contrast ventriculography. The overall systolic wall thickening in the normal subjects was $48\pm28\%$, in the normal segments of the patients $43\pm31\%$, in hypokinetic zones $6\pm18\%$, in akinetic zones $-4\pm24\%$, and in dyskinetic zones $-13\pm25\%$. Peshock et al. (117) reported a maximal systolic wall thickening of $60\pm18\%$ in 10 normal volunteers. In seven patients with regional wall abnormalities, cine NMR imaging showed a sensitivity of 94% and a specificity of 80% when correlated with biplane angiography. Lotan et al. (118) studied 59 patients with suspected coronary artery disease with both biplane cine NMR imaging and biplane cineangiography. In the right anterior oblique view, agreement was within one grade in 96% of 275 segments, and in the left anterior oblique view in 92% of segments. Pennell et al. (119) studied 17 patients with coronary artery disease both by cine NMR imaging and thallium tomography using the coronary arterial dilator dipyridamole as an alternative stress method.

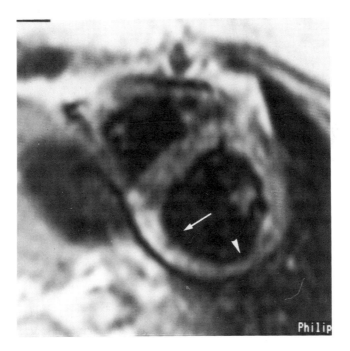

Figure 7
Short-axis NMR image of a patient with an acute inferior wall infarction after a previously sustained posterior wall infarction. There is increased signal intensity of the inferior wall (arrow), marked wall thinning of the posterior wall (arrowhead), and a clear dilatation of the left ventricle.

Newly developing wall motion abnormalities in nine patients occurred all at the site of the reversible thallium perfusion defects. This illustrates the feasibility of cine NMR imaging to perform stress imaging and to detect the functional sequelae of reversible myocardial ischemia. In conclusion, cine NMR imaging is very useful for the quantitative noninvasive assessment of global and regional myocardial function in patients with coronary artery disease.
Newer studies will focus on dobutamine as an alternative pharmacologic stress inducer.

2. Sequelae of acute myocardial infarction

NMR imaging is very well capable to detect long-term sequelae of myocardial infarction. Higgins et al. (120) showed that segmental wall thinning was highly indicative of a sustained myocardial infarction in 9 of 10 patients with chronic infarctions. McNamara and Higgins (121) observed regional wall thinning in 20 of 22 patients with prior infarctions; in 10 of 14 patients with sufficient residual wall thickness for measurement of T2-relaxation times, decreased signal intensities and shortened T2-values were measured at the site of the infarcted area. In a study by Krauss et al. (122), 19 acute infarct patients were studied by NMR imaging at discharge of whom 13 patients were reexamined 4-7 months later. In 10 patients infarct site and size did not change, and the T2 relaxation times remained prolonged particularly in the patients with anterior infarction. In three patients wall thinning prevented adequate measurement of T2-values. The finding of prolonged T2-values in chronically infarcted areas was also observed in animal experiments by Checkley et al. (123), who found high-signal areas at 10 days in infarcted mini-pig hearts. After 2 weeks no further change in signal intensity was detected, but myocardial thinning became more evident. These studies suggested that detection of infarcted areas is possible at the chronic phase of infarction both by altered signal intensities and morphologic appearance (Fig. 7).

Also complications of acute myocardial infarction including thromboembolism, ventricular aneurysm, ventricular septum perforation, and mitral regurgitation can be readily demonstrated by NMR imaging (70,124,125). The differentiation of thrombus and slowly moving blood may be demonstrated by - in case of a thrombus - the absence of even-echo rephasing, the presence of wall thinning, and the presence of a wall motion abnormality (Fig. 8). Left ventricular septal defect is clearly visualized by NMR as absence of muscular tissue in the septal area. Early detection of complications by NMR imaging may be very important for guiding proper patient management.

3. The evaluation of coronary artery bypass grafts

NMR imaging has been used to evaluate the patency of coronary artery bypass grafts. Using the spin-echo technique, the grafts appear as small circular structures with absence of luminal signal since blood moves rapidly through normal grafts. However, sternal clips used in bypass grafting can lead to small regions of signal drop-out that may be mistaken for patent grafts. There must be also sufficient flow to generate contrast between the graft lumen and the wall. Generally, multislice multiphase imaging is required to obtain the appropriate images for detecting rapid graft flow at contiguous levels in the same phase. In a study by Rubinstein et al. (126), using the multislice technique in 20 patients after bypass surgery, the overall sensitivity and specificity for evaluating bypass patency were 92% and 85% respectively.

Gomes et al. (127) studied 20 patients with patent bypass grafts and showed that 54 of 64 grafts (84%) were detected by NMR imaging. Jenkins et al. (128) assessed graft patency by NMR imaging in 22 patients and found 90% accuracy compared with contrast angiography.

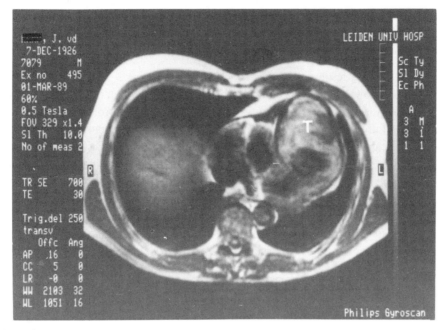

Figure 8
Transverse NMR imaging plane showing a left ventricular thrombus (T) occupying the whole left ventricle of a patient with a previously sustained large anterior wall infarction. Also aneurysmal formation of the antero-apical area can be observed. After surgical removal the largest diameter of the thrombus proved to be 7 cm.

Frija et al. (129) showed in 28 patients that NMR imaging after bypass surgery provided a correct diagnosis in 95% of cases. The major causes of diagnostic inaccuracies were hemostatic clips, in particular clips for internal mammary bypass grafts. While the spin-echo technique shows lack of signal intensity in vascular compartments with rapid blood flow, the cine NMR imaging technique depicts flowing blood as a bright signal. Therefore the presence of a bright visible intraluminal signal is indicative of graft patency. First results of cine NMR imaging by White et al. (130) for determination of bypass patency in 25 patients showed accuracies of 91% for patency and 72% for occlusion. A subsequent study by White et al. (131) in 10 patients showed for the determination of patency a sensitivity of 93%, a specificity of 86%, and an overall predictive accuracy of 89%. Aurigemma et al. (132) used cine NMR imaging in 20 operated patients with a total of 45 grafts and showed a sensitivity of 88%, a specificity of 100%, and an overall accuracy of 91%. Although these studies are preliminary, it has been presaged that a combined use of a spin-echo examination and cine NMR imaging will be the optimal approach for imaging bypass grafts. Furthermore, future flow-sensitive techniques are needed to exactly quantitating graft flow (133). Quantitation of bypass graft flow directly reflects distal runoff which seems more valuable than simply detecting bypass patency.

4. Visualization of the coronary arteries

The in plane spatial resolution of current NMR instruments is 3 x 1.5 mm, which is sufficient to allow the visualization of the major coronary arteries (134). Normal proximal and distal right coronary arteries and proximal left coronary arteries have been successfully imaged (Fig. 9). Left main coronary artery stenoses of more than 50% have been detected by NMR, and noninvasive characterization of coronary artery stenosis before and following angioplasty is currently under investigation. However, several factors make the imaging of the coronary arteries technically difficult. First, the position of the coronary arteries may vary due to motion from the respiratory tract and to heart-rate dependent changes in heart size which degrade NMR image quality. Second, because of the tortuous nature of the coronary arteries tomographic sections may be inadequate for diagnostic purposes. These problems can be overcome by using high-speed echo-planar imaging, the use of surface coils, and the three-dimensional imaging possibilities of NMR imaging. At this moment, echo-planar techniques have limited resolution, the appropriate surface coils have to be developed, and the use of the three-dimensional NMR potential increases the complexity and duration of the procedure. However, future technical developments will most probably enable successful NMR coronary arteriography within the next years.

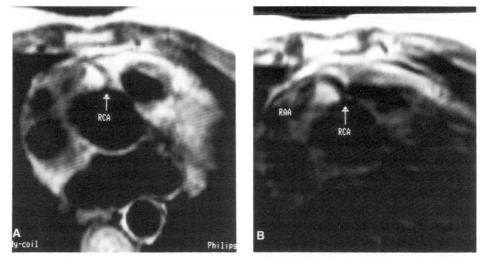

Figure 9
Transverse NMR image of the origin of the right coronary artery (RCA) using both a body coil (**Fig. 9A**) and a surface coil (**Fig. 9B**). The image quality is markedly improved with the surface coil. RAA=right atrial appendage.

Conclusion

At present, NMR imaging may provide useful information which is not readily available from other noninvasive conventional modalities such as echocardiography, radionuclide angiography, and computed tomography. The superb resolution, the inherent contrast, the three-dimensional nature, the lack of ionizing radiation, and its morphological imaging capabilities sufficiently justify the application of NMR imaging in cardiology. In particular in patients with coronary artery disease, the analysis of left ventricular mass and wall thickening, quantitation of cardiac volumes, tissue characterization and measurement of infarct size can be readily performed by NMR imaging. Although NMR imaging can be used without contrast media, the information it generates in ischemic heart disease will be increased by application of contrast agents like Gd-DTPA.

The definite judgments about the relative importance of NMR as an expensive diagnostic tool have still to be settled. For those clinical situations in which NMR imaging can replace the conventional techniques, these judgements should be based on additional prospective studies. For NMR imaging to have its most substantial impact in detecting coronary artery disease, future technical developments should allow to define accurate distribution of regional myocardial blood flow in order to assess the ischemic area at risk both at rest and during exercise, quantitative analysis of regional wall motion, and visualization of the coronary arteries. These advances include faster imaging sequences, automated quantitation algorithms, and three-dimensional angiography.

The early detection and visualization of coronary artery stenoses by NMR angiography would constitute a tremendous progress in cardiology and would far outweigh the cost inherent to the NMR procedure.

References

1. Kaufman L, Crooks L, Sheldon P, Hricak H, Herfkens R, Bank W. The potential impact of nuclear magnetic resonance imaging on cardiovascular diagnosis. Circulation 1983;67:251-7
2. Herfkens RJ, Higgins CB, Hricak H, Lipton MJ, Crooks LE, Lanzer P, Botvinick E, Brundage B, Sheldon PE, Kaufman L. Nuclear magnetic resonance imaging of the cardiovascular system: normal and pathologic findings. Radiology 1983;147:749-59
3. Florentine MS, Grosskreutz CL, Chang W, Hartnett JA, Dunn VD, Ehrhardt JC, Fleagle SR, Collins SM, Marcus ML, Skorton DJ. Measurement of left ventricular mass in vivo using gated nuclear magnetic resonance imaging. J Am Coll Cardiol 1986;8:107-12
4. Keller AM, Peshock RM, Malloy CR, Buja LM, Nunnaly R, Parkey RW, Willerson JT. In vivo measurement of myocardial mass using nuclear magnetic resonance imaging. J Am Coll Cardiol 1986;8:113-7
5. Caputo GR, Tscholakoff D, Sechtem U, Higgins CB. Measurements of canine left ventricular mass by using MR imaging. AJR 1987;148:33-8
6. Markiewicz W, Sechtem U, Kirby R, Derugin N, Caputo GC, Higgins CB. Measurement of ventricular volumes in the dog by nuclear magnetic resonance imaging. J Am Coll Cardiol 1987;10:170-7
7. Katz J, Milliken MC, Stray-Gundersen J, Buja LM, Parkey RW, Mitchell JH, Peshock RM. Estimation of human myocardial mass with MR imaging. Radiology 1988;169:495-8
8. Ostrzega E, Maddahi J, Honma H, Crues III JV, Resser KJ, Charuzi Y, Berman DS. Quantification of left ventricular myocardial mass in humans by nuclear magnetic resonance imaging. Am Heart J 1989;117:444-52
9. Friedman BJ, Waters J, Kwan OL, DeMaria AN. Comparison of magnetic resonance imaging and echocardiography in determination of cardiac dimensions in normal subjects. J Am Coll Cardiol 1985;5:1369-76
10. Longmore DB, Klipstein RH, Underwood SR, Firman DN, Hounsfield GN, Watanabe M, Bland C, Fox K, Poole-Wilson PA, Rees RSO, Denison D, McNeilly AM, Burman ED. Dimensional accuracy of magnetic resonance in studies of the heart. Lancet 1985;i:1360-2
11. Byrd III BF, Schiller NB, Botvinick EH, Higgins CB. Normal cardiac dimensions by magnetic resonance imaging. Am J Cardiol 1985;55: 1440-2
12. Shapiro EP, Rogers WJ, Beyar R, Soulen RL, Zerhouni EA, Lima JAC, Weiss JL. Determination of left ventricular mass by magnetic resonance imaging in hearts deformed by acute infarction. Circulation 1989;79:706-11
13. Mögelvang J, Thomsen C, Mehlsen J, Bräckle G, Stubgaard M, Henriksen O. Evaluation of left ventricular volumes measured by magnetic resonance imaging. Eur Heart J 1986;7:1016-21
14. Mögelvang J, Stubgaard M, Thomsen C, Henriksen O. Evaluation of right ventricular volumes measured by magnetic resonance imaging. Eur Heart J 1988;9:529-33
15. Stratemeier EJ, Thompson R, Brady TJ, Miller SW, Saini S, Wismer GL, Okada RD, Dinsmore RW. Ejection fraction determination by MR imaging: comparison with left ventricular angiography. Radiology 1986;158:775-7
16. Buckwalter KA, Aisen AM, Dilworth LR, Mancini GB, Buda AJ. Gated cardiac MRI: Ejection-fraction determination using the right anterior oblique view. AJR 1986;147:33-7
17. Van Rossum AC, Visser FC, Van Eenige MJ, Valk J, Roos JP. Magnetic resonance imaging of the heart for determination of ejection fraction. Int J Cardiol 1988;18:53-63
18. Van Rossum AC, Visser FC, Sprenger M, Van Eenige MJ, Valk J, Roos JP. Evaluation of magnetic resonance imaging for determination of left ventricular ejection fraction and comparison with angiography. Am J Cardiol 1988;62:628-33
19. Just H, Holubarsch C, Friedburg H. Estimation of left ventricular volume and mass by magnetic resonance imaging: comparison with quantitative biplane angiocardiography. Cardiovasc Intervent Radiol 1987;10:1-4
20. Underwood SR, Rees RSO, Savage PE, Klipstein RH, Firmin DN, Fox KM, Poole-Wilson PA, Longmore DB. Assessment of regional left ventricular function by magnetic resonance. Br Heart J 1986;56:334-40
21. Fisher MR, von Schulthess GK, Higgins CB. Multiphasic cardiac magnetic resonance imaging: normal regional left ventricular wall thickening. AJR 1985;145:27-30

22. Sechtem U, Sommerhoff BA, Markiewicz W, White RD, Cheitlin MD, Higgins CB. Regional left ventricular wall thickening by magnetic resonance imaging: evaluation in normal persons and patients with global and regional dysfunction. Am J Cardiol 1987;59:145-51

23. Akins EW, Hill JA, Sievers KW, Conti CR. Assessment of left ventricular wall thickness in healed myocardial infarction by magnetic resonance imaging. Am J Cardiol 1987;59:24-8

24. Sechtem U, Pflugfelder PW, White RD, Gould RG, Holt W, Lipton MJ, Higgins CB. Cine MR imaging: potential for the evaluation of cardiovascular function. AJR 1987;148:239-46

25. Sechtem U, Pflugfelder PW, Gould RG, Cassidy MM, Higgins CB. Measurement of right and left ventricular volumes in healthy individuals with cine MR imaging. Radiology 1987;163:697-702

26. Utz JA, Herfkens RJ, Heinsimer JA, Bashore T, Califf R, Glover G, Pelc N, Shimakawa A. Cine MR determination of left ventricular ejection fraction. AJR 1987;148:839-43

27. Buser PT, Auffermann W, Holt WW, Wagner S, Kircher B, Wolfe C, Higgins CB. Noninvasive evaluation of global left ventricular function with use of cine nuclear magnetic resonance. J Am Coll Cardiol 1989;13:1294-300

28. Pflugfelder PW, Sechtem UP, White RD, Higgins CB. Quantification of regional myocardial function by rapid cine MR imaging. AJR 1988;150:523-9

29. Crooks LE, Barker B, Chang H, Feinber D, Hoenninger JC, Watts JC, Arakawa M, Kaufman L, Sheldon PE, Botvinick E, Higgins CB. Magnetic resonance imaging strategies for heart studies. Radiology 1984;153:459-65

30. Beyar R, Shapiro EP, Graves WL, Rogers WJ, Guier WH, Carey GA, Soulen RL, Zerhouni EA, Weisfeldt ML, Weiss JL. Quantification and validation of left ventricular wall thickening by a three-dimensional volume element magnetic resonance imaging approach. Circulation 1990;81:297-307.

31. Rzedzian RR, Pykett IL. Instant images of the human heart using a new, whole-body MR imaging system. AJR 1987;149:245-50

32. Chapman B, Turner R, Ordidge RJ,Cawley M, Coxon R, Glover P, Mansfield P. Real-time movie imaging from a single cardiac cycle by NMR. Magn Reson Med 1987;5:246-54

33. Zerhouni EA, Parish DM, Rogers WJ, Yang A, Shapiro EP. Human heart: tagging with MR Imaging - A method for noninvasive assessment of myocardial motion. Radiology 1988;169:59-63.

34. Axel L, Dougherty L. Heart wall motion: improved method of spatial modulation of magnetization for MR Imaging. Radiology 1989;172:349-50

35. Akins EW, Hill JA, Fitzsimmons JR, Pepine CJ, Willams CM. Importance of imaging plane for magnetic resonance imaging of the normal left ventricle. Am J Cardiol 1985;56:366-72

36. Dinsmore RE, Wismer GL, Levine RA, Okada RD, Brady TJ. Magnetic resonance imaging of the heart: positioning and gradient angle selection for optimal imaging planes. AJR 1984;143:1135-42

37. Dinsmore RE. Quantitation of cardiac dimensions from ECG-synchronized MRI studies. Cardiovasc Intervent Radiol 1987;10:356-64

38. Kaul S, Wismer GL, Brady TJ, Johnston DL, Weyman AE, Okada RD, Dinsmore RE. Measurement of normal left heart dimensions using optimally oriented MR images. AJR 1986;146:75-9

39. Soulen R, Budinger TF, Higgins CB. Magnetic resonance imaging of prosthetic heart valves. Radiology 1985;154:705-7

40. Randall PA, Kohman LJ, Scalzetti EM, Szeverenyi NM, Panicek DM. Magnetic resonance imaging of prosthetic cardiac valves in vitro and in vivo. Am J Cardiol 1988;62:973-6

41. Erlebacher JA, Cahill PT, Pannizzo F, Knowles RJR. Effect of magnetic resonance imaging on DDD pacemakers. Am J Cardiol 1986;57:437-40

42. Roy OZ. Technical note: Summary of cardiac fibrillation thresholds for 60 Hz currents and voltages applied directly to the heart. Med Biol Eng Comput 1980;18:657-62

43. Johnston DL, Mulvagh SL, Cashion RW, O'Neill PG, Roberts R, Rokey R. Nuclear magnetic resonance imaging of acute myocardial infarction within 24 hours of chest pain onset. Am J Cardiol 1989;64:172-9

44. Higgins CB, Herfkens R, Lipton MJ, Sievers R, Sheldon P, Kaufman L, Crooks LE. Nuclear magnetic resonance imaging of acute myocardial infarction in dogs: alterations in magnetic relaxation times. Am J Cardiol 1983;52:184-8

45. Williams ES, Kaplan JI, Thatcher F, Zimmerman G, Knoebel SB. Prolongation of proton spin lattice relaxation times in regionally ischemic tissue from dog hearts. J Nucl Med 1980;21:449-53

46. Pflugfelder PW, Wisenberg G, Prato FS, Carroll SE, Turner KL. Early detection of canine myocardial infarction by magnetic resonance imaging in vivo. Circulation 1985;71:587-94

149

47. Wesbey G, Higgins CB, Lanzer P, Botvinick E, Lipton M. Imaging and characterization of acute myocardial infarction in vivo by gated nuclear magnetic resonance. Circulation 1984;69:125-30

48. Pflugfelder PW, Wisenberg G, Prato FS, Turner KL, Carroll SE. Serial imaging of canine myocardial infarction by in vivo nuclear magnetic resonance. J Am Coll Cardiol 1986;7:843-9

49. Ratner AV, Okada RD, Newell JB, Pohost GM. The relationship between proton nuclear magnetic resonance relaxation parameters and myocardial perfusion with acute coronary arterial occlusion and reperfusion. Circulation 1985;71:823-28

50. Johnston DL, Brady TJ, Ratner AV, Rosen BR, Newell JB, Pohost GM, Okada RD. Assessment of myocardial ischemia with proton magnetic resonance: effects of a three hour coronary occlusion with and without reperfusion. Circulation 1985;71:595-601

51. Slutsky RA, Brown JJ, Peck WW, Stritch G, Andre MP. Effects of transient coronary ischemia and reperfusion on myocardial edema formation and in vitro magnetic relaxation times. J Am Coll Cardiol 1984;3:1454-60

52. Aisen AM, Buda AJ, Zotz RJ, Buckwalter KA. Visualization of myocardial infarction and subsequent coronary reperfusion with MRI using a dog model. Magn Reson Imaging 1987;5:399-404

53. Johnston DL, Liu P, Rosen BR, Levine RA, Beaulieu PA, Brady TJ, Okada RD. In vivo detection of reperfused myocardium by nuclear magnetic resonance imaging. J Am Coll Cardiol 1987;9:127-35

54. Miller DD, Johnston DL, Dragotakes D, Newell JB, Aretz T, Kantor HL, Brady TJ, Okada RD. Effect of hyperosmotic mannitol on magnetic resonance relaxation parameters in reperfused canine myocardial infarction. Magn Reson Imaging 1989;7:79-88

55. Tscholakoff D, Higgins CB, Sechtem U, Caputo G, Derugin N. MRI of reperfused myocardial infarct in dogs. AJR 1986;146:925-30

56. Canby RC, Reeves RC, Evanochko WT, Elgavish GA, Pohost GM. Proton nuclear magnetic resonance relaxation times in severe myocardial ischemia. J Am Coll Cardiol 1987;10:412-20

57. Buda AJ, Aisen AM, Juni JE, Gallagher KP, Zotz RJ. Detection and sizing of myocardial ischemia and infarction by nuclear magnetic resonance imaging in the canine heart. Am Heart J 1985;110: 1284-90

58. Rokey R, Verani MS, Bolli R, Kuo LC, Ford JJ, Wendt RE, Schneiders NJ, Bryan RN, Roberts R. Myocardial infarct size quantification by MR imaging early after coronary artery occlusion in dogs. Radiology 1986;158:771-4

59. Bouchard A, Reeves RC, Cranney G, Bishop SP, Pohost GM, Bischoff P. Assessment of myocardial infarct size by means of T2-weighted 1H nuclear magnetic resonance imaging. Am Heart J 1989;117:281-9

60. Wisenberg G, Prato FS, Carroll SE, Turner KL, Marshall T. Serial nuclear magnetic resonance imaging of acute myocardial infarction with and without reperfusion. Am Heart J 1988;115:510-8

61. Caputo GR, Sechtem U, Tscholakoff D, Higgins CB. Measurement of myocardial infarct size at early and late time intervals using MR imaging: An experimental study in dogs. AJR 1987;149:237-43

62. Johnston DL, Homma S, Liu P, Weilbaecher DG, Rokey R, Brady TJ, Okada R. Serial changes in nuclear magnetic resonance relaxation times after myocardial infarction in the rabbit: relationship to water content, severity of ischemia, and histopathology over a six-month period. Magn Reson Med 1988;8:363-79

63. McNamara MT, Higgins CB, Schechtmann N, Botvinick E, Lipton MJ, Chatterjee K, Amparo EG. Detection and characterization of acute myocardial infarction in man with the use of gated magnetic resonance. Circulation 1985;71:717-24

64. Johnston DL, Thompson RC, Liu P, Dinsmore RE, Wismer GL, Saini S, Kaul S, Rosen BR, Brady TJ, Okada R. Magnetic resonance imaging during acute myocardial infarction. Am J Cardiol 1986;57:1059-65

65. Fisher MR, McNamara MT, Higgins CB. Acute myocardial infarction: MR evaluation in 29 patients. AJR 1987;148:247-51

66. Ahmad M, Johnson RF, Fawcett HD, Schreiber MH. Magnetic resonance imaging in patients with unstable angina: comparison with acute myocardial infarction and normals. Magn Reson Imaging 1988;6:527-34

67. Been M, Smith MA, Ridgway JP, Brydon JWE, Douglas RHB, Dean KM, Best JJK, Muir AL. Characterisation of acute myocardial infarction by gated magnetic resonance imaging. Lancet 1985;ii:348-50

68. Been M, Smith MA, Ridgway JP, Douglas RHB, DeBono DP, Best JJK, Muir Al. Serial changes in the T1 magnetic relaxation parameter after myocardial infarction in man. Br Heart J 1988;59:1-8

150

69. Postema S, De Roos A, Doornbos J, Krauss XH, Blokland JAK. Recent myocardial infarction: detection and localization by magnetic resonance imaging and thallium scintigraphy. J Med Imaging 1989;3:68-74

70. Krauss XH, Van der Wall EE, Doornbos J, Blokland JAK, Postema S, De Roos A, Van der Laarse A, Manger Cats V, Van Voorthuisen AE, Bruschke AVG. The value of nuclear magnetic resonance imaging in patients with a recent myocardial infarction; comparison with planar thallium-201 scintigraphy. Cardiovasc Interv Radiol 1989;12:119-24

71. Krauss XH, Van der Wall EE, Doornbos J, Van der Laarse A, Blokland JAK, Bloem JH, Van Dijkman PRM, Bruschke AVG. Nuclear magnetic resonance imaging of myocardial infarct size and cardiac function. Eur Heart J 1988;9(Suppl A1):340(Abstr)

72. Filipchuk NG, Peshock RM, Malloy CR, Corbett JR, Rehr RB, Buja LM, Jansen DE, Redish GR, Gabliani GI, Parkey RW, Willerson JT. Detection and localization of recent myocardial infarction by magnetic resonance imaging. Am J Cardiol 1986;58:214-9

73. White RD, Cassidy MM, Cheitlin MD Emilson B, Ports TA, Lim AD, Botvinick EH, Schiller NB, Higgins CB. Segmental evaluation of left ventricular wall motion after myocardial infarction: Magnetic resonance imaging versus echocardiography. Am Heart J 1988;115:166-75

74. White RD, Holt WW, Cheitlin MD, Cassidy MM, Ports TA, Lim AD, Botvinick EH, Higgins CB. Estimation of the functional and anatomic extent of myocardial infarction using magnetic resonance imaging. Am Heart J 1988;115:740-8

75. Wisenberg G, Finnie KJ, Jablonsky G, Kostuk WJ, Marshall T. Nuclear Magnetic resonance and radionuclide angiographic assessment of acute myocardial infarction in a randomized trial of intravenous streptokinase. Am J Cardiol 1988;62:1011-6

76. Johns JA, Leavitt MB, Newell JB, Yasuda T, Leinbach RC, Gold HK, Finkelstein D, Dinsmore RE. Quantitation of acute myocardial infarct size by nuclear magnetic resonance imaging. J Am Coll Cardiol 1990;15:143-9

77. Matheijssen NAA, De Roos A, Van der Wall EE, Doornbos J, Van Dijkman PRM, Bruschke AVG, Van Voorthuisen AE. Acute myocardial infarction: comparison of T2-weighted and T1-weighted Gadolinium-DTPA enhanced MR Imaging. Magn Reson Imaging 1991;17:460-9

78. Brown JJ, Higgins CB. Myocardial paramagnetic contrast agents for MR imaging. AJR 1988;151:865-72

79. Tweedle MF, Eaton SM, Eckelman WC, Gaughan GT, Hagan JJ, Wedeking PW, Yost FJ. Comparative chemical structure and pharmacokinetics of MRI contrast agents. Invest Radiol 1988;23(suppl 1):S236-9

80. Weinmann H-J, Brasch RC, Press W-R, Wesbey GE. Characteristics of Gadolinium-DTPA complex: a potential NMR contrast agent. AJR 1984; 142:619-24

81. Brasch RC, Weinmann H-J, Wesbey GE. Contrast-enhanced NMR Imaging: animal studies using Gadolinium-DTPA complex. AJR 1984;142:625-30

82. Elster AD, Jackels SC, Allen NS, Marrache RC. Europeum-DTPA: A Gadolinium-DTPA analogue traceable by fluorescence microscopy. AJNR 1989; 10:1137-44

83. Koenig SH, Spiller M, Brown III RD, Wolf GL. Relaxation of water protons in the intra- and extracellular regions of blood containing Gd-DTPA. Magn Reson Med 1986;3:791-5

84. Meyer D, Schaefer M, Bonnemain B. Gd-DOTA, a potential MRI contrast agent current status of physicochemical knowledge. Invest Radiol 1988;23(suppl 1):S232-5

85. Schouman-Claeys E, Frija G, Revel D, Doucet D, Donadieu A-M. Canine acute myocardial infarction: in vivo detection by MRI with gradient echo technique and contribution of Gd-DOTA. Invest Radiol 1988;23(suppl 1):S254-7

86. Ogan MD, Schmiedl U, Moseley ME, Grodd W, Paajanen H, Brasch RC. Albumin labeled with Gd-DTPA: an intravascular contrast-enhancing agent for magnetic resonance blood pool imaging: preparation and characterization. Invest Radiol 1987;22:665-71

87. Schmiedl U, Sievers RE, Brasch RC, Wolfe CL, Chew WM, Ogan MD, Engeseth H, Lipton MJ, Moseley ME. Acute myocardial ischemia and reperfusion: MR imaging with albumin-Gd-DTPA. Radiology 1989;170:351-6

88. Schmiedl U, Ogan M, Paajanen H, Marotti M, Crooks LE, Brito AC, Brasch RC. Albumin labeled with Gd-DTPA as an intravascular, blood pool-enhancing agent for MR Imaging: biodistribution and imaging studies. Radiology 1987;162:205-10

151

89. Schmiedl U, Ogan MD, Moseley ME, Brasch RC. Comparison of the contrast-enhancing properties of albumin-(Gd-DTPA) and Gd-DTPA at 2.0T: an experimental study in rats. AJR 1986;147:1263-70

90. Wesbey GE, Higgins CB, McNamara MT, Engelstad BL, Lipton MJ, Sievers R, Ehman RL, Lovin J, Brasch RC. Effect of Gadolinium-DTPA on the magnetic relaxation times of normal and infarcted myocardium. Radiology 1984;153:165-9

91. McNamara MT, Higgins CB, Ehman RL, Revel D, Sievers R, Brasch RC. Acute myocardial ischemia: Magnetic resonance contrast enhancement with Gadolinium-DTPA. Radiology 1984;153:157-63

92. Runge VM, Clanton JA, Wehr CJ, Partain CL, James Jr AE. Gated magnetic resonance imaging of acute myocardial ischemia in dogs: application of multiecho techniques and contrast enhancement with Gd DTPA. Magn Reson Imaging 1985;3:255-66

93. Johnston DL, Liu P, Lauffer RB, Newell JB, Wedeen VJ, Rosen BR, Brady TJ, Okada RJ. Use of Gadolinium-DTPA as a myocardial perfusion agent: potential applications and limitations for magnetic resonance imaging. J Nucl Med 1987;28:871-7

94. Nishimura T, Yamada Y, Kozuka T, Nakatani T, Noda H, Takano H. Value and limitation of Gadolinium-DTPA contrast enhancement in the early detection of acute canine myocardial infarction. Am J Physiol Imaging 1987;2:181-5

95. Miller DD, Holmvang G, Gill JB, Dragotakes D, Kantor HL, Okada RD, Brady TJ. MRI detection of myocardial perfusion changes by Gadolinium-DTPA infusion during dipyridamole hyperemia. Magn Reson Med 1989;10:246-55

96. Tscholakoff D, Higgins CB, Sechtem U, McNamara MT. Occlusive and reperfused myocardial infarcts: effect of Gd-DTPA on ECG-gated MR imaging. Radiology 1986;160:515-9

97. McNamara MT, Tscholakoff D, Revel D, Soulen R, Schechtmann N, Botvinick E, Higgins CB. Differentiation of reversible and irreversible myocardial injury by MR imaging with and without Gadolinium-DTPA. Radiology 1986;158:765-9

98. Peshock RM, Malloy CR, Buja LM, Nunnally RL, Parkey RW, Willerson JT. Magnetic resonance imaging of acute myocardial infarction: gadolinium diethylenetriamine pentaacetic acid as a marker of reperfusion. Circulation 1986;74:1434-40

99. Wolfe CL, Moseley ME, Wikstrom MG, Sievers RE, Wendland MF, Dupon JW, Finkbeiner WE, Lipton MJ, Parmley WW, Brasch RC. Assessment of myocardial salvage after ischemia and reperfusion using magnetic resonance imaging and spectroscopy. Circulation 1989;80:969-82

100. Schaefer S, Malloy CR, Katz J, Parkey RW, Buja LM, Willerson JT, Peshock RM. Gadolinium-DTPA-enhanced nuclear magnetic resonance imaging of reperfused myocardium: Identification of the myocardial bed at risk. J Am Coll Cardiol 1988;12:1064-72

101. Nishimura T, Yamada Y, Hayashi M, Kozuka T, Nakatani T, Noda H, Takano H. Determination of infarct size of acute myocardial infarction in dogs by magnetic resonance imaging and Gadolinium-DTPA: comparison with indium-111 antimyosin imaging. Am J Physiol Imaging 1989;4:83-8

102. Boudreau RJ, Frick MP, Levey RM, Lund G, Sirr SA, Loken MK. The preliminary evaluation of Mn-DTPA as a potential contrast agent for nuclear magnetic resonance imaging. Am J Physiol Imaging 1986;1:19-25

103. Pomeroy OH, Wendland M, Wagner S, Derugin N, Holt WW, Rocklage SM, Quay S, Higgins CB. Magnetic resonance imaging of acute myocardial ischemia using a manganese chelate, Mn-DPDP. Invest Radiol 1989;24:531-6

104. Pflugfelder PW, Wendland MF, Holt WW, Quay SC, Worah D, Derugin N, Higgins CB. Acute myocardial ischemia: MR Imaging with Mn-TP. Radiology 1988;167:129-33

105. Saeed M, Wagner S, Wendland MF, Derugin N, Finkbeiner WE, Higgins CB. Occlusive and reperfused myocardial infarcts: differentiation with Mn-DPDP-enhanced MR Imaging. Radiology 1989;172:59-64

106. Goldman MR, Brady TJ, Pykett IL, Burt CT, Buonanno FS, Kistler JP, Newhouse JH, Hinshaw WS, Pohost GM. Quantification of experimental myocardial infarction using nuclear magnetic resonance imaging and paramagnetic ion contrast enhancement in excised canine hearts. Circulation 1982;66:1012-16

107. Schaefer S, Lange RA, Kulkarni PV, Katz J, Parkey RW, Willerson JT, Peshock RM. In vivo nuclear magnetic resonance imaging of myocardial perfusion using the paramagnetic contrast agent manganese gluconate. J Am Coll Cardiol 1989;14:472-80

152

108. Eichstaedt HW, Felix R, Dougherty FC, Langer M, Rutsch W, Schmutzler H. Magnetic Resonance Imaging (MRI) in different stages of myocardial infarction using the contrast agent Gadolinium-DTPA. Clin Cardiol 1986;9:527-35

109. Nishimura T, Kobayashi H, Ohara Y, Yamada N, Haze K, Takamiya M, Hiramori K. Serial assessment of myocardial infarction by using gated MR Imaging and Gd-DTPA. AJR 1989;153:715-20

110. De Roos A, Doornbos J, Van der Wall EE, Van Voorthuisen AE. MR imaging of acute myocardial infarction: Value of Gd-DTPA. AJR 1988;150:531-4

111. Van der Wall EE, Doornbos J, Postema S, Van Dijkman PRM, Manger Cats V, De Roos A, Bruschke AVG. Improved detection of myocardial infarction by Gadolinium-enhanced magnetic resonance imaging. Eur Heart J 1988; 9(Suppl A):340(Abstr)

112. Van Dijkman PRM, Doornbos J, De Roos A, Van der Laarse A, Postema S, Matheijssen NAA, Bruschke AVG, Van Voorthuisen EA, Manger Cats V, Van der Wall. Improved detection of acute myocardial infarction by magnetic resonance imaging using Gadolinium-DTPA. Int J Cardiac Imaging 1989;5:1-8

113. Van Dijkman PRM, Van der Wall EE, Doornbos J, Van der Laarse A, Postema S, De Roos A, Van Voorthuisen AE, Bruschke AVG. Improved assessment of acute myocardial infarction by magnetic resonance imaging and Gadolinium-DTPA. J Am Coll Cardiol 1989;13:49A (Abstr)

114. De Roos A, Van Rossum AC, Van der Wall EE, Postema S, Doornbos J, Matheijssen N, Van Dijkman PRM, Visser FC, Van Voorthuisen AE. Reperfused and nonreperfused myocardial infarction: diagnostic potential of Gd-DTPA-enhanced MR imaging. Radiology 1989;172:717-20

115. Van der Wall EE, Van Dijkman PRM, De Roos A, Doornbos J, Van der Laarse A, Manger Cats V, Van Voorthuisen AE, Matheijssen NAA, Bruschke AVG. Diagnostic significance of gadolinium-DTPA (diethylenetriamine penta-acetic acid) enhanced magnetic resonance imaging in thrombolytic therapy for acute myocardial infarction: its potential in assessing reperfusion. Br Heart J 1990;63:12-7

116. De Roos A, Matheijssen NAA, Doornbos J, Van Dijkman PRM, Van Voorthuisen AE, Van der Wall EE. Assessment of myocardial infarct size after reperfusion therapy using Gadolinium-DTPA-enhanced magnetic resonance imaging. Radiology 1990;176:517-21

117. Peshock RM, Rokey R, Malloy CM, McNamee P, Buja LM, Parkey RW, Willerson JT. Assessment of myocardial systolic wall thickening using nuclear magnetic resonance imaging. J Am Coll Cardiol 1989;14:653-9

118. Lotan CS, Cranney GB, Bouchard A, Bittner V, Pohost GM. The value of cine nuclear magnetic resonance imaging for assessing regional ventricular function. J Am Coll Cardiol 1989;14:1721-9

119. Pennell DJ, Underwood SR, Burman ED, Ell PJ, Swanton RH, Walker M, Longmore DB. Reversible ventricular wall motion abnormalities in coronary artery disease assessed by dipyridamole magnetic resonance imaging. Soc Magn Reson Med 1989;2:54(Abstr)

120. Higgins CB, Lanzer P, Stark D, Botvinick E, Schiller NB, Crooks L, Kaufman L, Lipton MJ. Imaging by nuclear magnetic resonance in patients with chronic ischemic heart disease. Circulation 1984;69:523-31

121. McNamara MT, Higgins CB. Magnetic resonance imaging of chronic myocardial infarcts in man. AJR 1986;146:315-20

122. Krauss XH, Van der Wall EE, Van der Laarse A, De Roos A, Doornbos J, Matheijssen NAA, Rietsema C, Van Voorthuisen AE, Bruschke AVG. Long-term follow-up of regional myocardial T2 relaxation times in patients with myocardial infarction evaluated with magnetic resonance imaging. Eur J Radiol 1990;11:110-9

123. Checkley D, Loveday BE, Waterton JC, Zhu XP, Isherwood I. Detection of myocardial infarction in the mini-pig using NMR imaging. Magn Reson Med 1987;5:201-16

124. Ahmad M, Johnson RF, Fawcett HD, Schreiber MH. Left ventricular aneurysm in short axis: a comparison of magnetic resonance, ultrasound and thallium-201 Spect images. Magn Reson Imaging 1987;5:293-300

125. Lalisang RR, Baur LHB, Van der Wall EE, De Roos A, Bruschke AVG. Left ventricular aneurysmectomy after myocardial infarction following detection of left ventricular thrombosis by magnetic resonance imaging. Magn Reson Imaging 1990;8:661-3

126. Rubinstein RI, Askenase AD, Thickman D, Feldman MS, Agarwal JB, Helfant RH. Magnetic resonance imaging to evaluate patency of aortocoronary bypass grafts. Circulation 1987;76:786-91

127. Gomes AS, Lois JF, Drinkwater DC, Corday SR. Coronary artery bypass grafts: visualization with MR imaging. Radiology 1987;162:175-9

128. Jenkins JPR, Love HG, Foster CJ, Isherwood I, Rowlands DJ. Detection of coronary artery bypass graft patency as assessed by magnetic resonance imaging. Br J Radiol 1988;61:2-4

129. Frija G, Schouman-Claeys E, Lacombe P, Bismuth V, Ollivier J-P. A study of coronary artery bypass graft patency using MR Imaging. J Comp Ass Tomography 1989;13:226-32

130. White RD, Caputo GR, Mark AS, Modin GW, Higgins CB. Coronary artery bypass graft patency: noninvasive evaluation with MR Imaging. Radiology 1987;164:681-6

131. White RD, Pflugfelder PW, Lipton MJ, Higgins CB. Coronary artery bypass grafts: evaluation of patency with cine MR imaging. AJR 1988: 150:1271-4

132. Aurigemma GP, Reichek N, Axel L, Schiebler M, Harris C, Kressel HY. Noninvasive determination of coronary artery bypass graft patency by cine magnetic resonance imaging. Circulation 1989;80:1595-602

133. Underwood SR, Firmin DN, Klipstein RH, Rees RSO, Longmore DB. Magnetic resonance velocity mapping: clinical application of a new technique. Br Heart J 1987;57:404-12

134. Paulin S, Von Schulthess GK, Fossel E, Krayenbuehl HP. MR imaging of the aortic root and proximal coronary arteries. AJR 1987;148:665-70

8.
Acute myocardial infarction:
Evaluation by nuclear imaging techniques

Summary

In recent years, nuclear cardiology techniques have been successfully applied in patients with acute myocardial infarction. These scintigraphic measurements have provided important diagnostic, therapeutic and prognostic information based on the extent of myocardial damage and the functional reserve of the left ventricle. In particular in the thrombolytic era, myocardial perfusion imaging and radionuclide angiography showed to be valuable methods to study the effects of reperfusion on the extent of myocardial damage. Nuclear magnetic resonance imaging, preferably with contrast enhancement, is one of the newly developed nuclear imaging techniques that have probably the greatest potential in accurately delineating myocardial infarct size and in the evaluation of left ventricular function. Radionuclide procedures, on the other hand, employ more biologically oriented tracers and are therefore capable to monitor biochemical changes in the course of acute myocardial infarction.

Introduction

Management of patients with infarction has become directed at strategies to salvage ischemic myocardium. Particularly in the thrombolytic era one wants to know the early and late benefits of reperfusion therapy. Myocardial infarction can be divided functionally into two phases: the acute phase of infarction when myocardial damage is evolving, and the recovery or convalescent phase, after the completed infarct. Acutely, one wishes know how much myocardium remains at risk, how much is permanently damaged, how much potentially reversibly damaged myocardium is present, the level of ventricular function, and the efficacy of any intervention employed in the early hours of the infarct. In the recovery phase, one wishes to define and determine myocardial functional reserve, the presence of ischemia, and the future risk and prognosis. In both phases, nuclear techniques can play an important role in providing the necessary data leading to an appropriate management strategy. The use of nuclear techniques in the recovery phase for functional characterization and risk stratification has become routine; the value of newer nuclear techniques for acutely distinguishing reversibly from irreversibly damaged myocardium and assessing the efficacy of intervention is currently under active investigation. More than one nuclear imaging procedure is presently available and a relative newcomer for studying myocardial infarction is magnetic resonance imaging which offers promise in view of its high spatial resolution and nonionizing character. These features make magnetic resonance imaging potentially very suitable to evaluate patients with myocardial infarction.

Myocardial perfusion scintigraphy

Thallium-201

Thallium-201 scintigraphy has been employed to detect and to localize acute myocardial infarction (1). Wackers et al. (2) were the first to show that thallium-201 defects could be detected in nearly all patients who were evaluated within six hours of the onset of symptoms. However, when more than 24 hours have elapsed following the onset of symptoms, the sensitivity of thallium-201 decreases, presumably as a result of spontaneous reperfusion and development of collateral flow to the infarcted area. The potential for estimating prognosis by thallium-201 scintigraphy in acute infarct patients has been reported by Silverman et al. (3). They attempted to quantify infarct size (Fig. 1), and observed that patients with a thallium-201 defect involving more than 40% of the left ventricular circumference identified a patient group with 62% mortality at 6 months, compared with a 6-month mortality of only 7% in patients with lower thallium-201 defect scores.

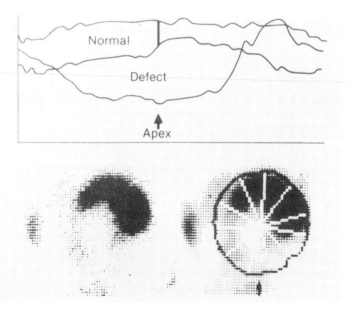

Figure 1
Scintigraphic (thallium-201) estimation of infarct size in a patient with a large anteroseptal infarction based on circumferential profile analysis. (Reproduced with permission from Silverman et al., 1980, Ref. 3)

Thallium-201 imaging in thrombolysis

In the era of thrombolytic therapy, thallium-201 scintigraphy has been used as a method of assessing efficacy of reperfusion. Schofer et al. (4) did find that patients who demonstrated improvement in regional wall motion in the infarct zone following successful thrombolysis had new thallium-201 uptake, and in patients with failed reperfusion, there was no change in either regional ejection fraction or thallium-201 uptake. However, immediate injection of the tracer after reperfusion overestimates the amount of viable tissue whereas, when thallium is injected more than 48 hours after reperfusion, this phenomenon is not observed (5). As a result, thallium-201 has no prominent role in the immediate assessment of reperfusion-related salvage but may be of use for follow-up studies. In this respect, Van der Wall et al. (6) demonstrated by thallium-201 exercise scintigraphy at 3 months after the acute event, that patients with reperfusion therapy showed a decrease in infarct size on thallium-201 images compared with those without reperfusion therapy, in particular in patients with an anterior infarction (Fig. 2).

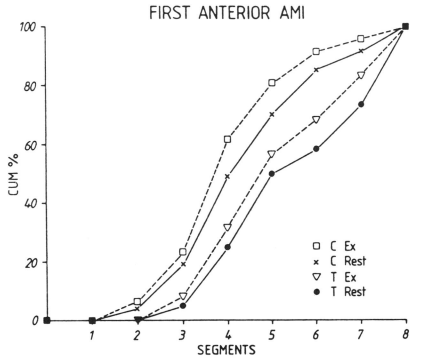

Figure 2
Cumulative percentage of normal thallium-201 segments in patients with a first anterior infarction. The number of normal segments is significantly higher in the patients with thrombolysis(T) compared to the control patients (C), both at rest and during exercise.

Predischarge thallium-201 imaging

Predischarge thallium imaging combined with exercise or with pharmacologic-induced vasodilatation, has proven to be useful to predict future cardiac events in patients recovering from acute myocardial infarction. The classic work on predischarge assessment was performed in 1983 by Gibson et al. (7), who assessed patients' prognosis before discharge by means of submaximal exercise testing, coronary angiography and thallium-201 scintigraphy. They then followed patients for 3 years to determine the subsequent event rate. A low- and high-risk pattern was defined for each of the 3 studies. Although the event rate in patients with a high-risk pattern was similar for exercise testing, coronary angiography and thallium-201 scintigraphy, the event rate in the low-risk group defined by thallium-201 (no redistribution, no defects in zones remote from the infarct zone and no lung uptake) was significantly lower (6%) than that observed in the low-risk group defined by exercise electrocardiography (27%), and coronary arteriography (22%). Thus, in patients with uncomplicated acute myocardial infarction who are nearing discharge, low-level stress Tl-201 scintigraphy appears to be clinically useful in guiding management. A variation of this approach for patients who cannot exercise involves a 4-minute intravenous infusion of dipyridamole followed by injection of thallium-201. Imaging then proceeds as it would after stress. The procedure can be used before discharge in patients with myocardial infarction and in patients with suspected coronary artery disease. Leppo et al. (8) were the first to report results of this technique in predicting new myocardial infarction or death in patients with acute myocardial infarction studied before discharge. The event rate within 1 year was only 6% in patients whose scans showed no thallium-201 redistribution compared with 33% in patients whose scans did show redistribution. The dipyridamole-thallium imaging technique thus identified a high-risk subset of patients and proved to be significantly more predictive of future events than submaximal exercise testing by electrocardiography alone. An extended variant of the dipyridamole approach is the combination with low-level exercise, as advocated by Laarman et al. (9). The conjunction with low-level exercise significantly improves the image quality.

Reinjection thallium-201 imaging

A major topic of interest at the current time is the value of 24-hour delayed imaging (10) and, in particular, reinjection of thallium-201 at rest following redistribution (11). Conventional exercise/redistribution thallium-201 imaging may overestimate the extent of infarction because it has been shown that seemingly persistent defects may fill in on 24-hour delayed images or after reinjection, indicating residual myocardial viability in presumed necrotic areas (10,11). This phenomenon is of major interest in patients after myocardial infarction, as in this group of patients one wishes to know whether the infarcted tissue is completely necrotic or still contains viable, potentially jeopardized, myocardial cells. This may have important implications for further patient management in terms of a more conservative approach in case of a definite necrotic area versus a more aggressive approach in case of remaining viable myocardial tissue.

Early predischarge thallium-201 scintigraphy

A recently proposed different and more challenging approach is to perform thallium-201 exercise testing already in the subacute phase after myocardial infarction i.e. within 3 days after the acute event. The rationale for this approach is early risk stratification of infarct patients and the potential early discharge of a subgroup of patients with negative findings, reducing health care costs. Topol et al. (12) studied 61 patients after reperfusion therapy for acute myocardial infarction who underwent a submaximal exercise test at 72 hours after the acute event. The exercise test was performed in conjunction with thallium-201 single photon emission computed tomography (SPECT). Of the 61 patients, 40 had no evidence of reversible ischemia by thallium-201 scintigraphy, and 17 patients showed reversible ischemic defects; 4 patients had equivocal results. At follow-up, 5 of 17 patients had an adverse clinical event versus none of 40 patients ($p<0.001$). This trial documented the safety and feasibility of thallium-201 exercise testing 3 days after infarction, and presaged the safety of early hospital discharge following a negative thallium-201 SPECT test. Pirelli et al. (13) suggested that utilization of dipyridamole thallium stress in the very early post-infarct setting might be preferable to conventional exercise thallium-201 scintigraphy. With dipyridamole thallium-201 imaging, the hazard of early exercise in producing complications, such as sudden circulatory collapse or infarct extension, can be avoided.

Technetium-99m SestaMIBI

To circumvent the radiophysical limitations of thallium-201 (low gamma-emission of 80 keV, long half-life of 72 hours), technetium-99m labeled isonitrile complexes have been developed. Technetium-99m methoxy-isobutyl-isonitrile (technetium-99m SestaMIBI) exhibits the best biological properties for clinical implications. Due to the short half-life (6 hours), dosages up to 10 times as much as thallium-201 can be administered, resulting in better counting statistics. Similar to thallium-201, technetium-99m SestaMIBI accumulates in the myocardium predominantly according to myocardial blood flow. In contrast to thallium-201, it has a slow washout with minimal myocardial redistribution. These features make technetium-99m SestaMIBI more suitable for SPECT imaging and allow more flexibility in the time for starting the imaging procedure following tracer injection, according to findings by Verzijlbergen et al. (14). The tracer is particularly useful for the immediate assessment of myocardial salvage in the reperfused regions without any delay in administration of thrombolytic therapy (15). Performing subsequent comparative studies after repeat injections, e.g. 1 to 4 days later, the zone of hypoperfusion representing the final infarct can be identified and compared to the perfusion defect of the initial risk zone (16) (Fig. 3). Verani et al. (17) showed that a 30% reduction of defect size was highly predictive of patency.

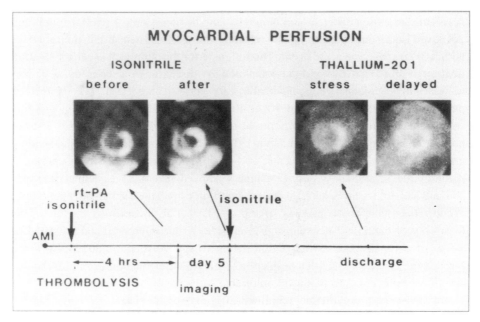

MYOCARDIAL PERFUSION

Figure 3

Images with technetium-99m SestaMibi (Tc-MIBI) injected before and after thrombolytic therapy. The images from Tc-MIBI injected before administration of tissue plasminogen activator (rt-PA) show a large septal defect. Images obtained after a second injection of Tc-MIBI (post-thrombolysis) show partial filling in of the defect. The predischarge low-level stress redistribution Tl-201 study showed evidence of some viable myocardium in the previously jeopardized zone. AMI= acute myocardial infarction. (Reproduced with permission from Kayden et al., 1988, Ref. 16).

In the future, technetium-99m SestaMIBI may be more effective than thallium-201 for predischarge assessment because it will enable simultaneous assessments of exercise ejection fraction and exercise myocardial perfusion. The predischarge routine of the future may well incorporate a first-pass analysis of ventricular function at rest, a delayed gated tomographic assessment of the size of the perfusion defect, and the performance of the first-pass and gated tomographic procedures with exercise.

Rubidium-82

Williams et al. (18) examined the use of the positron emitter rubidium-82 with planar positron imaging in the coronary care unit and clinical laboratory for detection of perfusion defects due to myocardial infarction. They studied 22 patients with myocardial infarction and the rubidium images showed similar sensitivity and specificity as for the thallium-201 and regional wall motion images.

Myocardial infarct-avid scintigraphy

Imaging of acute myocardial infarction with infarct-avid imaging agents allows definition of the zone of acute myocardial necrosis as an area of increased radioactivity ("hot spot"). A number of agents has been used, such as technetium-99m pyrophosphate and more recently indium-111 labeled antimyosin.

Technetium-99m pyrophosphate

Technetium-99m pyrophosphate was first introduced as a means of diagnosing acute myocardial infarction in 1974, and proved to be highly sensitive for the clinical diagnosis of acute infarct (19). Technetium-99m pyrophosphate forms a complex with calcium deposited in damaged myocardial cells. As myocardial uptake is flow dependent, the uptake is poor in the centre of low flow areas of a large infarct, where the uptake is predominantly epicardial. In experimental studies it was shown that technetium-99m pyrophosphate infarcts larger than 3 grams can be visualized by in vivo imaging (20). Especially right ventricular infarction can be easily diagnosed as reported by Braat et al. (21). The timing of the technetium-99m pyrophosphate study is of critical importance, and best results have been obtained 24-72 hours post-infarction by which ideally any intervention to salvage myocardium should have taken place (22). However, Hashimoto et al. (23), who performed early technetium-99m pyrophosphate imaging with SPECT, showed that positive images were very adequate in sizing myocardial infarction soon after coronary reperfusion as early as eight hours after the onset of infarction. Although the sensitivity of pyrophosphate imaging is high, the specificity is rather low since a number of different disease processes show radioisotope accumulation by the myocardium. Positive images have been observed in patients with myocardial trauma, ventricular aneurysm, and after radiation therapy (24). Additionally, the uptake of technetium-99m pyrophosphate in skeletal structures may restrict the proper assessment of myocardial infarction.

Indium-111 antimyosin

The development of easily applicable infarct-avid agents, that provide scintigrams which become abnormal within shorter periods with closer correlation between tissue uptake and severity of necrosis, is extremely important. Radiolabeled antimyosin (indium-111 antimyosin) is a monoclonal antibody that binds to cardiac myosin exposed upon cell death. Maximal uptake occurs in regions of lowest flow, and mostly in necrotic areas (Fig 4). Infarct size in grams can be calculated from transaxially reconstructed, normalized, and background corrected indium-111 antimyosin SPECT images (25). By performing dual-isotope SPECT imaging with indium-111 monoclonal antibodies and thallium-201, infarct size and percentage of infarcted myocardium can be estimated accurately (26). Furthermore, the antimyosin images can be then superimposed on the perfusion images to distinguish between viable and

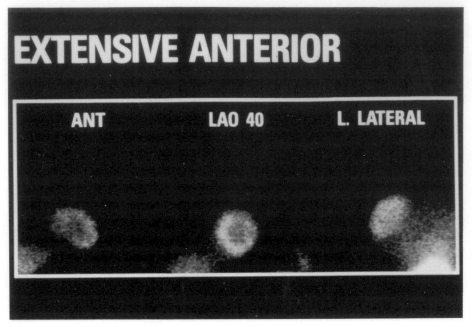

Figure 4
Indium-lll antimyosin scintigram of a patient with an extensive anterior infarction. Uptake of the tracer is clearly visible in the anteriorly localized myocardial areas. (Image courtesy of W. van Prooyen, Centocor, Leiden).

necrotic tissue.

Not only for detection of myocardial necrosis, but also for assessment of prognosis indium-111 antimyosin has proven to be valuable. Follow-up for evaluation of major cardiac events was conducted in a large multicenter study to relate the extent of antimyosin uptake to the major event rate (27). The incidence of cardiac events ranged from 5-8% in patients with negative or minimally positive scans, up to an event rate of about 40% in patients with extensive myocardial uptake of antimyosin. In a subsequent study, Johnson et al. (28) showed in 42 infarct patients that a mismatch pattern between thallium-201 defects and antimyosin uptake (i.e. regions with neither thallium-201 nor antimyosin uptake) identified patients at further ischemic risk. Van Vlies et al. (29), in patients following reperfusion therapy, showed that the level and extent of indium-111 antimyosin uptake could predict improvement of left ventricular wall motion. Drawbacks of indium-111 antimyosin are the blood pool contamination and interference from liver activity with indium-111, its suboptimal imaging characteristics (gamma-emission 170 and 247 keV, half-life 68 hours), and the late moment of reliable infarct definition at approximately 48 hours after infarction.

Biologically based scintigraphy

Carbon-11 palmitate, Fluorine-18 deoxyglucose

Radioactive tracers derived specifically for imaging on the basis of their known biologically activity have been studied extensively. Positron emitters as carbon-11 palmitate and fluorine-18 deoxyglucose, and the single photon agents such as radioiodinated free fatty acids and their analogs, are suitable for assessing infarct size and viable myocardial tissue (30,31). Positron emission tomography is valuable in delineating areas with reversible and irreversible injury, in assessing the feasibility of surgical revascularization, coronary angioplasty, or thrombolysis with respect to potentially salvageable tissue (32), (Fig. 5). The potential benefits of interventions could be evaluated more precisely in patients after myocardial infarction with advanced coronary disease and severely impaired ventricular function.

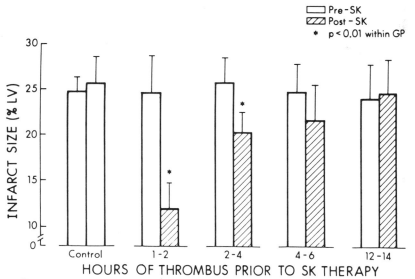

Figure 5

Histogram of tomographically estimated infarct size for control animals with sustained coronary occlusion (n=6), and animals with 1-2 (n=4), 2-4(n=6), 4-6 (n=4) and 12-14 hours of coronary occlusion prior to streptokinase(SK)(n=3). Repeat tomography was performed 90 minutes after SK. Significant decreases of apparent infarct size (or increases in metabolic activity in jeopardized myocardium) occurred only in animals subjected to reperfusion within four hours of occlusion. The results illustrate the utility of positron emission tomography for sequential characterization of myocardium before and after reperfusion. (Reproduced with permission from Bergmann et al., 1982, Ref. 32).

Clinical studies in infarct patients showed that areas with persistent thallium-201 perfusion defects have evidence of remaining metabolic activity in 47% of regions when studied with positron emission tomography, indicating overestimation of irreversible injury (33). The implication, derived from this finding, is that in areas with perfusion defects, if glucose activity remains, the region is viable (mismatch pattern);

conversely, if such activity is absent, the area is likely to be infarcted or necrotic (match pattern). In case of remaining viability, patients are more likely to benefit from therapeutical interventions than patients with definite necrotic myocardial areas. Although the assessment of a (mis)match pattern is unique to positron imaging, remaining myocardial viability can also be assessed by reinjection of thallium-201 immediately following the performance of the redistribution images, as stated before. Dilsizian et al. (11) demonstrated improved or normal thallium-201 uptake after reinjection in 49% of apparently fixed defects, observed at redistribution.

Iodine-123 fatty acids

Metabolic imaging has also been performed with single-photon radiopharmaceuticals using radioiodinated free fatty acids. These can be imaged by both planar and tomographic techniques. Van der Wall et al. (34) demonstrated regionally decreased uptake of I-123 labeled heptadecanoic in patients with acute myocardial infarction. In addition, altered fatty acid metabolism was demonstrated in the infarcted regions. Visser et al. (35), in acute infarct patients, showed restored fatty acid metabolism in myocardial areas that were sucessfully reperfused.

The role of metabolic imaging in guiding and evaluating therapeutic interventions for acute ischemic states will hopefully expand.

Radionuclide angiography

In the setting of acute myocardial infarction, radionuclide angiography can be used for diagnosis and quantification of infarct size, evaluation of complications such as ventricular septum defect, (false) aneurysm and mitral regurgitation, assessment of the effects of interventions such as thrombolysis, and assessment of prognosis. Among clinical and angiographic variables, global left ventricular ejection fraction at rest, a direct measure of left ventricular function, is the most important predictor of mortalility after acute myocardial infarction (36-38). Analysis of regional left ventricular function may be a more direct means of assessing the efficacy of thrombolytic therapy than global ejection fraction, since global left ventricular ejection fraction obtained early in the course of acute myocardial infarction reflects the function of both viable and nonviable myocardium and thus may not necessarily predict whether reperfusion will improve function. Global ejection fraction determined at predischarge remains however the most important measurable prognostic endpoint following infarction (38). A progressive increase in 1-year mortality rate occurs when left ventricular ejection fraction decreases below 40% (Fig. 6). Combined rest and exercise radionuclide angiography at the time of hospital discharge, is an attractive procedure for risk assessment after acute infarction because its provides noninvasive measurements of both the severity of left ventricular dysfunction and the presence of potentially ischemic myocardium. Corbett et al. (39) studied 75 infarct patients with a mean resting ejection fraction of 55% at predischarge. Failure to

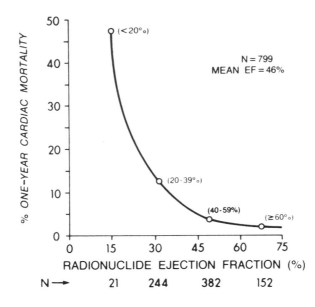

Figure 6
Relation of predischarge left ventricular ejection fraction to 1-year cardiac mortality in 799 patients with acute myocardial infarction. (Reproduced with permission from The Multicenter Post-infarction Research Group, 1983, Ref. 38).

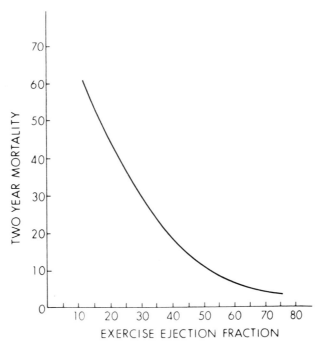

Figure 7
Life-table survival of patient population by exercise ejection fraction (EF). (Reproduced with permission from Morris et al., 1985, Ref. 40).

increase ejection fraction by 5% or more was associated with a significantly increased rate of reinfarction. Similarly, Morris et al. (40) found a significant association between the time to death and ejection fraction at rest and during exercise in 106 consecutive survivors of acute myocardial infarction (Fig. 7). In a large study conducted by the Interuniversity Cardiology Institute of the Netherlands (ICIN), it was shown that patients with anterior infarction following reperfusion therapy - studied at 2 days, 2 weeks, and 3 months after the acute onset - had significantly improved left ventricular function compared to conventionally treated patients (41,42) (Fig. 8).

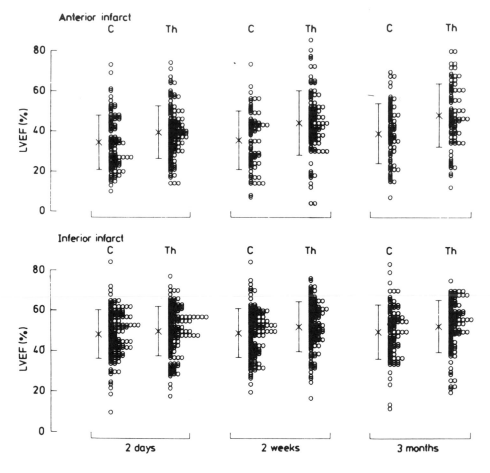

Figure 8
Distribution of left ventricular ejection fraction (LVEF) 2 days, 2 weeks and 3 months after admission in patients with anterior or anteroseptal infarction (top) and in patients with inferior wall infarction (bottom). Means and standard deviations are indicated C, conventional treatment; Th, patients allocated to thrombolytic treatment. In particular patients with anterior infarction showed significantly improved LVEF after reperfusion therapy. (Reproduced with permission from Res et al., 1986, Ref. 42).

Nuclear Magnetic Resonance Imaging

Magnetic resonance imaging has potential for quantifying and identifying areas of myocardial necrosis (43). Magnetic resonance imaging is a nonionizing high resolution tomographic technique providing good soft tissue contract, sharp delineation of the myocardium, and adequate characterization of myocardial tissue. The area of acute myocardial infarction can be visualized as a high signal intensity area associated with prolonged T2 relaxation times. By using contrast enhancement with gadolinium-DTPA the infarct can be located more precisely (44) (Fig. 9). In our institution infarct size could be determined by nuclear magnetic resonance imaging using gadolinium-DTPA in patients receiving streptokinase for acute myocardial infarction (45). Infarct size proved to be significantly smaller in patients with successful reperfusion in comparison with patients without reperfusion (46) (Fig. 10). Van Rossum et al. (47), in patients after thrombolysis, demonstrated that the dynamics of gadolinium-DTPA are useful for the noninvasive assessment of successful reperfusion.

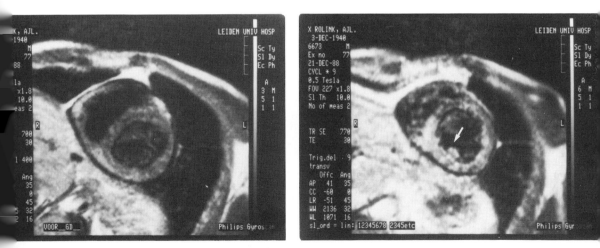

Figure 9A   **Figure 9B**

Magnetic resonance images before (9A) and after (9B) administration of the contrast agent Gadolinium-DTPA from a patient with an acute inferoposterior infarction. After administration of Gadolium-DTPA significant contrast enhancement is observed in the inferoposterior myocardial area (arrow). Summing up of the extent of contrast enhancement in the different tomographic slices covering the complete left ventricle, an estimate of infarct size can be obtained.

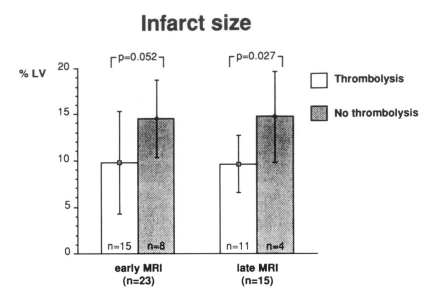

Figure 10
Following thrombolytic therapy a significant reduction of magnetic resonance imaging (MRI) determined infarct size is observed, in particular in patients with late MRI (5 weeks after the acute onset).

Similar to positron emission tomography, drawbacks of magnetic resonance imaging are expenses and the limited availability of magnetic resonance facilities. Although promising, the clinical value in assessing infarct size and the extent of myocardial salvage after thrombolytic therapy remains to be settled.

Conclusion

In the assessment and management of the patient with acute myocardial infarction, nuclear studies have a role in both the acute and convalescent phase. In the acute phase, areas of decreased flow can be assessed by resting perfusion imaging, and assessment of reperfusion and potential salvage of myocardium can be made qualitatively with delayed imaging. Thallium-201 and technetium-99m SestaMibi SPECT may provide additional quantification of infarct size, and possible quantitation of salvaged myocardium if serial studies are performed. Further studies are necessary to determine their role. Positron emission tomography is currently the only noninvasive technique that can identify and separate infarcted and ischemic myocardium on a metabolic basis. Whether the application of this expensive new technology to assessment of myocardial viability in patients with acute myocardial infarction will become practical for widespread use remains to be determined. In particular, reinjection of thallium-201 may circumvent the need for positron imaging in determining viability. In the convalescent phase, global and regional left ventricular function provide important prognostic information, and the results of exercise testing combined with either thallium perfusion imaging or ventricular function studies to assess myocardial reserve an be used for risk stratification and to determine the most appropriate management strategies. Magnetic resonance imaging has shown to be useful in assessing infarct size and in following the sequelae after acute interventions. Although offering a great potential, the clinical utility of magnetic resonance imaging in patients with acute myocardial infarction remains to be settled.

References

1. Niemeyer MG, Pauwels EKJ, Van der Wall EE, et al. Detection of multivessel disease in patients with sustained myocardial infarction by thallium 201 myocardial scintigraphy: No additional value of quantitative analysis. Am J Physiol Imaging 1989;4:105-14.
2. Wackers FJT, Busemann Sokole E, Samson G, et al. Value and limitations of thallium-201 scintigraphy in the acute phase of myocardial infarction. N Engl J Med 1976;295:1-5.
3. Silverman KJ, Becker LC, Bulkley BH, et al. Value of early thallium-201 scintigraphy for predicting mortality in patients with acute myocardial infarction. Circulation 1980;61:996-1003.
4. Schofer J, Mathey DG, Monty R, Bleifeld W, Strizke P. Use of dual intracoronary scintigraphy with thallium-201 and technetium-99m pyrophosphate to predict improvement in left ventricular wall motion immediately after intracoronary thrombolysis in acute myocardial infarction. J Am Coll Cardiol 1983;2:737-44.
5. De Coster PM, Melin JA, Detry J-M, Brasseur LA, Beckers C, Col J. Coronary artery reperfusion in acute myocardial infarction: assessment by pre- and post-intervention thallium-201 myocardial perfusion imaging. Am J Cardiol 1985;55:889-93.
6. Van der Wall EE, Res JCJ, Van den Pol R, et al. Improvement of myocardial perfusion after thrombolysis assessed by thallium-201 exercise scintigraphy. Eur Heart J 1988;9:828-35.
7. Gibson RS, Watson DD, Craddock GB, et al. Prediction of cardiac events after uncomplicated myocardial infarction; a prospective study comparing predischarge exercise thallium-201 scintigraphy and coronary angiography. Circulation 1983;68:321-36.
8. Leppo JA, O'Brien J, Rothendler JA, Getchell JD, Lee VW. Dipyridamole-thallium-201 scintigraphy in the prediction of future cardiac events after myocardial infarction. N Engl J Med 1984;310:1014-8.
9. Laarman GJ, Bruschke AVG, Verzijlbergen FJ, Bal ET, Van der Wall EE, Ascoop CA. Efficacy of intravenous dipyridamole with exercise in thallium-201 myocardial perfusion scintigraphy. Eur Heart J 1988;9:1206-14.
10. Kiat H, Berman DS, Maddahi J, et al. Late reversibility of tomographic myocardial thallium-201 defects: an accurate marker of myocardial viability. J Am Coll Cardiol 1988;12:1456-63.
11. Dilsizian V, Rocco T, Freedman NMT, Leon MB, Bonow RO. Enhanced detection of ischemic but viable myocardium by the reinjection of thallium after stress-redistribution imaging. N Engl J Med 1990;323:141-6.
12. Topol EJ, Juni JE, O'Neil WW, et al. Exercise testing three days after onset of acute myocardial infarction. Am J Cardiol 1987;60:958-62.
13. Pirelli S, Inglese E, Suppa M, Corrada E, Campolo L. Dipyridamole-thallium scintigraphy in the early post-infarction period. Eur Heart J 1988;9:1324-31.
14. Verzijlbergen JF, Cramer MJ, Niemeyer MG, Ascoop CAPL, Van der Wall EE, Pauwels EKJ. ECG-gated and static Technetium-99m-SESTAMIBI planar myocardial perfusion imaging; a comparison with Thallium-201 and study of observer variabilities. Am J Physiol Imaging 1990;5:60-7.
15. Santoro GM, Bisi G, Sciagra R, et al. Single photon emission computed tomography with technetium-99m hexakis 2-methoxyisobutyl isonitrile in acute myocardial infarction before and after thrombolytic treatment: assessment of salvaged myocardium and prediction of late functional recovery. J Am Coll Cardiol 1990;15:301-14.
16. Kayden DS, Mattera JA, Zaret BL, Wackers FJTh. Demonstration of reperfusion after thrombolysis with technetium-99m isonitrile myocardial imaging. J Nucl Med 1988;29:1865-7.
17. Verani MS, Jeroudi MO, Mahmarian JJ, et al. Quantification of myocardial infarction during coronary occlusion and myocardial salvage after reperfusion using cardiac imaging with technetium-99m 2-methoxyisobutyl isonitrile. J Am Coll Cardiol 1988;12:1573-81.
18. Williams KA, Ryan JW, Resnekov L, et al. Planar positron imaging of rubidium-82 for myocardial infarction: a comparison with thallium-201 and regional wall motion. Am Heart J 1989;118: 601-10.
19. Willerson JT, Parkey RW, Stokely EM, et al. Infarct sizing with technetium-99m stannous pyrophosphate scintigraphy in dogs and man; relationship between scintigraphic and precordial mapping estimates of infarct size in patients. Cardiovasc Res 1977;11:291-6.
20. Stokely EM, Buja M, Lewis SE, et al. Measurement of acute myocardial infarcts in dogs with 99m-Tc-stannous pyrophosphate scintigrams. J Nucl Med 1976;17:1-5.

21. Braat SH, Brugada P, De Zwaan C, Coenegracht JM, Wellens HJJ. Value of electrocardiogram in diagnosing right ventricular involvement in patients with an acute inferior wall myocardial infarction. Br Heart J 1983;49:368-72.

22. Olson HG, Lyons KP, Butman S, et al. Validation of technetium-99m stannous pyrophosphate myocardial scintigraphy for diagnosing acute myocardial infarction more than 48 hours old when serum creatine kinase-MB has returned to normal. Am J Cardiol 1983;52:245-51.

23. Hashimoto T, Kambara H, Fudo T, et al. Early estimation of acute myocardial infarct size soon after coronary reperfusion using emission computed tomography with technetium-99m pyrophosphate. Am J Cardiol 1987;60:952-7.

24. Wynne J, Holman BL. Acute myocardial infarct scintigraphy with infarct-avid radiotracers. Med Clin North Am 1980;64:119-25.

25. Antunes ML, Seldin DW, Wall RM, Johnson LL. Measurement of acute Q-wave myocardial infarct size with single photon emission computed tomography imaging of indium-111 antimyosin. Am J Cardiol 1989;63:777-83.

26. Johnson LL, Lerrick KS, Coromilas J, et al. Measurement of infarct size and percentage myocardium infarcted in a dog preparation with single photon computed tomography, thallium-201 and indium 111-monoclonal antimyosin Fab. Circulation 1987;76:181-90.

27. Johnson LL, Seldin DW, Becker LC, et al. Antimyosin imaging in acute transmural myocardial infarctions: results of a multicenter clinical trial. J Am Coll Cardiol 1989;13:27-35.

28. Johnson LL, Seldin DW, Keller AM, et al. Dual isotope thallium and indium antimyosin SPECT imaging to identify acute infarct patients at further ischemic risk. Circulation 1990;81:37-45.

29. Van Vlies B, Baas J, Visser CA, et al. Predictive value of indium-111 antimyosin uptake for improvement of left ventricular wall motion after thrombolysis in acute myocardial infarction. Am J Cardiol 1989;64:167-71.

30. Ter-Pogossian MM, Klein MM, Markham J, Roberts R, Sobel BE. Regional assessment of myocardial metabolic integrity in vivo by positron-emission tomography with C-11-labelled palmitate. Circulation 1980;61:242-55.

31. Sochor H, Schwaiger M, Schelbert HR, et al. Relationship between Tl-201, Tc-99m (Sn) pyrophosphate and F-18 2-deoxyglucose uptake in ischemically injured dog myocardium. Am Heart J 1987;114:1066-77.

32. Bergmann SR, Lerch RA, Fox KAA, et al. Temporal dependence of beneficial effects of coronary thrombolysis characterized by positron tomography. Am J Med 1982;73:573-81.

33. Brunken R, Schwaiger M, Grover-McKay M, Phelps ME, Tillisch J, Schelbert HR. Positron emission tomography detects tissue metabolic activity in myocardial segments with persistent thallium perfusion defects. J Am Coll Cardiol 1987;10:557-67.

34. Van der Wall EE, Den Hollander W, Heidendal GAK, Westera G, Majid PA, Roos JP. Dynamic scintigraphy with I-123 labelled free fatty acids in patients with myocardial infarction. Eur J Nucl Med 1981;6:383-9.

35. Visser FC, Westera G, Van Eenige MJ, Van der Wall EE, Heidendal GAK, Roos JP. Free fatty acid scintigraphy in patients with successful thrombolysis after myocardial infarction. Clin Nucl Med 1985;10;35-9.

36. Taylor GJ, Humphries JO, Mellits ED, et al. Predictors of clinical course, coronary anatomy and left ventricular function after recovery from acute myocardial infarction. Circulation 1980;62:960-70.

37. Sanz G, Castanar A, Betriu A, et al. Determinants of prognosis in survivors of myocardial infarction: a prospective clinical angiographic study. N Engl J Med 1982;306:1065-70.

38. Multicenter Postinfarction Research Group. Risk stratification and survival after myocardial infarction. N Engl J Med 1983;309:331-6.

39. Corbett JR, Dehmer GJ, Lewis SE, et al. The prognostic value of submaximal exercise testing with radionuclide ventriculography before hospital discharge in patients with recent myocardial infarction. Circulation 1981;64:535-41.

40. Morris KG, Palmeri ST, Califf RM, et al. Value of radionuclide angiography for predicting specific cardiac events after acute myocardial infarction. Am J Cardiol 1985;55:318-24.

41. Van der Wall EE, Res JCJ, Van Eenige MJ, et al. Effects of intracoronary thrombolysis on global left ventricular function assessed by an automated edge detection technique. J Nucl Med 1986;27:478-83.

42. Res JC, Simoons ML, Van der Wall EE, et al. Long term improvement in global left ventricular function after early thrombolytic treatment in acute myocardial infarction. Br Heart J 1986;56:414-21.

171

43. Bouchard A, Reeves RC, Cranney G, Bishop SP, Pohost GM, Bischoff P. Assessment of myocardial infarct size by means of T2-weighted 1H nuclear magnetic resonance imaging. Am Heart J 1989;117:281-9.

44. Nishimura T, Yamade Y, Hayashi M, et al. Determination of infarct size of acute myocardial infarction in dogs by magnetic resonance imaging and gadolinium-DTPA: comparison with indium-111 antimyosin imaging. Am J Physiol Imaging 1989;4:83-8.

45. De Roos A, Matheijssen NAA, Doornbos J, Van Dijkman PRM, Van Voorthuisen AE, Van der Wall EE. Assessment of myocardial infarct size after reperfusion therapy using gadolinium-DTPA enhanced magnetic resonance imaging. Radiology 1990;176:517-21.

46. Van Dijkman PRM, Van der Wall, De Roos, et al. Infarct size determined by gadolinium-DTPA enhanced magnetic resonance imaging in the evaluation of the efficacy of coronary thrombolysis. Neth J Cardiol 1990;3:95 (Abstract).

47. Van Rossum AC, Visser FC, Van Eenige MJ, et al. Value of gadolinium-diethylene-triamine penta-acetic acid dynamics in magnetic resonance imaging of acute myocardial infarction with occluded and reperfused coronary arteries after thrombolysis. Am J Cardiol 1990; 65:845-51.

9.
Infarct sizing by scintigraphic techniques and nuclear magnetic resonance imaging

Summary

Assessment of myocardial infarct size is the cornerstone in the evaluation of interventions designed to salvage myocardium, such as thrombolytic therapy and urgent coronary angioplasty. Enzymatic methods have probably the highest accuracy but can only be used in the very early phase of infarction. The electrocardiogram allows a reasonable estimate of infarct size but the confidence limits are wide, and in inferior wall infarction the estimates are unreliable. In recent years, radionuclide techniques have been successfully used to identify, localize, and determine infarct size in the course of acute myocardial infarction. These scintigraphic measurements have provided important diagnostic, therapeutic, and prognostic information based on the extent of myocardial damage. Nuclear magnetic resonance imaging, particularly with contrast enhancement, is one of the methods that have the greatest potential in accurately delineating myocardial infarct size. Nuclear medicine procedures, on the other hand, employ more biologically oriented tracers and offer prospects in view of their ability to monitor biochemical alterations as an effect of therapy in the course of myocardial infarction.

Introduction

Infarct size is a strong predictor of in-hospital complications as well as long-term prognosis in patients after acute myocardial infarction. Assessment of infarct size has become more important nowadays because of the introduction of therapeutic strategies to limit infarct size in the acute phase of myocardial infarction. Scintigraphic techniques for estimating infarct size have been developed and utilized in the past years particularly since the electrocardiogram is not quantitative for assessing the extent of damage and has limited ability for exactly localizing the site of the infarct. Methods based on myocardial enzyme release are accurate for infarct sizing, but only useful in the hyperacute phase of myocardial infarction.

Many nuclear cardiology studies have been performed for the detection, localization, and sizing of acute myocardial infarction, and for the evaluation of the effects of acute therapeutical interventions such as thrombolytic therapy and coronary angioplasty. A relative newcomer for studying infarct size is nuclear magnetic resonance imaging. This chapter addresses the current applications of both scintigraphic and magnetic resonance imaging techniques in determining myocardial infarct size.

Myocardial scintigraphy

Commonly, the major nuclear medicine procedures are divided into several categories which are either related to the use of radionuclide agents such as myocardial perfusion agents, infarct-avid imaging tracers, and metabolic markers, or to the various radionuclide procedures i.e. single photon emission computed tomography, positron emission tomography, and radionuclide angiography. Most of these agents and procedures have been applied for studying myocardial infarct size in patients with acute myocardial infarction.

MYOCARDIAL PERFUSION IMAGING

Thallium-201-chloride is at present the most widely used radiopharmaceutical for myocardial perfusion imaging. After intravenous administration, thallium-201 distributes in proportion to regional blood flow and myocardial infarction can be diagnosed by the visually estimated findings of a diminished tracer uptake i.e. a 'cold spot' lesion in regional myocardial areas. In 1976, Wackers et al. already showed that planar thallium-201 imaging is extremely sensitive (94%) for the detection of acute myocardial infarction when studies are performed within 24 hours of the acute onset. Regarding the assessment of infarct size, the same group of investigators demonstrated a good correlation between the thallium-201 defect size and the post-mortem findings in 23 patients who died from acute myocardial infarcts (r=0.91 for anterior infarcts, r=0.97 for inferior infarcts) (Wackers et al. 1977). The thallium defect size was measured by planimetry of both the perfusion defect and the left ventricular outline, and expressed as a percentage of the total left ventricular area. In addition, the autopsy studies showed thallium-201 scintigraphy to be unequivocally superior to electrocardiography in localizing and sizing myocardial infarcts. For example, infarcts that appeared to be inferior by electrocardiography may scintigraphically extend into the lateral and/or posterior walls.

The estimation of infarct size by thallium-201 scintigraphy has shown to be useful in assessing prognosis in acute infarct patients upon admission to the coronary care unit. Silverman et al. (1980) showed that survival in patients following myocardial infarction was strongly related to the initially measured thallium defect size. A quantitative score based on the thallium-201 image proved to be more predictive than conventional variables either alone or in combination. Tweddel et al. (1988). showed that infarct sizing acutely provides valuable information in patients with extensive infarcts in whom prognosis is poor. With the advent of thrombolytic therapy, thallium-201 is increasingly being employed as the method of assessing efficacy of reperfusion (Beller 1987). However, early in the postinfarct period a thallium perfusion defect is a composite of necrotic and ischemic myocardium, implying that only after resolution of peri-infarction ischemia, thallium defect size corresponds accurately to the actual infarct size (Schwartz et al. 1983). This finding is of major importance in the era of thrombolytic therapy with the goal to achieve early reperfusion of the infarct-related artery and to improve regional myocardial perfusion. Immediate administration of thallium-201 after reperfusion overestimates the amount of viable tissue due to hyperemic flow (DeCoster et al. 1985), but this phenomenon is not observed if thallium is injected more than 48 hours after reperfusion (Okada et al. 1986). As a result, thallium-201 has no prominent role in the immediate assessment of reperfusion-related salvage, but may be of use for follow-up studies. Several studies have now demonstrated that, when thallium-201 is injected more than 48 hours after the acute event, patients with successful reperfusion show a decrease in defect size on serial thallium images compared to those without successful reperfusion (Van der Wall et al. 1986; Heller et al. 1987).

Single photon emission computed tomography (SPECT)

SPECT imaging has been advocated to enhance the contrast between ischemic lesions and normally perfused myocardial zones, thereby increasing the sensitivity for detecting infarcted myocardial areas. The essence of SPECT is providing tomographic images by reconstruction from projections. Thallium-201 SPECT has been used to measure the mass of infarcted left ventricular myocardium as a percentage of total left ventricular mass or by applying a treshold method (Keyes et al. 1981; Wolfe et al. 1984). In an animal model, it has been shown that the volume of myocardium that is relatively hypoperfused following coronary artery occlusion can be reliably calculated from thallium-201 SPECT data (Caldwell et al. 1984). Prigent et al. (1986) demonstrated in dogs an excellent correlation (r=0.93) between SPECT defect size and the pathologic infarct size determined by staining with triphenyl tetrazolium chloride (TTC). Thallium SPECT estimates of myocardial infarct size also correlated well (r=0.89) with accumulated creatine kinase-MB fraction release in man (Tamaki et al. 1982). Mahmarian et al. (1988) found a high correlation between thallium-SPECT and enzymatic measurements in patients with acute myocardial infarction, particularly in those with anterior infarction (r=0.91). Based on these observations, thallium-201 tomography has been successfully used to assess the effect of streptokinase on infarct size in patients with acute myocardial infarction (Ritchie et al. 1984). By virtue of its ability to quantitate the volume of infarcted myocardium, the thallium-SPECT technique is more accurate than planar imaging for infarct sizing. Prigent et al. (1987) developed tomographic image-based algorithms for determination of the contribution of myocardial slices to the left ventricular mass in normal hearts, and successfully applied these algorithms for the assessment of infarct size. Also Parker (1989) described the merits of quantitative SPECT imaging although uncertainties in the reconstruction process remain. It may yet be expected that quantitative thallium-SPECT offers a great diagnostic and prognostic power in patients with acute myocardial infarction.

Technetium-99m Sestamibi

Technetium-99m labeled to hexakis-2-methoxy-2-methylpropyl-isonitrile (technetium-99m Sestamibi) is a new radiopharmaceutical that appears useful for myocardial perfusion imaging. The gamma-emission energy of technetium-99m Sestamibi is higher than thallium-201, which allows the improvement of image quality and augments the role of SPECT imaging. Similar to thallium-201, technetium-99m Sestamibi accumulates in normal myocardium in direct proportion to blood flow, but unlike thallium-201, it has a slow washout from the myocardium with minimal redistribution. Imaging can therefore be delayed for up to four to six hours and still provide information about the distribution of myocardial perfusion at the time of administration. This makes technetium-99m Sestamibi a very suitable agent for the immediate assessment of thrombolytic therapy without any delay in administration of thrombolytic therapy. Animal studies of permanent occlusion had already shown a close correlation (r=0.95) between pathologic infarct size and SPECT technetium-99m Sestamibi defect size (Verani et al. 1988). In patients with acute myocardial infarction receiving thrombolytic therapy, Wackers et al. (1988) reported that a change in defect size on the technetium-99m Sestamibi images before and after thrombolytic therapy provided information as to whether the infarct-related artery was open. With quantitative planar imaging before and 24 hours after thrombolytic therapy, it was shown that a 30% reduction of defect size was highly predictive of patency. Recently, Gibbons et al. (1989) showed that tomographic imaging with technetium-99m Sestamibi allowed the assessment of the area at risk in patients with acute myocardial infarction. Imaging was performed before and 6-14 days after therapy and in the patients who received thrombolytic therapy a significant decrease (-13%) in the extent of hypoperfused myocardium was observed compared to a nonsignificant increase (+4%) in the patients without thrombolytic therapy. Also Santoro et al. (1990) showed the usefulness of isonitrile tomography in demonstrating the size of myocardial damage and in assessing the extent of myocardial salvage after thrombolytic therapy in patients with acute myocardial infarction. Therefore, technetium-99m Sestamibi offers promise as a measurement tool for the evaluation of acute intervention strategies. For instance, this approach could be used to distinguish subgroups of acute infarct patients who remain on conservative treatment or who are candidates for urgent coronary angioplasty.

INFARCT-AVID IMAGING

Infarct-avid imaging refers to the accumulation of a radiopharmaceutical within a region of irreversibly injured myocardium and allows the visualization of a 'hot spot' at the site of the infarcted area. The most commonly used infarct-avid imaging agent is technetium-99m stannous pyrophosphate but also indium-111 antimyosin has been recently used for detection and quantification of acute myocardial infarction. Technetium-99m pyrophosphate may form a complex with the calcium deposited in damaged myocardial cells while indium-111 antimyosin shows a specific affinity for cardiac myosin and also only localizes in irreversibly injured myocardial cells.

Technetium-99m pyrophosphate

In experimental anterior myocardial infarcts involving more than three grams of myocardium, the extent of technetium-99m pyrophosphate activity on planar images correlated well with anatomic infarct size (Stokeley et al. 1976). Ko et al. (1977) observed a rather good correlation (r=0.74) between pyrophosphate uptake and the peak level of creatine kinase in patients with acute myocardial infarction. Lewis et al. (1984) used SPECT to measure technetium-99m pyrophosphate activity in dogs following coronary artery ligation. An excellent correlation (r=0.98) was observed between scintigraphic findings and anatomic infarct weight, although the correlation was weaker (r=0.81) for infarcts involving less than 10 grams of myocardium. Holman et al. (1982) and the group of Willerson (Corbett et al. 1984, Jansen et al. 1985) showed that SPECT imaging with technetium-99m pyrophosphate can accurately measure infarct size in patients with acute myocardial infarction. In these studies, the scintigrams did not become positive for 24-48 hours after the acute event by which time any intervention to salvage myocardium should have taken place. However, Hashimoto et al. (1987) showed that early positive acute technetium-99m pyrophosphate imaging with SPECT is a reliable and safe means of documenting early reperfusion and an effective method of sizing and localizing infarct soon after coronary reperfusion as early as eight hours after the onset of acute myocardial infarction.

Although the sensitivity of pyrophosphate imaging is high, the specificity is rather low since a number of different disease processes show radioisotope accumulation by the myocardium. Positive images with technetium-99m pyrophosphate have been observed in patients with ventricular aneurysm, myocardial trauma, and after radiation therapy (Wynne and Holman 1980). Another problem is that uptake of technetium-99m pyrophosphate in bone may restrict the accurate estimation of infarct size.

Indium-111 antimyosin

Radiolabeled antimyosin may be more useful than technetium-99m pyrophosphate in estimating infarct size because of its closer correlation between tissue uptake and severity of necrosis (Beller et al. 1977). In an experimental study by Johnson et al. (1987) the estimated infarct size from indium-111 antimyosin SPECT images showed an excellent correlation with TTC defined infarct size (r=0.95). Khaw et al. (1987) showed in dog hearts that the area of myocardial damage defined by pyrophosphate was approximately 1.5 times that delineated by TTC staining, whereas the area by antimyosin uptake was not significantly different from the region defined by TTC. In the first clinical study by Khaw et al. (1986), antimyosin and pyrophosphate imaging were used with both planar and SPECT techniques in patients with acute myocardial infarction. For antimyosin, the computed infarct size in grams showed a significant correlation (r=0.90) with peak creatine kinase. Infarct size by pyrophosphate SPECT proved to be 1.7 times larger than infarct size by antimyosin SPECT, suggesting that pyrophosphate may also accumulate in ischemic myocardial regions adjacent to the necrotic area. In a recent study, SPECT imaging with indium-111 antimyosin was reported to measure acute infarct size in man (Antunes et al. 1989). The results correlated well with left ventricular ejection fraction, peak creatine kinase-MB and thallium defect size (r=0.89). Infarct sizing by indium-111 antimyosin may be useful in patients with reperfusion, right ventricular infarction, left bundle branch block, and prior infarcts. Especially in such patients the peak creatine kinase-MB, the electrocardiogram, and left ventricular ejection fraction are not very helpful to estimate the extent of myocardial damage. Similar to pyrophospate imaging, the specificity of indium-111 antimyosin is suboptimal as myocardial uptake of labeled antimyosin has been described in patients with acute myocarditis (Yasuda et al. 1987) and in allograft hearts with evidence of transplant rejection (Addonizio et al. 1987). Other drawbacks are the blood pool contamination with indium-111, the far from ideal imaging characteristics of indium-111, and the late moment of optimal infarct definition at approximately 48 hours after infarction. The late positive scintigrams limit the use of indium-111 antimyosin for serial assessment of acute interventions. A more rapidly localizing monoclonal antibody against antimyosin would offer advantages. Such biological properties may justify the use of technetium-99m, involving better imaging characteristics than indium-111.

POSITRON EMISSION TOMOGRAPHY (PET)

Positron emission tomography offers the advantage of studying tracers that can be incorporated into natural substrates (e.g. carbon-11 labeled to palmitate as a marker of fatty acid metabolism). After reconstruction, the concentration of tracer in each myocardial slice or region can be measured. The PET technique using carbon-11 palmitate appeared to be capable of assessing infarct size in patient with acute myocardial infarction (Ter-Pogossian et al. 1980). Infarct size was determined by geometric reconstruction of the tomographic slices, and regions with 50% of less than maximal palmitate uptake were considered regions of acute infarct. The areas were planimetered and within each slice the areas with infarct were summed to derive the total mass of infarcted myocardium. This value correlated closely (r=0.92) with enzymatic infarct size obtained from creatine kinase curves. Geltman et al. (1982) showed with quantitative PET measurements that patients with Q-wave infarctions had significantly larger infarcts than patients with non-Q-wave infarctions (50±8 versus 19±4 PET gramequivalents, respectively). Bergmann et al. (1982)

determined infarct size in dogs using the PET technique and assessed the uptake of C-11 palmitate by the reperfused myocardium after administration of streptokinase. Uptake increased by 76% when reperfusion was carried out within two hours of occlusion, as opposed to 15% two to four hours after occlusion. This finding indicates that restoration of myocardial metabolism occurs already very soon after reperfusion emphasizing the need for early institution of thrombolytic therapy. Further experimental PET studies using the metabolic marker fluorine-18 deoxyglycose indicated that the degree of improvement of thallium defect is a measure of viable myocardium (Sochor et al. 1987; Melin et al. 1988). Clinical PET studies using metabolic markers showed that myocardial regions with outspoken thallium perfusion defects may still have evidence of metabolic activity (Brunken et al. 1987; Tamaki et al. 1988), implying that perfusion imaging alone may overestimate infarct size. Although PET imaging may be more useful for quantitating infarct size and differentiating viable from nonviable myocardium than thallium-201 imaging (Piérard et al. 1990), the overall clinical utility of this expensive technology in risk stratification after myocardial infarction remains to be settled. At present, PET is still a research tool and will have few applications in the acute phase of myocardial infarction.

RADIONUCLIDE ANGIOGRAPHY (RNA)

Radionuclide angiography is an accurate, noninvasive method for evaluation of left ventricular function at rest and during exercise. Both left ventricular ejection fraction and wall motion abnormalities can be readily assessed in patients with acute myo-cardial infarction. Although left ventricular ejection fraction is an indirect measure of infarct size, in animal studies the ejection fraction determined 24 hours after coronary artery ligation proved to be linearly related to infarct size (Schneider et al. 1985). Also in man, a favorable correlation of radionuclide angiographic estimates of infarct size and release of creatine kinase-MB fraction (r=-0.81) has been observed (Morrison et al. 1980). In a study conducted by the Interuniversity Cardiology Institute Netherlands (ICIN) with the aim to investigate the effects of streptokinase on radionuclide left ventricular function, it was demonstrated that the enzymatically determined reduction of infarct size in the treated group went along with a significant improvement of left ventricular ejection fraction (Res et al. 1986, Van der Wall et al. 1986).

However, similar to thallium-201, a resting radionuclide angiogram cannot distinguish between acutely infarcted myocardium, myocardial scar, and myocardial ischemia. Moreover, in the presence of a prior infarction the degree of functional depression reflects the total extent of scar and not the most recent event, which limits the accuracy of estimating acute myocardial infarct size by this technique. The major value of radionuclide angiography in the setting of acute myocardial infarction is currently the assessment of left ventricular ejection fraction at discharge, -being the most important single predictor of mortality after myocardial infarction-, and the evaluation of the effects of acute interventions over time.

NUCLEAR MAGNETIC RESONANCE IMAGING (MRI)

Apart from scintigraphic techniques for evaluation of infarct size, magnetic resonance imaging has emerged as a new diagnostic technique to study the extent of anatomical and functional abnormalities in patients with acute myocardial infarction. (Fig.1) Magnetic resonance imaging is a non-ionizing high-resolution tomographic technique providing high soft-tissue contrast, sharp delineation of the myocardium, and adequate characterization of myocardial tissue. The signal intensity of the images is both dependent on the hydrogen density and on the relaxation times (i.e. T1 or longitudinal relaxation time, T2 or transverse relaxation time) of the myocardial tissue. Signal intensity increases with a higher hydrogen density, shortening of T1, and lengthening of T2 relaxation time.

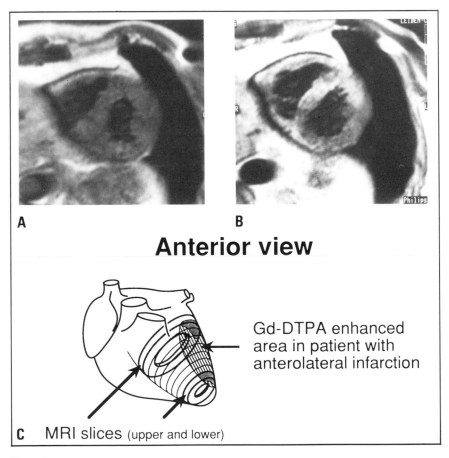

A

B

Anterior view

Gd-DTPA enhanced area in patient with anterolateral infarction

C MRI slices (upper and lower)

Figure 1
Short-axis magnetic resonance images of a patient with an anterior infarction before (left) and after (right) administration of the contrast agent Gd-DTPA. After Gd-DTPA administration, increased signal intensity is observed in the anterior area. By summation of the areas with significant contrast enhancement (> mean signal intensity + 2SD), an estimate of infarct size is obtained (lower figure).

Relaxation times

Both experimental and clinical experience using magnetic resonance imaging for direct anatomic estimation of infarct size are still limited. First studies were done in dog hearts and showed that the relaxation times T1 and in particular T2 were usually prolonged in disease states which are characterized by edematous changes that occur in regions with acute myocardial ischemia or infarction (Tscholakoff et al. 1986). Measurements of the relative size (percentage left ventricle) of an acute myocardial infaction based on regional changes in T2 relaxation times in the myocardium following experimental coronary artery occlusion have correlated closely with postmortem estimates of infarct size both at three days (r=0.98) and 21 days (r=0.94) after coronary artery occlusion (Caputo et al. 1987). Rokey et al. (1986) showed in dog hearts that the T2 values derived from infarcted regions clearly discriminated between infarcted (T2=126±22 msec) and normal myocardium (T2=88±10 msec). In addition, estimates of infarct size by magnetic resonance imaging compared well with TTC staining of the infarcted region over a wide range of infarct sizes. Buda et al. (1985) demonstrated in an excised canine heart occlusion-reperfusion model that magnetic resonance imaging overestimates infarct size and corresponds best to the area including both infarction and the surrounding ischemic region. The overestimation of infarct size by magnetic resonance imaging was recently confirmed by Ryan et al. (1990) who studied dogs three hours after reperfusion and observed a mediocre correlation between signal intensity and the TTC stained area (r=0.69). This overestimation may occur because magnetic resonance imaging reflects risk area rather than infarct zone. Bouchard et al. (1989) experimentally demonstrated that infarct size could be assessed based on different T2 relaxation times between infarcted and normal tissue after 1 week of coronary artery occlusion, although infarct size was still slightly overestimated. Wisenberg et al. (1988a) showed in dogs that the evaluation of T2 is not suitable for early assessment of infarct size but delineates the extent of an infarction only by day 21. This finding was corroborated in patients three weeks after acute myocardial infarction in whom infarct size could reliably be assessed. In addition, a significant reduction in infarct size was measured in those patients who had received streptokinase acutely (Wisenberg et al. 1988b).

Anatomic features

Given the relatively limited clinical reliability of the tissue relaxation parameters for infarct sizing in the acute phase, the extent of regional wall thinning may offer greater potential as a measure of infarct size in patients with either a recent or remote infarction. In a recent clinical study performed by White et al. (1989) in acute infarction patients, infarct size was estimated based on regional left ventricular wall thinning observed on magnetic resonance images. Relative infarction size was calculated from both the cumulative volume of regionally thinned left ventricular wall and the total myocardial volume of the left ventricle. These measurements were made by manual planimetry of endsystolic images of sequential anatomic levels of the left ventricle (five or six levels of 10 mm or 11 mm thickness) and by use of a modification of the method of Simpson. The resulting values for relative infarct size correlated inversely with left ventricular ejection fraction determined by either radionuclide angiography or biplanar contrast angiography (r=-0.99). Johns et al. (1990) recently showed in 20 patients 9±3 days after myocardial infarction a good correlation (r=0.84) between mean infarct volume assessed by nuclear magnetic resonance imaging and the quantitated left ventricular segment that was hypokinetic at contrast angiography.

Contrast agents

Despite the ability to generate images with varying image contrast using the relaxation parameters T1 and T2, it is far from easy to detect abnormalities in tissue physiology in the early stage of myocardial ischemia. As a result, paramagnetic contrast agents have been developed and one of these agents, Gadolinium (Gd)-DTPA, can be safely used to provide contrast in nuclear magnetic resonance images of patients with acute myocardial infarction. Gd-DTPA shortens both T1 and T2 relaxation times in irreversibly damaged myocardial tissue. The effect on T1 relaxation time is predominant, and therefore T1-weighted images will show enhanced signal intensity in acutely infarcted myocardium after administration of Gd-DTPA.

In an experimental study by Nishimura et al. (1989) infarct size measured by magnetic resonance imaging and Gd-DTPA was compared with Indium-111 antimyosin imaging. Gd-DTPA showed significant contrast enhancement of the infarcted area because of greater T1 shortening, and the extent of Gd-DTPA contrast enhancement expressed the infarct size almost precisely (r=0.86). In a study by our own institution in 21 patients who received streptokinase for acute myocardial infarction, we determined infarct size by nuclear magnetic resonance imaging and Gd-DTPA (0.2 mmol/kg i.v.)(De Roos et al. 1990). Nine contiguous slices (10 mm thick), perpendicular to the long axis of the left ventricle were obtained and for every slice the area with enhanced signal intensity (>mean of normal myocardium + 2SD) was considered to be infarcted. These areas were summed for all slices after which infarct size was calculated and expressed as a percentage of the total left ventricular volume (Fig. 1). Infarct size proved to be significantly less in those patients in whom reperfusion was achieved compared to the patients without reperfusion (8±5% versus 15±4%, respectively) (See also Chapter 9).

In this way employed, nuclear magnetic resonance imaging may be helpful in assessing infarct size and to follow the sequelae after acute interventions. Especially in the present thrombolytic era, there is an obvious need for future studies using nuclear magnetic resonance imaging for quantitating infarct size in patients with acute myocardial infarction. Similar to PET, drawbacks are the expenses, the limited availibity of magnetic resonance imaging machines, and the immobility of the apparatus which prevents patients to be studied within 24 hours after the acute event. Although offering a great potential, the clinical utility of magnetic resonance imaging in patients with acute myocardial infarction has still to be settled.

Conclusion

Estimation of infarct size is a prerequisite for evaluating the effects of interventions in patients with acute myocardial infarction (Rigo and DeLandsheere, 1989). The advent of thrombolytic therapy requires accurate techniques for infarct sizing both in the acute and in the follow-up phase of myocardial infarction. The present nuclear cardiology techniques provide reliable estimates for delineation of infarct size not only in the acute phase, but also in the subacute phase and further course of myocardial infarction. Whereas technetium-99m Sestamibi (preferably with SPECT) allows the immediate distinction between patients with successful and failed thrombolysis, the large majority of radionuclide agents (thallium-201, infarct-avid agents) and nuclear cardiology techniques (RNA, PET, MRI) have shown to be of optimal use more than 24 hours after the acute event. Consequently, both the early results and the sequelae of acute interventions can be determined by these techniques. The estimation of infarct size at different time phases after infarction is a unique property of the nuclear cardiology techniques and enhances their prognostic application to stratify patients into low and high risk patients based on the extent of myocardial damage.

References

1. Addonizio LJ, Michler RE, Marboe C, Esser PE, Johnson LL, Seldin DW, Gersony WM, Alderson PO, Rose EA, Cannon PJ (1987) Imaging of cardial allograft rejection in dogs using Indium-111 monoclonal antimyosin Fab. J Am Coll Cardiol 9:555-64.
2. Antunes ML, Seldin DW, Wall RM, Johnson LJ (1989) Measurement of acute Q-wave myocardial infarct size with single photon emission computed tomography imaging of indium-111 antimyosin. Am J Cardiol 63:777-83.
3. Beller GA (1987) Role of myocardial perfusion imaging in evaluating thrombolytic therapy for acute myocardial infarction. J Am Coll Cardiol 9:661-8.
4. Beller GA, Khaw BA, Haber E, Smith TW (1977) Localization of radiolabeled cardiac myosin-specific antibody in myocardial infarcts: comparison with technetium-99m pyrophosphate. Circulation 55:74-8.
5. Bergmann SR, Lerch RA, Fox KAA, Ludbrook PA, Welch MJ, Ter-Pogossian MM, Sobel BE (1982) Temporal dependence of beneficial effects of coronary thrombolysis characterized by positron tomography. Am J Med 73:573-81.
6. Bouchard A, Reeves RC, Cranney G, Bishop SP, Pohost GM, Bischoff P (1989) Assessment of myocardial infarct size by means of T2-weighted 1H nuclear magnetic resonance imaging. Am Heart J 117:281-9.
7. Brunken R, Schwaiger M, Grover-McKay M, Phelps ME, Tillisch J, Schelbert HR (1987) Positron emission tomography detects tissue metabolic activity in myocardial segments with persistent thallium perfusion defects. J Am Coll Cardiol 10:557-67.
8. Buda AJ, Aisen AM, Juni JE, Gallagher KP, Zotz RJ (1985) Detection and sizing of myocardial ischemia and infarction by nuclear magnetic resonance imaging in the canine heart. Am Heart J 110:1284-90.
9. Caldwell JH, Williams DL, Harp GD, Stratton JR, Ritchie JL (1984) Quantitation of size of relative

myocardial perfusion defect by single-photon emission computed tomography. Circulation 70:1048-56.

10. Caputo GR, Sechtem U, Tscholakoff D, Higgins CB (1987) Measurement of myocardial infarct at early and late time intervals using MR imaging: an experimental study in dogs. Am J Rontgenol 149:237-43.

11. Corbett JR, Lewis SE, Wolfe CL, Jansen DE, Lewis M, Rellas JS, Parkey RW, Rude RE, Buja LM, Willerson JT (1984) Measurement of myocardial infarct size by technetium pyrophosphate single-photon tomography. Am J Cardiol 54:1231-36.

12. DeCoster PM, Melvin JA, Detry J-MR, Brasseur LA, Beckers C, Col J (1985) Coronary artery reperfusion in acute myocardial infarction: assessment by pre- and post-intervention thallium-201 myocardial perfusion imaging. Am J Cardiol 55:889-93.

13. Geltman EM, Biello D, Welch MJ, Ter-Pogossian MM, Roberts R, Sobel BE (1982) Characterization of nontransmural myocardial infarction by positron-emission tomography. Circulation 65:747-55.

14. Gibbons RJ, Verani MS, Behrenbeck T, Pellikka PA, O'Connor MK, Mahmarian JJ, Chesebro JH, Wackers FJ (1989) Feasibility of tomographic 99mTc-hexakis-2-methoxy-2-methylpropyl-isonitrile imaging for the assessment of myocardial area at risk and the effect of treatment in acute myocardial infarction. Circulation 80:1277-86.

15. Hashimoto T, Kambara H, Fudo T, Tamaki S, Nohara R, Takatsu Y, Hattori R, Tokunaga S, Kawai C (1987) Early estimation of acute myocardial infarct size soon after coronary reperfusion using emission computed tomography with technetium-99m pyrophosphate. Am J Cardiol 60:952-7.

16. Heller GV, Parker A, Silverman K, Royal H, Kolodny G, Paulin S, Braunwald E, Markis J (1987) Intracoronary thallium-201 scintigraphy after thrombolytic therapy for acute myocardial infarction compared with 10 and 100 day intravenous thallium-201 scintigraphy. J Am Coll Cardiol 9:300-7.

17. Holman BL, Goldhaber SZ, Kirsch CM, Polak JF, Friedman BJ, English RJ, Wynne J (1982) Measurement of infarct size using single photon emission computed tomography and technetium-99m pyrophosphate: A description of the method and comparison with patient prognosis. Am J Cardiol: 50:503-11.

18. Jansen DE, Corbett JR, Wolfe CL, Lewis SE, Gabliani G, Filipchuk N, Redish G, Parkey RW, Buja LM, Jaffe AS, Rude R, Sobel BE, Willerson JT (1985) Quantification of myocardial infarction: a comparison of single photon-emission computed tomography with pyrophosphate to serial plasma MB-creatine kinase measurements. Circulation 72:327-33.

19. Johns JA, Leavitt MB, Newell JB, Yasuda T, Leinbach RC, Gold HK, Finkelstein D, Dinsmore RE (1990) Quantification of myocardial infarct size by nuclear magnetic resonance imaging. J Am Coll Cardiol 15:143-9.

20. Johnson LL, Lerrick KS, Coromilas J, Seldin DW, Esser PD, Zimmerman JM, Keller AM, Alderson PO, Bigger JT, Cannon PJ (1987) Measurement of infarct size and percentage myocardium infarcted in a dog preparation with single photon-emission computed tomography, thallium-201 and indium 111-monoclonal antimyosin Fab. Circulation 76:181-90.

21. Keyes JW Jr, Brady TJ, Leonard PF, Svetkoff DB, Winter SM, Rogers WL, Rose EA (1981) Calculation of viable and infarcted myocardial mass from thallium-201 and emission computed tomography. J Nucl Med 22:339-43.

22. Ko P, Kostuk WJ, Deatrich D (1977) Technetium pyrophosphate scanning in the detection of acute myocardial infarction: clinical experience. Can Med Assoc J 116:260-6.

23. Khaw BA, Gold HK, Tsunehiro Y, Leinbach RC, Kanke M, Fallon JT, Barlai-Kovach M, Strauss HW, Sheehan F, Haber E (1986) Scintigraphic quantification of myocardial necrosis in patients after intravenous injection of myosin-specific antibody. Circulation 74:501-8.

24. Khaw BA, Strauss HW, Moore R, Fallon JT, Yasuda T, Gold HK, Haber E (1987) Myocardial damage delineated by Indium-111 antimyosin Fab and Technetium-99m pyrophosphate. J Nucl Med 28:76-82.

25. Lewis SE, Devous MD Sr, Corbett JR, Izquerdo C, Nicod P, Wolfe CL, Parkey RW, Buja LM, Willerson JT (1984) Measurement of infarct size in acute canine myocardial infarction by single-photon emission computed tomography with technetium-99m pyrophosphate. Am J Cardiol 54:193-9.

26. Mahmarian JJ, Pratt CM, Borges-Neto S, Cashion WR, Roberts R, Verani MS (1988) Quantification of infarct size by 201TI single-photon emission computed tomography during acute myocardial infarction in humans. Circulation 78:831-9.

27. Melin JA, Wijns W, Keyeux A, Gurné O, Cogneau M, Michel C, Bol A, Robert A, Charlier A, Pouleur H (1988) Assessment of thallium-201 redistribution versus glucose uptake as predictors of viability

184

after coronary occlusion and reperfusion. Circulation 77:927-34.

28. Morrison J, Coromilas J, Munsey D, Robbins M, Zema M, Chiaramida S, Reiser P, Scherr L (1980) Correlation of radionuclide estimates of myocardial infarction size and release of creatine kinase-MB in man. Circulation 62:277-87.

29. Nishimura T, Yamada Y, Hayashi M, Kozuka T, Nakatani T, Noda H, Takano H. (1989) Determination of infarct size of acute myocardial infarction in dogs by magnetic resonance imaging and Gadolinium-DTPA: Comparison with indium-111 antimyosin imaging. Am J Physiol Imag 4:83-8.

30. Okada RD, Pohost GM (1984) The use of pre-intervention and post intervention thallium imaging for assessing the early and late effects of experimental coronary arterial reperfusion in dogs. Circulation 69:1153-9.

31. Parker JA (1989) Quantitative SPECT: basic theoretical considerations. Sem Nucl Med 19:3-12.

32. Piérard LA, De Landsheere CM, Berthe C, Rigo P, Kulbertus HE (1990) Identification of viable myocardium by echocardiography during dobutamine infusion in patients with myocardial infarction after thrombolytic therapy: comparison with positron emission tomography. J Am Coll Cardiol 15: 1021-31.

33. Prigent F, Maddahi J, Garcia EV, Resser K, Lew AS, Berman DS (1987) Comparative methods for quantifying myocardial infarct size by thallium-201 SPECT. J Nucl Med 28:325-33.

34. Prigent F, Maddahi J, Garcia EV, Satoh Y, VanTrain K, Berman DS (1986) Quantification of myocardial infarct size by thallium-201 single-photon emission computed tomography: Experimental validation in the dog. Circulation 74:852-61.

35. Res JCJ, Simoons ML, Van der Wall EE, Van Eenige MJ, Vermeer F, Verheugt FWA, Wijns W, Braat S, Remme WJ, Serruys PW, Roos JP (1986) Long term improvement in global left ventricular function after early thrombolytic treatment in acute myocardial infarction. Br Heart J 56:414-21.

36. Rigo P, De Landsheere C (1989) Radionuclide imaging in the assessment of cardiac disease. Curr Opin Cardiol 4:824-33.

37. Ritchie JL, Davis KB, Williams DL, Caldwell J, Kennedy JW (1984) Global and regional left ventricular function and tomographic radionuclide perfusion: The Western Washington Intracoronary Streptokinase In Myocardial Infarction Trial. Circulation 70:867-75.

38. Rokey R, Verani M, Bolli R, Kuo LC, Ford JJ, Wendt RE, Schneiders NJ, Bryan RN, Roberts R (1986) Myocardial infarct size quantification by MRI Imaging early after coronary artery occlusion in dogs. Radiology 158:771-4.

39. De Roos A, Matheijssen NAA, Doornbos J, Van Dijkman PRM, Van Voorthuisen AE, Van der Wall EE (1990) Assessment of myocardial infarct size after reperfusion therapy using Gadolinium-DTPA enhanced magnetic resonance imaging. Radiology 76:517-21

40. Ryan T, Tarver RD, Duerk JL, Sawada SG, Hollenkamp NC (1990) J Am Coll Cardiol 15:1355-64.

41. Santoro GM, Bisi G, Sciagra R, Leoncini M, Fazzini PF, Meldolesi U (1990) Single photon emission computed tomography with technetium-99m hexakis 2-methoxyisobutyl isonitrile in acute myocardial infarction before and after thrombolytic treatment: assessment of salvaged myocardium and prediction of late recovery. J Am Coll Cardiol 15:310-4.

42. Schneider RM, Chu A, Akaishi M, Weintraub WS, Morris KG, Cobb FR (1985) Left ventricular ejection fraction after acute coronary occlusion in conscious dogs: Relation to the extent and site of myocardial infarction. Circulation 72:632-8.

43. Schwartz JS, Ponto RA, Forstrom LA, Bache RJ (1983) Decrease in thallium-201 image defect size after permanent coronary occlusion. Am Heart J 106:1083-8.

44. Silverman KJ, Becker LC, Bulkley BH, Burow RD, Mellits ED, Kallman CH, Weissfeldt ML (1980) Value of early thallium-201 scintigraphy for predicting mortality in patients with acute myocardial infarction. Circulation 61:996-1003.

45. Sochor H, Schwaiger M, Schelbert HR, Huang SC, Ellison D, Hansen H, Selin C, Parodi O, Phelps M (1987) Relationship between TI-201, Tc-99m (Sn) pyrophosphate and F-18 2-deoxyglucose uptake in ischemically injured dog myocardium. Am Heart J 114:1066-77.

46. Stokely EM, Buja M, Lewis SE, Devous MD Sr, Corbett JR, Wolfe CL, Buja LM, Willerson JT (1976) Measurement of acute myocardial infarcts in dogs with 99mTc-stannous pyrophosphate scintigrams. J Nucl Med 17:1-5.

47. Tamaki N, Yonekura Y, Senda M, Yamashita K, Koide H, Saji H, Hashimoto T, Fudo T, Kambara H, Kawai C, Konishi J (1988) Value and limitation of stress thallium-201 single photon emmission computed tomography: Comparison with nitrogen-13 ammonia positron tomography. J Nucl Med

29:1181-88.

48. Tamaki S, Nakajima H, Murakami T, Yui Y, Kambara H, Kadota K, Yoshida A, Kawai C, Tamaki N, Mukai T, Ishii Y, Torizuka K (1982) Estimation of infarct size by myocardial emission computed tomography with thallium-201 and its relation to creatine kinase-MB release after myocardial infarction in man. Circulation 66:994-1001.

49. Ter-Pogossian MM, Klein MM, Markham J, Roberts R, Sobel BE (1980) Regional assessment of myocardial metabolic integrity in vivo by positron-emission tomography with C-11-labeled palmitate. Circulation 61:242-55.

50. Tscholakoff D, Higgins CB, Sechtum U, Caputo G, Derugin N (1986) MRI of reperfused infarcts in dogs. Am J Rontgenol 146:925-30.

51. Tweddel AC, Martin W, McGhie I, Hutton I (1988) Infarct size can be measured acutely in developing myocardial infarction. Br Heart J 2:29 (Abstract).

52. Van der Wall EE, Res JCJ, Van Eenige MJ, Verheugt FWA, Wijns W, Braat S, de Zwaan C, Remme WJ, Vermeer F, Reiber JHC Simoons ML (1986) Effects of intracoronary thrombolysis on global left ventricular function assessed by an automated edge detection technique. J Nucl Med 27:478-83.

53. Van der Wall EE, Res JCJ, Van den Pol R, Vermeer F, Van der Laarse A, Braat S, Fioretti P, Krauss XH, Verheugt FWA, Simoons ML (1988) Improvement of myocardial perfusion after thrombolysis assessed by thallium-201 exercise scintigraphy. Eur Heart J 9:828-35.

54. Verani MS, Jeroudi MO, Mahmarian JJ, Boyce TM, Borges-Neto S, Patel B, Bolli R (1988) Quantification of myocardial infarction during coronary occlusion and myocardial salvage after reperfusion using cardiac imaging with technetium-99m hexakis 2-methoxyisobutyl isonitrile. J Am Coll Cardiol 12;1573-81.

55. Wackers FJTh, Becker AE, Samson G, Busemann Sokole E, Van der Schoot JB, Vet AJT, Lie KI, Durrer D, Wellens HJJ (1977) Location and size of acute transmural myocardial infarction estimated from thallium-201 scintiscans. A clinicopathologic study. Circulation 56:72-8.

56. Wackers FJTh, Busemann Sokole E, Samson G, Van der Schoot JB, Lie KI, Liem KL, Wellens HJJ (1976) Value and limitations of thallium-201 scintigraphy in the acute phase of myocardial infarction. N Engl J Med 295:1-5.

57. Wackers FJ, Gibbons R, Kayden D, Pellika P, Behrenbeck T, Verani M, Mahmarian J, Zaret B (1988) Serial planar Tc-99m isonitrile imaging for early noninvasive identification of reperfusion after thrombolysis. Circulation 78:(suppl. II)II-130 (Abstract).

58. White RD, Holt WW, Cheitlin MD, Cassidy MM, Ports TA, Liu AD, Botvinick EH, Higgins CB (1988) Estimation of the functional and anatomic extent of myocardial infarction using magnetic resonance imaging. Am Heart J 115:740-8.

59. Wisenberg G, Prato FS, Carroll SE, Turner KL, Marshall T (1988a) Serial nuclear magnetic resonance imaging of acute myocardial infarction with and without reperfusion. Am Heart J 1115:510-8.

60. Wisenberg G, Finnie KJ, Jablonsky G, Kostuk WJ, Marshall (1988b) Nuclear magnetic resonance and radionuclide angiographic assessment of acute myocardial infarction in a randomized trial of intravenous streptokinase. Am J Cardiol 62:1011-6.

61. Wolfe CL, Corbett JR, Lewis SE, Buja LM, Willerson JT (1984) Determination of left ventricular mass by single-photon emission computed tomography with thallium-201. Am J Cardiol 53:1365-68.

62. Wynne J, Holman BL (1980) Acute myocardial infarct scintigraphy with infarct-avid radiotracers. Med Clin North Am 64: 119-25.

63. Yasuda T, Palacios IF, Dec W, Fallon JT, Gold HK, Leinbach RC, Strauss HW, Khaw BA, Haber E (1987) Indium 111-monoclonal antimyosin antibody imaging in the diagnosis of acute myocarditis. Circulation 76:306-11.

10.
Metabolic imaging in cardiology with radioisotope techniques and magnetic resonance spectroscopy

Introduction

The regional, noninvasive assessment of myocardial functional integrity with the aim to distinguish normal from abnormal myocardial areas is highly desirable in patients with cardiac disease. Therefore attempts have been made to determine the metabolic integrity of the myocardium quantitatively with radioactively labeled metabolic substrates. Human cardiac disease such as coronary artery disease, hypertensive heart disease and various forms of cardiomyopathy, is mostly diagnosed and treated in a more progressive stage when structural and anatomical derangements are already present. However, disease starts at the biochemical level and it is very likely that structural abnormalities are preceded by metabolic disorders of the myocardium. Since it became apparent that free fatty acids (FFA) are the primary substrates of the myocardium under normal physiological circumstances, a lot of investigative work has been performed to label FFA with appropriate radionuclides and to study the metabolic processes of the normal and abnormal heart. Also glucose can be labeled with various radioisotopes to study the myocardial carbohydrate metabolism under different pathological conditions. Fatty acids and glucose can be labeled with single-photon and positron-emitting agents as well and they provide, in a different way, important information of cardiac metabolism. In particular in patients with coronary artery disease, labeled metabolic substrates have been proven a valuable aid for the detection of ischemic myocardial areas. Not only by visual inspection of the obtained images, but also by the measurement of metabolic turnover rates, it has been shown that metabolic tracers may adequately localize specific myocardial areas with diminished perfusion and metabolism. Although metabolic imaging has no worldwide application - mostly due to expensive equipment facilities or difficult labeling techniques - its clinical relevance is growing and it will play a vital role in the early diagnosis and treatment of patients with cardiac disease.

A rather new recently developed technique is nuclear magnetic resonance (NMR) spectroscopy. With this technique, spectroscopic analysis of myocardial tissue can be performed which provides valuable information of cardiac metabolism. For instance, by analysis of the phosphorus spectrum, the amount of adenosinetriphosphate (ATP) can be assessed in healthy and diseased myocardial tissue. Its clinical value, however, has yet to be determined and until now no studies have been reported on spectroscopic analysis of adult human hearts. It is to be expected that nuclear magnetic resonance spectroscopy, if successfully applied to human cardiac disease, will have a major impact on clinical cardiology.

Both radioisotope imaging techniques and nuclear magnetic resonance spectroscopy will undergo rapid further development in the study of myocardial metabolism.

I. INSTRUMENTATION

Gamma camera

The currently used gamma cameras can grosso modo be divided into 1) the conventional gamma camera, and 2) the positron camera. The conventional gamma camera is very well suited for routine procedures in large number of patients, because of wide availability of gamma-emitting tracers and its relative low cost. A drawback is the difficulty of exactly quantitating radionuclide concentrations in tissue because of attenuation of radioactivity as a function of the distance between organ and camera.

Positron camera

The positron camera is a less widely available and rather expensive type of camera, and is therefore mostly employed as a research tool. It has one or multiple rings of detectors arranged in opposing pairs around the patient. Only positron-emitting tracers can be detected on the basis of positron-electron annihilation. Positrons are positively charged electrons which travel only a very short distance (less than 1 mm) to encounter an electron. When the positron and the electron combine, both are annihilated and the energy of the two particles is converted to two high energy photons (511 keV) that are emitted 180° apart in opposite directions. Major advantages of this approach include accurate tomographic localization of regional events in the myocardium, adequate correction for photon attenuation and therefore more reliable reflection of the quantity of activity within the heart than is obtained with conventional camera systems.

Nuclear magnetic resonance instrument

Every modern NMR-instrument consists of at least five important major parts. First, the magnet which has to generate a very homogeneous magnetic field. Most magnets are liquid helium-cooled superconducting solenoids (a coil of wire in the form of a cylinder) with a field strength that may vary from 0.1 to 2.0 Tesla. Second, the transmitter that transmits the radiofrequency power of the short pulses of radiowaves to an antenna. Third, the coil i.e. the antenna that transmits the radiofrequency power to the patient. The coil either totally surrounds the patient or is put on its surface as a flat surface coil, depending on whether information is required from the whole patient or from a selected region. Fourth, the receiver which gains the signal that is picked up by the coil. Fifth, the computer which is used for data processing and also for operating the entire system.

Technical aspects

Several future technical challenges must be overcome for the appropriate clinical applications of NMR spectroscopy to come to fruition. Spatial-localization methods must by optimized to acquire high-resolution spectra from within well-defined regions of myocardium without contamination from surrounding structures. In addition, the proper balance must be attained among several factors that affect the NMR signal-to-noise ratio. In order to achieve clinical usefulness, spectra must be acquired from within relatively small volumes of myocardium, necessitating stringent limitations on voxel size, with accompanying loss of signal. This can partially be compensated for with multiple signal averaging; however, the acquistition time must be kept within reasonable limits for patient compliance. The MR-signal-to-noise ratio also is enhanced at higher magnetic field strengths. However, for spectroscopy to be practical and cost-effective in the clinical arena, is most likely will need to be integrated with MR imaging at field strengths no greater than 2 T.

II. METABOLIC TRACERS

Radiolabeled substrates

In general, metabolic isotope tracers should meet the following requirements. 1) They should be highly specific of a given metabolic pathway, 2) They must not change the physiological behaviour of the metabolic substrates, 3) They have to allow adequate external detection by currently available imaging devices (gamma or positron cameras), and 4)
The metabolic tracers should have clinical application. These conditions are best fulfilled by radionuclides with chemical identities akin to those of physiological substrates such as carbon, nitrogen, and oxygen. Regarding FFA, the positron-emitter carbon-11 (^{11}C) has been shown to label adequately with palmitate. An added advantage of ^{11}C is its short half-life of 20 minutes, allowing repeated measurements to be made at short intervals, which can be of great importance in intervention procedures. However, the speed of the catabolic process in the myocardium places severe constraints on the time of measurement. For instance, after entry in the heart, 11_C-palmitate is catabolized to produce CO_2 within 30 seconds.
Several analogs of FFA have been synthesized with the gamma-emitting iodine labels. In particular ^{123}I (half-life 13.2 hours) may be very well tagged to FFA and can easily be detected with any commercial available gamma camera. A relative drawback of the ^{123}I-FFA is the release of the iodine label into the circulation during beta-oxidation in the myocardium, resulting in a substantial amount of background activity which needs to be corrected for by a special subtraction method.
Regarding kinetics of the labeled FFA, most studies have shown that they clear from the myocardium in a biexponential fashion, indicating tracer distribution between at least two different pools. This clearance pattern reflects the distribution of FFA

between immediate oxidation (rapid turnover phase) and the intermediate storage in the endogenous lipid pool (slow turnover phase).

Both ^{11}C-palmitate and ^{123}I-FFA have been applied for the detection of coronary artery disease and they show decreased turnover of FFA in ischemic myocardial regions indicating impaired myocardial FFA metabolism in those areas. To avoid the background activity of the iodinated FFA, analogs were synthesized with a phenyl ring at the omega position of the molecule. This prevents release of the iodine label into the circulation, but leads to increase in residence time of the fatty acid in the myocardium which may complicate the measurements of the FFA turnover.

Other labeled iodinated FFA have been obtained by inserting a methyl radical in the beta-position of the molecule. This inhibits beta-oxidation and the FFA are therefore trapped in the myocardium resulting in residence half-times of more than 5 hours. These compounds are very suitable for studies of regional distribution and can be used to study aberrations in myocardial FFA metabolism under normal flow conditions.

Glucose analogs can be labeled either with ^{11}C or preferably with fluor-18 (2-^{18}F-deoxyglucose). The residence time of 2-^{18}F-deoxyglucose in the myocardium is increased since this agent reaches a specific step in the catabolic process where it is recognized as different from the native substance. Therefore, it remains in the cell for a prolonged interval to over 90 minutes and the use of this analog provides a measurement of exogenous glucose utilization. The clinical value of 2-^{18}F-deoxyglucose is at the moment not very well established, but it may have a supplementary role to perfusion markers for the detection of important coronary artery disease. For instance in ischemic myocardial regions, where glucolysis is inhibited, a mismatch pattern can be observed i.e. the discrepancy between perfusion (cold spot) and glucose utilization (hot spot) in the same region. This phenomenon has become a hallmark of potentially reversible myocardial ischemia and denotes viability of myocardium recovering from ischemia. In this way used, 2-^{18}F-deoxyglucose could play an important role in determining myocardial viability after administration of thrombolytic therapy.

Atomic nuclei

NMR spectroscopy employs atomic nuclei for evaluation of cardiac metabolism. Many atomic nuclei behave, due to a property known as spin, as tiny bar magnets. When placed in a magnetic field, the tiny nuclear magnets will orient themselves either parallel or anti-parallel to the magnetic field. When the object is irradiated with a radiofrequency pulse, transitions between the two orientations can be induced. After the pulse the nuclei relax back to their equilibrium orientation and emit a weak radiofrequency signal. The frequency at which this resonance process occurs is directly proportional to the magnetic field strength and depends also on the type of nucleus. The nuclei of most interest for metabolic imaging are hydrogen (^{1}H), fluor-19 (^{19}F), phosphorus-31 (^{31}P), sodium-23 (^{23}Na), and carbon-13 (^{13}C). Since the

NMR signal is in principle proportional to the number of nuclei, that are present in the observed volume, it is evident that the NMR-technique is a powerful tool for nondestructive, quantitative determinations of myocardial metabolites and can be used to follow the metabolism of an individual heart during a series of interventions. Until now most NMR spectroscopic studies have been performed with ^{31}P. The range of biological phosphorus containing compounds is wider compared to the other nuclei and its number is limited, which makes the ^{31}P spectra easily to interpret. The metabolic consequences of global and regional ischemia have been intensively investigated with ^{31}P NMR, and the fast decrease of the phosphocreatine level at the onset of ischemia, followed by a slower decrease of the ATP level has been well documented. The question of which element will emerge as the most clinically useful for NMR spectroscopy of the heart remains unanswered. ^{31}P NMR spectroscopy has been studied the most widely and is currently the closest to clinical use. ^{1}H MR spectroscopy, with its high sensitivity and access to a wide range of metabolites, has received increasing interest in recent year and is a promising area for further investigation. NMR spectroscopy with ^{13}C, ^{23}Na, ^{39}K, and ^{19}F offers additional opportunities for studying myocardial metabolism that may yield clinical applications in the future.

III. CURRENT STATUS

In recent years three general publications have been appeared, which have very well set the stage of myocardial metabolic imaging.
The first is a special issue of the European Journal of Nuclear Medicine (1), which covers the symposium called "Assessment of myocardial metabolism by cardiac imaging ", that was held in Vienna, October 1985. All different imaging modalities, except for NMR, are extensively described and the most recent experimental and clinical data are presented. The second is a very nice review article which appeared April 1987 in the Seminars of Nuclear Medicine (2) by H.R. Schelbert. This paper highlights the most important radionuclides for today cardiac imaging, and most emphasis has been laid on metabolic tracers both with positron emission tomography and conventional imaging techniques. The third is the book called " Noninvasive imaging of cardiac metabolism " (3) by E.E. van der Wall, which appeared in the spring of 1987. This book compiles the various aspects of metabolic imaging including the NMR technique, and gives a recent state of the art in this field.

Labeling methods and new tracers

Two short communications by Mertens et al. (4,5) have been appeared in the European Journal of Nuclear Medicine on labeling methods and on new tracers. The first (4) describes a high-yield method for labeling 17-I-heptadecanoic acid with ^{123}I, and a clinical evaluation in 5 normal subjects and in 29 patients is given. It was found that the addition of thiosulfate to the reaction medium avoids the formation of side-products and increases the yield considerably to 80% carrier-free iodinated heptade-canoic acid. In this way synthesized, background correction for free iodine is probably not necessary for differentiation between clinical classes. By the same group, a potential myocardial tracer was proposed by a new high yield ^{123}I radioiodi-nation method, based on the Cu(I) assisted isotopic exchange in an ethanol water mixture (5). This tracer, 15(p-I-phenyl)-9-methyl pentadecanoic acid, can be obtained with an overall yield of 77%. The labeling method allows for the first time kit labeling of phenyl fatty acids.

Kinetics

In an article by Schön et al. (6) myocardial fatty acid metabolism was studied by the measurement of the kinetics of ^{123}I-heptadecanoic acid in 8 dog hearts. They investigated the influence of myocardial oxygen consumption and blood flow on extraction and time-activity curve of the compound. It was shown that the extraction fraction was not influenced by myocardial oxygen consumption or blood flow. It was also observed that, with increased myocardial oxygen consumption, the half-time of the early phase was prolonged and the clearance of ^{123}I activity became slower. The half-time of the late phase, which is associated with storage in lipid pools, was independent of oxygen consumption and blood flow.

It was concluded that the kinetics of ^{123}I-heptadecanoic acid are different from previous studies with the more physiologic tracer ^{11}C-palmitate. Therefore, metabolic turnover rates from the myocardium cannot be measured form the early phase of the time-activity curve. Accordingly, this study suggests that the significance of measuring turnover rates of ^{123}I-heptadecanoic acid for clinical purposes will be very questionable.

Effect of substrates

Three papers dealt with the influence of substrate administration on myocardial metabolism studied with radiolabeled FFA. The first paper, by Bianco et al. (7), reported the effects of glucose and insulin infusion on myocardial extraction of a radioiodinated methyl-substituted fatty acid. They studied 8 dogs with 14-iodophenyl-betamethyl-tetradecanoic acid (BMTDA) and they found that the mean extraction fraction at baseline raised from 0.38 to 0.44 after hyperglycemia plus insulin. It was concluded that glucose and insulin infusion results in increased first-pass extraction of BMTDA, indicating an insulin-mediated augmented transport of the compound. Therefore, BMTDA may be useful for the detection of regional alterations in FFA utilization by radionuclide imaging techniques. In the next article, Duwel et al. (8) studied the influence of glucose on the myocardial time-activity curve after injection of 17-[123]I- heptadecanoic acid in 9 patients with coronary artery disease. In contrast with earlier observations - both with radioiodinated FFA and ^{11}C-palmitate - no influence of glucose on the disappearance curve was noticed. In the third article, Schelbert et al. (9) studied the effects of oral glucose on myocardial metabolism with ^{11}C-palmitate in five normal subjects and in 16 patients with chronic left ventricular dysfunction (mean left ventricular ejection fraction 36±12%). During the control period the clearance half-times did not differ between the normal subjects and the patients. After glucose administration the myocardial half-time values of the normal subjects increased with 46%, while in the patients a variable response was noted. In nine patients the half-time values increased with 72%, and in seven patients the values decreased with 36%. This paradoxic response was unrelated to the etiology of the disease and could not be explained.

The authors hypothesize that the ability of the normal heart to resort to alternate substrates may be abnormal in myocardial disease.

Myocardial viability

Kennedy at al. (10) studied the myocardial uptake and clearance of ^{123}I-phenyl-pentadecanoic acid at rest and during exercise in 15 normal volunteers and in 18 patients with known coronary artery disease. The volunteers showed uniform segmental left ventricular activity and uniform clearance of the myocardium after exercise. In contrast, the patients showed initially increased segmental activity but delayed clearance from the regions supplied by significantly narrowed coronary arteries. It was concluded that exercise scintigraphy with ^{123}I-phenyl- pentadecanoic acid allows the noninvasive identification of segmental metabolic abnormalities associated with severe coronary artery disease.

Camici et al. (11) studied regional myocardial perfusion and metabolism with rubidium-82 ([82]Rb) and 2-^{18}F-deoxyglucose at rest in 10 normal volunteers and in 12 patients with coronary artery disease and stable angina pectoris. Five volunteers and eight patients was also studied at maximal exercise. In patients at rest, the myocardial uptake of the two tracers did not differ significantly from that measured in normal subjects. All eight patients showed reduced segmental [82]Rb uptake during exercise, which returned to normal uptake values about 10 minutes after exercise. In seven of eight patients, it was observed that the regions with reduced [82]Rb uptake during exercise were characterized by increased uptake of 2-^{18}F-deoxyglucose in corresponding regions.

The authors conclude that myocardial glucose transport and phosphorylation seem to be enhanced in the postischemic myocardium of patients with exercise-induced ischemia.

Myocardial infarction

Schwaiger et al. (12) studied regional myocardial blood flow and glucose metabolism in 13 patients with acute myocardial infarction within 72 hours using the flow marker nitrogen-13(^{13}N)-ammonia and 2-^{18}F-deoxyglucose. Also two-dimensional echocardiography and radionuclide angiography were performed on the day of the tomographic study and 6 weeks later. Interestingly, they noticed that patients with persistent wall motion abnormalities had a concordant decrease in flow and glucose metabolism. In contrast, patients with improved wall motion over time showed the characteristic mismatch pattern i.e. diminished uptake of ^{13}N-ammonia but increased uptake of 2-^{18}F-deoxyglucose in similar regions. This study suggests therefore that the combined evaluation of blood flow and glucose utilization provides a noninvasive means to distinguish necrotic from potentially viable myocardial tissue in patients with acute myocardial infarction. However, the pathophysiologic mechanism of increased uptake of labeled glucose in ischemic mycardium remains to be elucidated. Stoddart et al. (13) studied the prognostic value of ^{123}I-heptadecanoic acid in 20 patients within six days of acute myocardial infarction by the measurement of half-time values from different myocardial regions. Also radionuclide angiography was performed within six days, which was repeated after six months. The mean value of the half-times from infarcted regions was significantly shorter than that of normal myocardium, but there was no clear-cut relation between the acutely assessed half-time values and improvement of left ventricular function after six months. These findings reduced the ability of the use of half-times of ^{123}I-heptadecanoic acid as a valuable prognostic indicator for longterm left ventricular function. They suggest that improved background subtraction techniques may be needed for scintigraphy with radioiodinated FFA to become of practical significance.

Therapeutic interventions

Stoddart et al. (14) extended his studies with ^{123}I-heptadecanoic acid to six patients before and after successful percutaneous transluminal coronary angioplasty. All patients underwent maximal exercise testing and the half-times, measured before angioplasty from myocardial areas supplied by an artery with a stenosis of more than 90%, were longer than the half-times from normal regions. However, after angioplasty no significant change of the half-time values from the same regions was observed. This implies that the use of half-time values after ^{123}I-heptadecanoic acid is highly questionable as a good parameter for the assessment of myocardial metabolism after percutaneous transluminal coronary angioplasty.

Cardiomyopathies

In a report by Eisenberg et al. (15), 20 patients with dilated cardiomyopathy were studied with ^{11}C-palmitate in an attempt to differentiate nonischemic from ischemic cardiomyopathy. Regions of homogeneously severely depressed tracer accumulation were observed in eight of 10 patients with ischemic but in none of 10 patients with nonischemic cardiomyopathy. In addition, the patients with ischemic cardiomyopathy showed homogeneous tracer distribution, while in the nonischemic patients marked heterogeneity of ^{11}C-palmitate distribution was observed. These findings support the hypothesis that multiple myocardial infarction underlie the process of dilated cardiomyopathy in patients with coronary artery disease. It was concluded that the use of ^{11}C-palmitate allows differentiation of ischemic from nonischemic cardiomyopathy.

IV. MAGNETIC RESONANCE SPECTROSCOPY

The excitement surrounding NMR spectroscopy arises from its ability to monitor the metabolism of intact organs noninvasively, thereby potentially detecting pathologic processes earlier and with greater sensitivity than other diagnostic techniques.

Most of the research on cardiac NMR spectroscopy has been directed toward myocardial ischemia. Spectroscopic investigators of ischemia and infarction have ranged from analyses of myocardial tissue samples to image-guided in vivo studies of intact animals and humans. Several experimental studies appeared on examination of cardiac metabolites with ^{31}P NMR. In a study by Kantor et al. (16), cyclic changes in ATP and phosphocreatine (PC) levels were assessed in the dog heart. A special ^{31}P NMR catheter coil was placed in the apex of the right ventricle and was used to monitor the high energy phosphates at four points in the cardiac cycle. No changes in the PC/ATP ratio were noted in any of the four points of the cardiac cycle, suggesting that a variation in free adenosine diphosphate (ADP) could not be detected. This is a surprising finding since ADP has been considered as the key intermediate in the regulation of myocardial oxidative phosphorylation.

In a next study by Hoerter et al. (17), adult rat hearts were used to study the effects of sodium-potassium inhibition and sodium-calcium exchange alterations on the tissue content of high energy phosphates, all measured by ^{31}P NMR. The sodium-potassium pump was inhibited by a reduction of potassium in the perfusate and was associated with a rapid decrease in ATP and PC. When the amount of extracellular calcium was reduced, a normal metabolic profile persisted after reduction of potassium. This study emphasizes the role of the sodium-potassium pump in maintaining the cell calcium gradient and underscores the importance of calcium in the regulation of cardiac metabolism. In the third study by Markiewicz et al. (18), ^{31}P NMR was used to evaluate the effects of verapamil on mitochondrial function in syrian hamsters with cardiomyopathy. After treatment with verapamil significantly higher ATP levels were observed compared to the untreated animals, indicating markedly improved mitochondrial function in the group receiving verapamil.

A growing body of literature is coming up with respect to clinical studies with NMR spectroscopy (19-24). The latter studies have noninvasively shown metabolic alterations due to exercise, ischemia, congestive heart failure, cardiomyopathies, and left ventricular hypertrophy, thus confirming the feasibility of clinical cardiac NMR spectroscopy.

Thrombolytic therapy, coronary angioplasty, and other means of reestablishing blood flow to ischemic myocardium have become increasingly prevalent in recent years. The success of these techniques underscores the clinical need for a reliable method to assess myocardial viability (22), the effects of reperfusion, and the recovery of myocardial physiologic function after reestablishment of coronary blood flow. Although NMR spectroscopy may be usefull in the regard, the task is complicated by the fact that ischemic regions of myocardium are histologically heterogeneous, containing cells with different degrees of ischemic damage. NMR spectroscopy may be useful to quantify and characterize ischemic myocardium in relatively stable patients with coronary artery disease, particularly those in whom the severity of disease is out of proportion to clinical symptoms (21). Other potential clinical applications include the examination of patients with cardiomyopathies (24) and patients on cardiotoxic drug therapy. Spectroscopy also may be useful in the detection of rejection of cardiac allografts and for evaluating and guiding therapeutic protocols for a variety of cardiac abnormalities (23).

Conclusion

Metabolic imaging
Myocardial metabolic imaging has become a valuable and essential adjunct to standard diagnostic techniques like coronary angiography, echocardiography, and in particular to the routine radionuclide imaging techniques. Almost any kind of cardiac disease has metabolic forerunners and they can only be detected by the described metabolic imaging modalities. Both conventional imaging and positron emission tomography provide indispensable supplementary information of cardiac metabolism. Although the operational costs for positron emission tomography have been major limitations for its widespread application, the information obtained is unique and of more clinical relevance than initially has been thought. Also the radioiodinated fatty acids can be used on a routine basis in clinical practice, but they are still most apt for pure imaging purposes since the mechanism of the kinetics is poorly understood. Therefore, the use of the metabolic clearance rates of the radioiodinated fatty acids has no straightforward clinical importance at the moment (25). Based on the most recent observations it seems justifiable to suggest that the pendulum is swinging towards the use of positron emission tomography for adequate detection and interpretation of cardiac metabolic abnormalities.

Magnetic resonance spectroscopy
The usefulness of MR spectroscopy as a research tool has been well established. The clinical status of cardiac MR spectroscopy is currently investigational, and its eventual clinical role is largerly speculative. However, research in this area has prgressed in an encouraging manner. Exploring the potential of NMR spectroscopy to aid the treatment of patients with cardiac disease presents an exciting challenge for future research.

References

1. Sochor H, Ogris E, Pachinger O, Kaindl F. Assessment of myocardial metabolism by cardiac imaging. An international symposium. Vienna, Austria, October 1985. Eur J Nucl Med 1986, 12: S1-S75.
2. Schelbert HR. Current status and prospects of new radionuclides and radiopharmaceuticals for cardiovascular nuclear medicine. Seminucl Med 1987; 17: 145-81.
3. Van der Wall EE. Noninvasive imaging of cardiac metabolism, 1987.
   Editor: van der Wall EE, Publisher: Martinus Nijhoff, Dordrecht, The Netherlands.
4. Mertens J, Vanryckeghem W, Bossuyt A. Fast low-temperature preparation of carrier-free 17-123I-heptadecanoic acid applied for liver and heart scintigraphy. Eur J Nucl Med 1986;11: 361-2.
5. Mertens J, Eersels J, Van Ryckeghem W. New high yield Cu(I) assisted 123I radioiodination of 15(p-I-phenyl)-9-methyl pentadecanoic acid. Eur J Nucl Med 1987; 13: 159-60.
6. Schön HR, Senekowitsch R, Berg D, Schneidereit M, Reidel G, Kriegel H, Pabst HW, Blömer H. Measurement of myocardial fatty acid metabolism: kinetics of Iodine-123 heptadecanoic acid in normal dog hearts. J Nucl Med 1986;27: 1449-55.
7. Bianco JA, Elmaleh DR, Leppo JA, King MA, Moring A, Livni E, Espinoza E, Alpert JS, Straus HW. Effect of glucose and insulin infusion on the myocardial extraction of a radioiodinated methyl-substituted fatty acid. Eur J Nucl Med 1986; 12: 120-4.
8. Duwel CMB, Visser FC, van Eenige MJ, van der Lugt HAM, Roos JP. The influence of glucose on the myocardial time-activity curve during 17-iodo-123 heptadecanoic acid scintigraphy. Nucl Med Commun 1986;8: 207-15.
9. Schelbert HR, Henze E, Sochor H, Grossman RG, Huang SC, Barrio JR, Schwaiger M, Phelps ME. Effect of substrate availability on myocardial C-11 palmitate kinetics by positron emission tomography in normal subjects and patients with ventricular dysfunction. Am Heart J 1986; 111: 1055-64.
10. Kennedy PL, Corbett JR, Kulkarni PV, Wolfe CL, Jansen DE, Hansen CL, Buja LM, Parkey RW, Willerson JT. Iodine 123-phenylpentadecanoic acid myocardial scintigraphy: usefulness in the identification of myocardial ischemia. Circulation 1986; 74: 1007-15.
11. Camici P, Araujo LI, Spinks T, Lammertsma AA, Kaski JC, Shea MJ, Selwyn AP, Jones T, Maseri A. Increased uptake of 18F-flourodeoxyglucose in postischemic myocardium of patients with exercise-induced angina. Circulation 1986; 74: 81-88.
12. Schwaiger M, Brunken R, Grover-McKay M, Krivokapich J, Child J, Tillisch JH, Phelps ME, Schelbert HR. Regional myocardial metabolism in patients with acute myocardial infarction assessed by positron emission tomography. J Am Coll Cardiol 1986; 8: 800-8.
13. Stoddart PGP, Papouchado M, Wilde P. Prognostic value of 123-iodo-heptadecanoic acid imaging in patients with acute myocardial infarction. Eur J Nucl Med 1987; 12: 525-8.
14. Stoddart PGP, Papouchado M, Jones JV, Wilde P. Assessment of percutaneous transluminal coronary angioplasty with 123-iodo-heptadecanoic acid. Eur J Nucl Med 1987; 12: 605-8.
15. Eisenberg JD, Sobel BE, Geltman EM. Differentiation of ischemic from nonischemic cardiomyopathy with positron emission tomography. Am J Cardiol 1987;59: 1410-4.
16. Kantor HL, Briggs RW, Metz KR, Balaban RS. Gated in vivo examination of cardiac metabolites with 31P nuclear magnetic resonance. Am J Physiol 1986;251: H171-H175.
17. Hoerter JA, Miceli MV, Renlund DG, Jacobus WE, Gerstenblith G, Lakatta EG. A phosphorus-31 nuclear magnetic resonance study of the metabolic, contractile, and ionic consequences of induced calcium alterations in the isovolumic rat heart. Circ Res 1986;58: 539-51.
18. Markiewicz W, Wu SS, Parmley WW, Higgins CB, Sievers R, James TL, Wikman-Coffelt J, Jasmin G. Evaluation of hereditary syrian hamster cardiomyopathy by 31P nuclear magnetic resonance spectroscopy: improvement after acute verapamil therapy. Circ Res 1986;59:597-604.
19. Brown JJ, Mirowitz SA, Sandstrom JC, Perman WH. MR Spectroscopy of the heart. AJR 1990;155:1-11.
20. Conway MA, Bristow JD, Blackledge MJ, Rajagopalan B, Radda GK. Cardiac metabolism during exercise in healthy volunteers measured by 31P magnetic resonance spectroscopy. Br Heart J 1991;65:25-30.
21. Weiss RG, Bottomley PA, Hardy CJ, Gerstenblith G. Regional myocardial metabolism of high-energy phosphates during isometric exercise in patients with coronary artery disease. N Engl J Med 1990;323:1593-600.

22. Wroblewski LC, Aisen AM, Swanson SD, Buda AJ. Evaluation of myocardial viability following ischemic and reperfusion injury using phosphorus 31 nuclear magnetic resonance spectroscopy in vivo. Am Heart J 1990;120:31-9.

23. Mancini DM, Schwartz M, Ferraro N, Seestedt R, Chance B, Wilson JR. Effect of dobutamine on skeletal muscle metabolism in patients with congestive heart failure. Am J Cardiol 1990;65:1121-6.

24. Schaefer S, Gober JR, Schwartz GG, Twieg DB, Weiner MW, Massie B. In vivo phosphorus-31 spectroscopic imaging in patients with global myocardial disease. Am J Cardiol 1990;65:1154-61.

25. Van der Wall EE. Myocardial imaging with radiolabeled free fatty acids: applications and limitations. Eur J Nucl Med 1986;12:S11-S15.

11.
Alternative stress methods in the evaluation of coronary artery disease

Summary

Bicycle exercise and treadmill exercise are the commonest devices used in evaluating coronary artery disease. However, not all patients are capable of performing a maximal exercise test due to orthopedic, vascular or pulmonary disease, poor physical condition and motivation. Alternative tests as a reliable substitute for the more conventional methods have been proposed, such as right atrial pacing, arm ergometry, handgrip test, cold pressure test, inotropic stimulation and stress echocardiography. In particular, pharmacologic stress testing with dipyridamole (and recently with adenosine and dobutamine) in combination with radionuclide techniques has gained much interest. This chapter will consider the usefulness and role of alternative stress testing to provoke myocardial ischemia, with emphasis on pharmacologic stress testing in conjunction with thallium-201 myocardial perfusion scintigraphy.

Introduction

The bicycle and treadmill are the commonest devices used in the performance of multistage or maximal stress testing, although any exercise device which stresses large muscle groups may be employed. While both are useful, certain differences should be recognized. Hemodynamic stress including rate-pressure product and systolic blood pressure is slightly greater at any given submaximal whole body oxygen consumption for bicycle than for treadmill exercise tests [1]. Maximum myocardial oxygen consumption is slightly greater (10%) with the treadmill.

The use of the bicycle has several advantages. The patient's chest and forelimbs are in relatively stable position; the surface electrode noise may be less than on the treadmill, allowing better during-exercise recording of the electrocardiogram and it may be easier to record blood pressure responses. There is a relatively smaller influence of the patient's body weight on exercise capacity. The bicycle requires less space in the laboratory and is usually less expensive than the treadmill. A disadvantage of bicycle testing can be incoordination and leg fatigue limiting exercise capacity, especially in patients unfamiliar with bicycle pedalling. Treadmill testing has a number of advantages because of the possibility to adjust the speed and grade of walking to the agility of the patient.

Studies during dynamic exercise have evaluated alterations in electrocardiography, patterns of myocardial perfusion with radioisotopes like thallium-201, and regional and global left ventricular function with radionuclide ventriculography. By using scintigraphic techniques it is possible to make diagnosis more accurate than by exercise electrocardiography alone [2,3].

In some patients exercise with leg muscles cannot adequately be performed because of anxiety, poor motivation, peripheral vascular disease, chronic obstructive pulmonary disease, or neuromuscular skeletal disorders.

Numerous diagnostic tests requiring an increase in cardiac work have been developed. Although dynamic supine or upright exercise has been the most commonly employed stress test, there has been increasing interest in alternative means for detecting coronary artery disease. Some of these are of great interest, because of their simplicity and lack of patient motion, facilitating the recording of concomitant radionuclide or echocardiographic recordings. In addition, these tests may be independent of patient motivation and effort [4,5].

Right atrial pacing

With this technique myocardial oxygen demand is enhanced by increasing cardiac heart rate and it therefore allows assessment of cardiac stress without voluntary muscular exercise. The pacing technique, either pacing the right atrium via a vein or via the oesophagus, is not totally "noninvasive".

The hemodynamics of conventional exercise and atrial pacing differ substantially. At equivalent heart rates afterload is much lower with atrial pacing than with conventional exercise. Several studies have questioned the efficacy of atrial pacing in the evaluation of the ischemic response. Pacing has been shown to be less sensitive of myocardial ischemia than bicycle or treadmill exercise [6]. The presence or absence of ischemic ST-T segment changes during pacing may be an unreliable indicator of the status of the coronary circulation. False positives and false negatives occur more commonly with this technique than with the treadmill exercise when studied in the same group of patients [7,8]. Its major value is in a research setting, although it may be useful in patients who are unable to perform standard exercise tests. Myocardial perfusion with thallium-201 can also be assessed during atrial pacing [9,10].

Dynamic exercise of the upper limbs

Forelimb ergometry is an attractive alternative for patients with lower limb impairment as it is readily available, quite easy to perform and it offers a controlled, noninvasive method for gradually increasing myocardial oxygen demand to provoke ischemia [11]. However, comparing forelimb ergometry with treadmill testing, it was found that forelimb ergometry using the ST-T response alone was significantly less sensitive than treadmill testing [12]. Thallium scintigraphy in conjunction with arm exercise has proven useful in enhancing the detection of coronary artery disease [11]. Previous studies showed that during dynamic exercise of the upper part of the arms with a bicycle ergometer, the total peripheral vascular resistance declines, but that the mean arterial pressure increases moderately. The maintenance of the systemic pressure during exercise depends on the increase in cardiac output and vasoconstriction of the resistance vessels in the non-exercising vascular beds [13]. There is an increase in the tone of the resistance vessels in the nonactive vascular beds and this probably explains why exercise performed with small muscle groups is attended with a greater increase in mean arterial pressure than in patients with larger muscles, like leg muscles. Arm exercise is generally accompanied by smaller increase in cardiac output than leg exercise, there is less dilatation of the vascular bed and also the ischemic responses are less.

Isometric handgrip test

This procedure consists of squeezing a dynamometer at from one fourth to three fourths of the maximum hand strength and sustaining this for as long as possible [14]. Handgrip exercise increases the heart rate and systolic blood pressure in normal subjects and in patients with coronary artery disease [5,15].

Although the mean ejection fraction of groups of normal subjects does not alter, individual normal subjects may have a decline of 5% or more [15,16]. Thus the normal ejection fraction response to handgrip is heterogeneous, with some subjects having an increase and others having a decrease. The mechanism of the decrease in ejection fraction in some patients may be increased afterload or changes in coronary arterial tone [5,17]. In patients with coronary artery disease, there is generally an increase in left ventricular end-diastolic volume, end-systolic volume, and end-diastolic pressure, while the ejection fraction either decreases slightly or remains unchanged.

Isometric handgrip testing is used mostly in conjunction with radionuclide ventriculography, showing wall motion abnormalities as predictor of coronary artery disease, or with intravenous dipyridamole [5,17,18]. However, the hemodynamic abnormalities noted during handgrip exercise are less pronounced than during dynamic exercise. Kerber et al. [19] compared the isometric with the dynamic exercise and concluded that the isometric test was an insufficient way of initiating ischemia. Although the isometric test is useful in certain situations, its efficacy as a diagnostic stress test appears to be limited.

Cold pressure test

The autonomic response to exposure to cold results in coronary vasoconstriction in patients with coronary artery disease but not in patient with normal coronary vessels. Normally cold pressure stimulation has been demonstrated to produce an increase in mean coronary flow because of the increase in double product, without a change in coronary vascular resistance. In patients with coronary artery disease, on the contrary, coronary vascular resistance increases and coronary flow decreases [14,20]. Malacoff et al. demonstrated that in response to cold pressure testing, the regional myocardial blood flow increased in healthy persons, while it decreased in regions distal to coronary artery stenosis [21]. Additionally cold pressure testing has been found to precipitate Prinzmetal's angina [22]. In this situation there may be an alteration in the coronary flow because of cold pressure induced narrowing of the large epicardial coronary arteries, perhaps by the alpha-adrenergic stimulation [23]. Suggesting that cold pressure testing may result in a decrease in coronary blood flow, it was found useful for the detection of coronary artery stenosis in combination with thallium-201 scintigraphy or radionuclide ventriculography [24,25].

Inotropic stimulation

Inotropic stimulation with drugs like isoprenaline, dopamine or dobutamine has been used as a method of testing for ischemia [4,26,27]. Mannering et al. [28] proposed the dobutamine stress test as an excellent alternative to exercise testing requiring only simple, familiar equipment. The dobutamine stress test may also prove to be of value when combined with other forms of cardiac imaging, such as radionuclide studies [27]. The double product was found to be lower during dobutamine administration since although the systolic blood pressure increased to a comparable extent during dobutamine infusion, the increase in heart rate was less than during exercise. The ischemia produced during dobutamine infusion therefore seems to be caused predominantly by an increase in the inotropic state rather than through an increase in heart rate (as it is during exercise). It has to be mentioned that arrhythmias can be induced, however, so that the test may not be suitable in patients with a tendency to arrhythmias. At present, inotropic stimulation (mostly performed with dobutamine) falls into the category of pharmacological stress testing (see below).

Stress echocardiography

Echocardiography can be performed during or after exercise testing as well as during alternative testing [29]. It must be emphasised, however, that in many patients detailed echocardiographic analysis of wall motion is not feasible and also that assessment of wall motion is subjective. Considerable expertise is needed to detect small changes in wall motion and such changes are probably not reliable enough to be of much value in practice. In cases in which there are considerable changes, however, useful conclusions may be drawn [30]. During upright bicycle or treadmill exercise this technique is limited by the availability of acoustic windows. One is usually limited to only apical or subcostal examinations with this type of study. The technique that seems to be promising at the moment is the immediate postexercise echocardiogram [31]. The major disadvantage of the immediate postexercise approach is the fact that ischemia ceases and the wall motion reverts to normal shortly after stress discontinues. Abnormal wall motion, however, is the first event to occur with ischemia and the last to recover. Thus one has several minutes in which to record the abnormality. It should be stressed that the commonly performed thallium stress test also involves a postexercise examination, but the images reflect the myocardial status at peak exercise. Because of technical problems with physical exercise, other investigators have utilized handgrip, cold pressure or right atrial pacing in conjunction with echocardiography [32-34].

Pharmacological stress testing

Dipyridamole, infused at a rate of 0.14 mg/min for 4 minutes, is used as a vasodilatory agent in conjunction with thallium-201 myocardial perfusion imaging, and is particularly useful in patients who are physically unable to perform exercise, such as patients with neurologic, orthopedic, chronic pulmonary or peripheral vascular disease [35,36]. It was shown by Gould et al. [37] to be a good method for non-invasively assessing the regional coronary flow reserve and the physiologic significance of moderate stenoses of the coronary arteries. Dipyridamole is a potent vasodilator, primarily of the small coronary arterioles with minor systemic effects.
The side effects are usually mild and include headaches, nausea, dizziness, and mild chest pain. Sometimes severe side effects occur such as severe nausea, vomiting, hypotensive reactions, notable ST-T segment depression, and severe chest discomfort [38-41]. The pharmacologic effects can completely be blocked by aminophylline.
It has been reported in studies using dipyridamole as a stress technique, that angina is significantly less common and less severe than with exercise stress in the same patients [42]. ST-T segment depression as evidence of myocardial ischemia occurs [43,44], but is less frequent during imaging with dipyridamole than during exercise stress testing [35,45].

TABLE I Results of Studies with Intravenous Dipyridamole-Thallium Imaging.					
		No. Patients			
Study	Year	CAD	No CAD	Sensitivity	Specificity
Albro et al[45]	1978	51	11	67%	91%
Leppo et al[46]	1982	40	20	93%	80%
Francisco et al[47]	1982	51	35	80-90%	67-96%
Okada et al[82]	1983	23	7	91%	100%
Schmoliner et al[83]	1983	60	0	90%	NA
Socher et al[84]	1984	149	45	92%	81%
Taillefer et al[63]	1986	39	11	79-85%	86-100%
Lam et al[85]	1988	110	32	84-86%	70-75%
Laarman et al[48]	1988	81	20	78%	86%
CAD = coronary artery disease; NA = not available.					

Many investigators have shown that thallium imaging after dipyridamole infusion is highly sensitive and specific for coronary artery disease [35,46-48] (Table I). Gould et al. [37] showed that the quality of the myocardial perfusion images of thallium injected during coronary vasodilatation induced by dipyridamole was equal to images during maximal exercise.

There are substantial differences between exercise increased coronary blood flow and those due to pharmacological vasodilation. Exercise stress testing has been reported to increase coronary flow one to three times in man [49-51]. The effectiveness of exercise as a stimulus for coronary flow is dependent on the level of work achieved. Dipyridamole has been reported to increase coronary blood flow up to five times normal [37,52]. The uptake of thallium is linearly proportional to flow at resting levels and at decreased flows to zero, but at higher flow rates, especially when the increased flow is secondary to coronary vasodilatation, the uptake is not linearly related to flow. Strauss et al. [53] have reported that the percent alteration in myocardial uptake of thallium by tissue counting was 40 to 50% of the increase in coronary flow over resting values using microspheres under circumstances of pronounced coronary vasodilatation. Also Gould et al. [37] found that the maximal thallium uptake by tissue counting during peak coronary vasodilatation after dipyridamole was only 50 to 60% higher than the control levels. While thallium uptake increases as coronary blood flow increases, this relationship is not linear and cannot be used as an absolute (quantitative) index of flow changes. Thus, the diagnostic technique that utilizes the maximal stimulus for coronary blood flow and a myocardial imaging agent that is linearly related to flow should be the most sensitive indicator of a significant coronary artery stenosis. Studies in dogs have shown that a flow differential between a normal and stenotic coronary artery of about 2 to 1 is required before a definite defect is noted in the thallium image [37]. This has very important implications when exercise is the stimulus for increasing coronary blood flow. The development of angina pectoris during exercise may limit exercise at a sufficiently low level that the coronary blood flow to normal myocardium does not increase enough to produce a regional perfusion defect by thallium imaging. Therefore it is suggested that dipyridamole images may reflect higher coronary flows than with exercise and may be a better stress test [35,54].

As dipyridamole causes an increase in myocardial uptake of thallium, it causes an increase in the myocardium-to-background count ratio. In studies with thallium stress testing the myocardial-to-background thallium ratio is 2 to 1, whereas that found in studies using dipyridamole infusion is slightly higher: 2.6 to 1 [42]. Dipyridamole thallium scintigraphy in combination with exercise stress testing has been used, with significantly higher myocardium-to-background ratios (4 or 5 to 1) [48]. An explanation can be the decreased splanchnic activity during exercise. The major advantage of intravenous dipyridamole imaging is that the procedure can be performed in patients who are unable to undergo maximal exercise testing. The major disadvantage is the lack of additional information provided by the electrocardio-graphic response to exercise.

Table II Comparison Between Dipyridamole and Exercise-thalium-201 Imaging Studies.								
		No. Patients				**Dipyridamole**		**Exercise**	
Study	**Year**	**CAD**	**No CAD**	**Protocol**	**SN**	**SP**	**SN**	**SP**
Timmis et al[86]	1980	20	0	IV	85%	NA	90%	NA
Narita et al[87]	1981	35	15	IV	69%	100%	71%	100%
Machecourt et al[88]	1981	58	10	IV	90%	90%	90%	80%
Josephson et al[35]	1982	30	3	IV	85%	64%	84%	68%
Wilde et al[56]	1982	12	3	IV	100%	100%	83%	100%
Gould et al[64]	1986	48	10	PO	48%	90%	60%	90%
Huikuri et al[89]	1988	81	12	IV	96%	75%	94%	NA

* Exercise protocol performed on 35 patiens with CAD only.
CAD = coronary artery disease; NA = not available; SN = sensitivity; SP = specificity.

Dipyridamole and exercise

The use of mild exercise along with dipyridamole has been evaluated by several investigators [17,40,48, 55-59] (Table II).

Isometric handgrip
Brown et al. [17] found a 68% increase in coronary sinus flow with the combination of isometric handgrip and dipyridamole as compared with i.v. dipyridamole alone. A study by Rossen et al. [55], using dipyridamole combined with handgrip exercise. demonstrated no significant change in coronary flow reserve as measured with a coronary Doppler catheter. They suggested that their results differed from Brown et al. [17] because of limitations intrinsic to coronary sinus thermodilution technique. Furthermore, they proposed that the addition of isometric handgrip to dipyridamole testing might well improve the accuracy of the technique as a result of factors other than a change in coronary flow.

Treadmill/bicycle exercise
Mild exercise produces an increase in heart rate and systolic pressure, which could increase myocardial oxygen demand. Increased heart rate may cause a decrease in coronary perfusion distal to a stenosis, and increased adrenergic tone may exacerbate coronary constriction. Casale et al. [59] compared the effects of intravenous dipyridamole with and without simultaneous low level treadmill exercise. They found a significant increase in peak heart rate and blood pressure when treadmill exercise was performed along with intravenous dipyridamole. Fewer noncardiac side effects were noted in the exercise group. There was a significant increase in the target-to-background thallium count ratio in the exercise group, accounting for a higher quality thallium image.
Laarman et al. [40,48], using low level exercise combined with intravenous dipyridamole thallium imaging, reported improved diagnostic accuracy over dipyridamole thallium imaging alone.

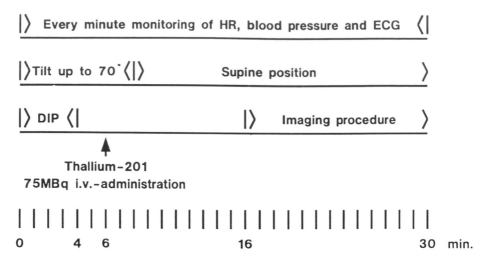

|⟩ Every minute monitoring of HR, blood pressure and ECG ⟨|

|⟩Tilt up to 70˚⟨|⟩ Supine position ⟩

|⟩ DIP ⟨| |⟩ Imaging procedure ⟩

↑
Thallium–201
75MBq i.v.–administration

| | | | | | | | | | | | | | | | | | | | | | | | | | | | | | | | | |
0   4   6   16   30   min.

Figure 1
This figure shows the protocol of the dipyridamole thallium-201 test. The patient is administered 0.14 mg. intravenous dipyridamole (Persantin®, Boehringer Ingelheim) per kg body weight per minute in a large anticubal vein for four minutes. Two minutes after completion of the administration of the dipyridamole, 75 MBq (2mCi) TI-201 is administered intravenously. During the first 30 minutes blood pressure, heart rate (HR) and electrocardiogram (ECG) are registered every minute. In case of occurrence of serious angina pectoris and (or) symptomatic hemodynamic changes, 125-250 mg aminophylline is administered intravenously as an antidote. Ten minutes after TI-201 injection, myocardial imaging is started in the three standard projections. After 4 hours the redistribution scintigrams are obtained in similar projections. The duration of imaging per view is 10 minutes. (Laarman GJ, Thallium-201 myocardial scintigraphy after dipyridamole infusion. Thesis, 1988).

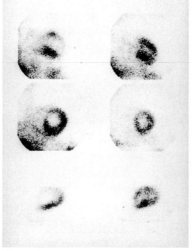

Figure 2
This is an example of dipyridamole TI-201 infusion testing in a 41-year old male with typical angina pectoris. After dipyridamole the patient experienced angina pectoris and the electrocardiogram did not show ST-segments changes. TI-201 scintigraphy revealed reversible perfusion defects in the myocardial segment related to the distribution of the LAD. Coronary arteriography showed a proximal stenosis of 99% in the LAD, while the RCA and LCX were normal. (Laarman GJ, Thallium-201 myocardial scinti-graphy after dipyridamole infusion. Thesis, 1988).

206

There were no significant differences in accuracy between visual and quantitative analysis. Walker et al. [57] compared a combined oral dipyridamole-treadmill/thallium protocol to standard treadmill/ thallium testing. Patients who did not have severe angina or ST-T segment changes 45 minutes after administration of 300 mg oral dipyridamole were exercised on a treadmill to a symptom-limited endpoint. They found a sensitivity of 89% for dipyridamole exercise testing in detecting coronary artery disease, compared with 76% in the exercise imaging group. Moreover, there were more thallium-201 defects seen in the dipyridamole-exercise group as well as a higher myocardial-to-background thallium ratio, resulting in visually superior thallium images in that group.

Table III Adverse Events reported by Patients Who Underwent Intravenous Dipyridamole-Thallium Imaging.

Adverse Events	Patients (n)	%
Chest pain	770	19.7
Headache	476	12.2
Dizziness	460	11.8
ST-T changes on ECG	292	7.5
Ventricular extrasystoles	204	5.2
Nausea	180	4.6
Hypotension	179	4.6
Flushing	132	3.4
Tachycardia	127	3.2
Pain (nonspecified)	102	2.6
Dyspnea	100	2.6
Blood pressure lability	61	1.6
Hypertension	59	1.5
Paresthesia	49	1.3
Fatigue	45	1.2
Dyspepsia	38	1.0

Values are for adverse events reported by at least 1.0% of total (100%) number of patients (3911) studied.
(Reproduced with permission from Circulation [41]).

Side effects of dipyridamole

The side-effect profile of dipyridamole in 3,911 patients studied by 64 investigators was recently reported by Ranhosky et al. [41] (Table III). Overall, serious side effects were uncommon. There were two nonfatal and two fatal myocardial infarctions; three of these four patients had a history of unstable angina. These were the only reported cases of myocardial infarction or death in the literature for intravenous or oral dipyridamole-thallium testing. There was one report of ventricular fibrillation in a patient following infusion of intravenous dipyridamole that converted to sinus rhythm after precordial thump [60]. Other cardiac side effects such as ST-T depression, angina, and arrhythmias (including ventricular premature complexes) may occur. ST-T depression occurs far less frequently than thallium perfusion defects but is probably a marker for myocardial ischemia due to coronary steal [61]. Inverted U-waves associated with ischemia have also been reported [62]. Chest pain alone is not a reliable marker for ischemia.

Noncardiac side effects such as headaches, flushing, dizziness, lightheadedness, nausea, or epigastric pain are not uncommon. These side effects occur with similar frequency in both the intravenous and oral protocols. Wheezing as a result of acute bronchospasm was not reported in any of the oral dipyridamole studies, [57-58,63-67] but it was reported in six patients (0.15%) with intravenous dipyridamole [41]. Most side effects subside without any treatment. Intravenous aminophylline can be administered if needed for reversal of more serious side effects. Dipyridamole testing is contraindicated in patients with a history of severe asthma or other bronchospastic lung diseases.

Risk stratification

Dipyridamole thallium-201 imaging provides an ideal screening method prior to elective vascular surgery in patients with peripheral vascular disease. These patients, whether symptomatic with angina or not, have a high incidence of coronary artery disease and, because of their peripheral vascular disease, are not candidates for exercise testing. Several studies have shown that patients with no transient perfusion defects on dipyridamole-thallium imaging have a low risk of perioperative events (death and nonfatal acute myocardial infarction). However, the risk of events increases by 6- to >20-fold in patients who have transient perfusion abnormalities [54,68-73].

Because only approximately one-third of such patients with reversible perfusion defects have subsequent events, the need for coronary arteriography and coronary artery revascularization before elective peripheral vascular surgery should be based on a number of factors, including the severity and extent of perfusion abnormalities, symptoms, and the presence or absence of associated electrocardiographic changes. In some patients, cardiac catherization and coronary revascularization may be necessary. In others, the surgical technique may be modified into a more conservative procedure, and more thorough monitoring before, during, and after surgery is necessary. In a study by Eagle et al. [73], clinical characteristics were useful in predicting postoperative events. Thus, none of 23 patients without a history of angina, myocardial infarction, congestive heart failure, diabetes, or Q-waves on the electrocardiogram had events, while 10 of 27 patients with one or more of these risk factors had events (death, infarction, or unstable angina pectoris). Therefore, it is possible that dipyridamole-thallium imaging is unnecessary in the low-risk group, while coronary arteriography may be indicated in high-risk patients who have reversible defects by dipyridamole imaging.

Leppo et al. [74] and Gimple et al. [75] found predischarge dipyridamole-thallium imaging after acute myocardial infarction to be at least as predictive for serious cardiac events as submaximal exercise testing. Younis et al. [76] found that the presence of a reversible thallium defect with dipyridamole-thallium testing and the extent of coronary artery disease were the only significant predictors of future cardiac events. Dipyridamole-thallium imaging was also studied for risk stratification after thrombolysis and coronary angioplasty [77]. Eichhorn et al. [78] found improved uptake of thallium in myocardial regions supplied by successfully dilated coronary arteries, and Jain et al. [79] suggested that the presence of a reversible thallium defect after oral dipyridamole-thallium imaging in post-coronary angioplasty patients identified those at high risk for restenosis.

Dipyridamole-thallium imaging is also useful in differentiating between ischemic and nonischemic cardiomyopathy [80]. In children, dipyridamole-thallium testing is useful in assessing the acute effects of Kwasaki disease, as well as its course during and after medical therapy [81].

Adenosine thallium-201 imaging

Although dipyridamole thallium-201 scintigraphy has traditionally been used for alternative stress testing, there may be several reasons why adenosine may be a preferable agent. First, dipyridamole acts by blocking the reuptake and transport of adenosine, which is the effective substance responsible for coronary vasodilation. Second, exogenous adenosine has a very short half-life (<2 seconds), which explains its very short duration of action as well as the brief, self-limiting duration of its side effects. Third, the adenosine infusion is controllable and may be increased or decreased as desired. Fourth, the coronary vasodilation induced by doses of adenosine of 140 µg/kg/minute may be more profound than that induced by the standard dipyridamole dose.

Verani and Mahmarian [90] studied nearly 1,000 patients and showed the adenosine thallium-201 test to be practical and well tolerated, with high sensitivity (87%) and specificity (94%) for detecting coronary artery disease. Iskandrian et al. [95] showed, using adenosine thallium-201 tomography, a sensitivity of 87% for one-vessel disease, 92% for two-vessel disease, and 98% for three-vessel disease. Side effects were mild and transient. The use of the reinjection technique enhanced the ability to detect reversible defects. In summary, the present experience of adenosine thallium-201 scintigraphy has demonstrated that this is a safe, well-tolerated, convenient, and accurate test for the diagnosis of coronary artery disease.

Conclusion

Many alternative approaches for conventional exercise testing have been applied. Pharmacological stress testing has emerged as the most reliable tool in patients unable to exercise. Dipyridamole thallium scintigraphy, with or without slight exercise, approves to be a useful and safe diagnostic tool in coronary artery disease. The sensitivity and specificity is quite comparable with those reported for thallium scintigraphy in combination with exercise. New pharmacological agents such as adenosine and dobutamine have still to find their way in clinical cardiology. With these alternative approaches at hand, it should be realized that conventional exercise should always be considered as the first option in the individual patient. Changes in hemodynamic and electrocardiographic parameters and the knowledge of the endurance of the patient are provide important information, not gained by alternative stress methods. Yet, in patients unable to perform maximal exercise, pharmacologic stress testing is indispensable.

References

1. Niederberger M, Bruce RA, Kusumi F, Whitkanak S. Disparities in ventilatory and circulatory responses to bicycle and treadmill exercise. Br Heart J 1974; 36:377-82.
2. Borer JS, Kent KM, Bacharach SL, et al. Sensitivity, specificity and predictive accuracy of radionuclide cineangiography during exercise in patients with coronary artery disease: Comparison with exercise electrocardiography. Circulation 1979;60:572-80.
3. Beller GA, Gibson RS Sensitivity, specificity, and prognostic significance of noninvasive testing for occult or known coronary disease. Progr Cardiovasc Dis 1987;241-70.
4. Manca C, Bianchi G, Effendy FN, Bolognesi R, Cucchuni F, Visioli O. Comparison of five different stress testing methods in the ECG diagnosis of coronary artery disease. Cardiology 1979;64:325-32.
5. Stratton JR, Halter JB, Hallstrom AP, Caldwell JH, Ritchie JL. Comparative plasma catecholamine and hemodynamic responses to handgrip, cold pressure and supine bicycle exercise testing in normal subjects. J Am Coll Cardiol 1983; 2:93-104.
6. Rios JC, Hurwitz LE. Electrocardiographic responses to atrial pacing and multistage treadmill exercise testing. Am J Cardiol 1974;33:661-7.
7. Keleman MN, Gillilan RE, Bouchard RJ, Heppner RL, Warbasse JR. Diagnosis of obstructive coronary disease by maximal exercise and atrial pacing. Circulation 1973;48:1227-33.
8. Fortuin MJ, Weiss JL. Exercise stress testing. Circulation 1977; 56:699-712.
9. McKay RG, Aroesty JM, Heller GV, et al. The pacing stress test re-examined: Correlation of pacing-induced hemodynamic changes with the amount of myocardium at risk. J Am Coll Cardiol 1984;3:1469-81.
10. Heller GV, Aroesty JM, Parker JA, et al. The pacing stress test: Thallium-201 myocardial imaging after atrial pacing. Diagnostic value in detecting coronary artery disease compared with exercise testing. J Am Coll Cardiol 1984;3:1197-204.
11. Balady GJ, Weiner DA, Rothendler JA, et al. Arm exercise-thallium imaging testing for the detection of coronary artery disease. J Am Coll Cardiol 1987; 9:84-8.
12. Balady GJ, Weiner DA, McCabe CH, et al. Value of arm exercise testing in detecting coronary artery disease. Am J Cardiol 1985;55:37-9.
13. Astrand PO, Ekblom B, Messin R, et al. Intra-arterial blood pressure during exercise with different muscle groups. J Appl Physiol 1965; 20:253-6.
14. Ellestad MH. Stress testing. Philadelphia. F.A. Davis Company, 1986:175-6.
15. Laird WP, Fixler D, Huffines FN. Cardiovascular response to isometric exercise in normal adolescents. Circulation 1979;59:651-8.

16. Peter CA, Jones RH. Effect of isometric handgrip and dynamic exercise in left ventricular function. J Nucl Med 1980; 21:1131-8.

17. Brown BG, Josephson MA, Peterson RB, et al. Intravenous dipyridamole combined with isometric handgrip for near maximal acute increase in coronary flow in patients with coronary artery disease. Am J Cardiol 1981;48:1077-85.

18. Bodenheimer MM, Banka VS, Fooshee, Gillespie JA, Helfant RH. Detection of coronary heart disease using radionuclide determined regional ejection fraction at rest and during handgrip exercise: correlation with coronary angiography. Circulation 1978;58:640-8.

19. Kerber RE, Miller RA, Najjar SM. Myocardial ischemic effects of isometric, dynamic and combined exercise in coronary artery disease. Chest 1975;67:388-94.

20. Mudge GH Jr, Grossman W, Mills RM Jr, et al. Reflex increase in coronary vascular resistance in patients with ischemic heart disease. N Engl J Med 1976;295:1333-7.

21. Malacoff RF, Mudge GH, Holman BL, et al. Effect of cold pressor test on regional myocardial blood flow in patients with coronary artery disease. Am Heart J 1983;106:78-84.

22. Endo M, Kanda L, Hosoda S. Prinzmetal's variant form of angina pectoris: Re-evaluation of mechanisms. Circulation 1975;52:33-7.

23. Epstein SE, Cannon RO, Talbot TL. Hemodynamic principles in the control of coronary blood flow. Am J Cardiol 1985;56:4E-10E.

24. Ahmad M, Dubiel JP, Haibach H. Cold pressor thallium-201 myocardial scintigraphy in the diagnosis of coronary artery disease. Am J Cardiol 1982;50:1253-7.

25. Jordan LJ, Borer JS, Zullo M, et al. Exercise versus cold temperature stimulation during radionuclide cineangiography: Diagnostic accuracy in CAD. Am J Cardiol 1983;51:1091-7.

26. Wisenberg G, Zawadowski AG, Gerbhardt VA, et al. Dopamine: its potential for inducing ischemic left ventricular dysfunction. J Am Coll Cardiol 1985;6:84-92.

27. Mason JR, Palac RT, Freeman ML, et al. Thallium scintigraphy during dobutamine infusion: non-exercise dependent screening test for coronary disease. Am Heart J 1984;107:481-5.

28. Mannering D, Cripps T, Leech G, et al. The dobutamine stress test as an alternative to exercise testing after acute myocardial infarction. Br Heart J 1988;59:521-6.

29. Robertson WS, Feigenbaum H, Armstrong WF, Dillon JC, O'Donnell J, McHenery PW. Exercise echocardiography: a clinically practical addition in the evaluation of coronary artery disease. J Am Coll Cardiol 1983;2:1085-91.

30. Iliceto S, D'Ambrosio G, Sorino M, et al. Comparison of post exercise and transesophageal atrial pacing two-dimensional echo-cardiography for detection of coronary artery disease. Am J Cardiol 1986;57:547-53.

31. Berberich SN, Zager JRS, Plotnick GD, Fisher ML. A practical approach to exercise echocardio-graphy: immediate postexercise echocardiography. J Am Coll Cardiol 1984;3:284-90.

32. Mitamura H, Ogawa S, Hori S, Yamazaki H, Handa S, Nakamura Y. Two dimensional echocardio-graphic analysis of wall motion abnormalities during handgrip exercise in patients with coronary artery disease. Am J Cardiol 1981;48:711-9.

33. Gondi B, Nanda NC. Gold pressor test during two dimensional echocardiography: usefulness in detection of patients with coronary disease. Am Heart J;1984;107:278-85.

34. Kondo S, Meerbaum S, Sakamaki T, et al. Diagnosis of coronary stenosis by two dimensional echocar-diographic study of dysfunction of ventricular segments during and immediately after pacing. J Am Coll Cardiol 1983;2:689-98.

35. Josephson MA, Brown BG, Hecht HS, Hopkins J, Pierce CD, Peterson RB. Noninvasive detection and localization of coronary stenoses in patients: comparison of resting dipyridamol and exercise thallium-201 myocardial perfusion imaging. Am Heart J 1982;103:1008-18.

36. Ruddy TD, Gill JB, Finkelstein DM, et al. Myocardial uptake and clearance of thallium-201 in normal Subjects: comparison of dipyridamole-induced hyperemia with exercise stress. J Am Coll Cardiol 1987; 10:547-56.

37. Gould KL. Noninvasive assessment of coronary stenoses by myocardial perfusion imaging during pharmacologic coronary vasodilation. I. Physiologic basis and expirimental validation. Am J Cardiol 1978;41:267-78.

38. Homma S, Gilliland Y, Guiney TE, Strauss HW, Boucher CA. Safety of intravenous dipyridamole for stress testing with thallium imaging. Am J Cardiol 1987;59:152-4.

39. Laarman GJ, Niemeyer MG, van der Wall EE, et al. Dipyridamole thallium testing: noncardiac side effects, cardiac effects, electrocardiographic changes and hemodynamic changes after dipyridamole infusion with and without exercise. Int J Cardiol 1988;20:231-8.

40. Laarman GJ, Bruschke AVG, Verzijlbergen JF, et al. Thallium-201 scintigraphy after dipyridamole infusion with low level exercise. II. Quantitative analysis vs visual analysis. Eur Heart J 1990;11:162-72.

41. Ranhosky A, Kempthorne-Rawson J. and the Intravenous Dipyridamole-thallium Imaging Study Group. The safety of intravenous dipyridamole thallium myocardial perfusion imaging. Circulation 1990;81:1205-9.

42. Gould KL. Pharmacologic intervention as an alternative to exercise stress. Sem Nucl Med 1987;17:121-30.

43. Laarman GJ, Verzijlbergen FJ, Ascoop CA. Ischemic ST-segment changes after dipyridamole infusion. Int J Cardiol 1987;14:384-6.

44. Chambers CE, Brown KA. Dipyridamole-induced ST segment depression during thallium-201 imaging in patients with coronary artery disease: angiographic and hemodynamic determinants. J Am Coll Cardiol 1988;12:37-41.

45. Albro PC, Gould KL, Westcott RJ, Hamilton GW, Ritchie JL, Williams DL. Noninvasive assessment of coronary stenoses by myocardial imaging pharmacologic coronary vasodilatation. III. Clinical trial. Am J Cardiol 1978; 42:751-60.

46. Leppo J, Boucher CA, Okada RD, et al. Serial thallium-201 myocardial imaging after dipyridamole infusion: diagnostic utility in detecting coronary stenoses and relationship to regional wall motion. Circulation 1982;66:649-57.

47. Francisco DA, Collins SM, Go RT, et al. Tomographic thallium-201 myocardial perfusion scintigrams after maximal coronary artery vasodilation with intravenous dipyridamole. Circulation 1982;66:370-9.

48. Laarman GJ, Bruschke AVG, Verzijlbergen FJ, Bal ET, van der Wall EE, Ascoop CAPL. Efficacy of intravenous dipyridamole with exercise in thallium-201 myocardial perfusion scintigraphy. Eur Heart J 1988;9:1206-14.

49. Parker JO, West RO, DiGiogi S. The effect of nitroglycerin on coronary blood flow and the hemodynamic response to exercise in coronary artery disease. Am J Cardiol 1971;27:59-65.

50. Klocke FJ. Coronary blood flow in men. Progr Cardiovasc Dis 1976; 19:117-66.

51. Bache RJ, Dymek DJ. Local and regional regulation of coronary vascular tone. Progr Cardiovasc Dis 1981; 24:191-212.

52. Wilson RF, Laughlin DE, Ackell PH, et al. Transluminal, subselective measurement of coronary artery blood flow velocity and vasodilator reserve in man. Circulation 1985;72:82-92.

53. Strauss HW, Harrison K, Langan JK, et al. Thallium-201 for myocardial imaging. Relation of thallium-201 to regional myocardial perfusion. Circulation 1975;51:641-45.

54. Young DZ, Guiney TE, McKusich KA, et al. Unmasking potential myocardial ischemia with dipyridamole-thallium imaging in patients with normal submaximal exercise thallium tests. Am J Noninvasive Cardiol 1987;1:11-4.

55. Rossen JD, Simoetti I, Marcus ML, Winniford MD. Coronary dilation with standard dose dipyridamole and dipyridamole combined with handgrip. Circulation 1989;79:566-72.

56. Wilde P, Walker P, Watt I, Russell Rees J, Rhys Davies E. Thallium myocardial imaging: recent experience using a coronary vasodilator. Clin Radiol 1982;33:43-50.

57. Walker PR, James MA, Wilde RPH, Wood CH, Russell Rees J. Dipyridamole combined with exercise for thallium-201 myocardial imaging. Br Heart J 1986;55:321-9.

58. Beer SG, Heo J, Kong B, Lyons E, Iskandrian AS. Use of oral dipyridamole SPECT thallium-201 imaging in detection of coronary artery disease. Am Heart J 1989;55:321-9.

59. Casale PN, Guiney TE, Strauss HW, Boucher CA. Simultaneous low-level treadmill exercise and intravenous dipyridamole stress thallium imaging. Am J Cardiol 1988;62:799-802.

60. Bayliss J, Pearson M. Sutton GC. Ventricular dysrhythmias following intravenous dipyridamole during "stress" myocardial imaging. Br J Radiol 1983;56:686.

61. Zhu YY, Lee W, Botvinick E, Chatterjee K, Danforth J, Ports T. The clinical and pathophysiologic implications of pain, ST abnormalities, and scintigraphic changes induced during dipyridamole infusion: their relationships to the peripheral hemodynamic response. Am Heart J 1988;116:1071-80.

62. Galli M, Bosimini E, Campi A, Tavazzi L. Dipyridamole-induced negative U waves: scintigraphic evidence of severe anterior myocardial ischemia. Am Heart J 1989;118:616-9.

212

63. Taillefer R, Lette J, Phaneuf DC, Leveille J, Lemire F, Essaimbie R. Thallium-201 myocardial imaging during pharmacologic coronary vasodilation: comparison of oral and intravenous administration of dipyridamole. J Am Coll Cardiol 1986;8:76-83.

64. Gould KL, Sorenson SG, Albro P, Caldwell JH, Chaudhuri T, Hamilton GW. Thallium-201 myocardial imaging during coronary vasodilatation induced by oral dipyridamole. J Nucl Med 1986;27:31-6.

65. Homma S, Callahan RJ, Ameer B, et al. Usefulness of oral dipyridamole suspension for stress-thallium imaging without exercise in the detection of coronary artery disease. Am J Cardiol 1986;57:503-8.

66. Segall GM, Davis MJ. Variability of serum drug level following a single oral dose of dipyridamole. J Nucl Med 1988;29:1662-7.

67. Borges-Neto S, Mahmarian JJ, Jain A, Roberts R, Verani MS. Quantitative thallium-201 single-photon emission computed tomography after dipyridamole for assessing the presence, anatomic location, and severity of coronary artery disease. J Am Coll Cardiol 1988;11:962-9.

68. Boucher CA, Brewster DC, Darling RC, Okada RD, Strauss HW, Pohost GM. Determination of cardiac risk by dipyridamole-thallium imaging before peripheral vascular surgery. N Engl J Med 1985;312:389-94.

69. Leppo JA, Plaza J, Gionet M, Tumolo J, Parakos JA, Cutler BS. Noninvasive evaluation of cardiac risk before elective vascular surgery. J Am Coll Cardiol 987;9:269-76.

70. Brewster DC, Okada RD, Strauss HW, Abbott WM, Darling RC, Boucher CA. Selection of patients for preoperative coronary angiography: use of dipyridamole stress thallium myocardial imaging. J Vasc Surg 1985;2:504-10.

71. Cutler BS, Leppo JA. Dipyridamole-thallium-201 scintigraphy to detect coronary artery disease before abdominal aortic surgery. J Vasc Surg 1987;5:91-100.

72. Levinson JR, Boucher CA, Coley CM, Guiney TE, Strauss HW, Eagle KA. Usefulness of semiquantitative analysis of dipyridamole-thallium-201 redistribution for improving risk strafication before vascular surgery. Am J Cardiol 1990;66:406-10.

73. Eagle KA, Singer DE, Brewster DC, Darling RC, Mulley AG, Boucher CA. Dipyridamole-thallium scanning in patients undergoing vascular surgery. Optimizing preoperative evaluation of cardiac risk. JAMA 1987;257:2185-9.

74. Leppo JA, O'Brien J, Rothendler JA, Getchell JD, Lee VW. Dipyridamole-thallium-201 scintigraphy in the prediction of future cardiac events after acute myocardial infarction. N Engl J Med 1984;310:1014-8.

75. Gimple LW, Hutter AM, Guiney TE, Boucher CA. Prognostic utility of predischarge dipyridamole-thallium imaging compared to pre-discharge submaximal exercise electrocardiography and maximal exercise thallium imaging after uncomplicated acute myocardial infarction. Am J Cardiol 1989;64:1243-8.

76. Younis LT, Byers S, Shaw L, Barth G, Goodgold H, Chaitman BR. Prognostic value of itravenous dipyridamole-thallium scintigraphy after an acute myocardial ischemic event. Am J Cardiol 1989;64:161-4.

77. Lette J, Laverdiere M, Cerino M, Waters D. Is dipyridamole-thallium imaging preferable to submaximal exercise thallium testing for risk strafification after thrombolysis? Am Heart J 1990;119:671-2.

78. Eichhorn EJ, Konstam MA, Salem DN, et al. Dipyridamole-thallium-201 imaging pre- and post-coronary angioplasty for assessment of regional myocardial ischemia in humans. Am Heart J 1989;117:1203-9.

79. Jain A, Mahmarian JJ, Borges-Neto S, et al. Clinical significance of perfusion defects by thallium-201 single-photon emission tomography following oral dipyridamole early after coronary angioplasty. J Am Coll Cardiol 1988;11:970-6.

80. Eichhorn EJ, Kusinski EJ, Lewis SM, Hill TC, Emond LH, Lelands OS. Usefulness of dipyridamole-thallium-201 perfusion scanning for distinguishing ischemic from nonischemic cardiomyopathy. Am J Cardiol 1988;62:945-51.

81. Nienaber CA, Spielmann RP, Hausdorf G. Dipyridamole-thallium-201 tomography documenting improved myocardial perfusion with therapy in Kawasaki disease. Am Heart J 1988;116:1575-79.

82. Okada RD, Lim YL, Rothendler J, Boucher CA, Block PC, Pohost GM. Split-dose thallium-201 dipyridamole imaging: a new technique for obtaining thallium images before and immediately after an intervention. J Am Coll Cardiol 1983;5:1302-10.

83. Schmoliner R, Dudczak R, Kronik G, et al. Thallium-201 imaging after dipyridamole in patients with coronary multi-vessel disease. Cardiology 1983;70:145-51.

84. Sochor H, Pachinger O, Ogris E, Probst P, Kaindl F. Radionuclide imaging after coronary vasodilation: myocardial scintigraphy with thallium-201 and radionuclide angiography after administration of dipyridamole. Eur Heart J 1984;5:500-9.

85. Lam JV, Chaitman BP, Glaencor M, et al. Safety and diagnostic accuracy of dipyridamole-thallium imaging in the elderly. J Am Coll Cardiol 1988;11: 585-9.

86. Timmis AD, Lutkin JE, Fenney LJ, et al. Comparison of dipyridamole and treadmill exercise for enhancing thallium-201 perfusion defects in patients with coronary artery disease. Eur Heart J 1980;1:275-80.

87. Narita M, Kurihara T, Usami M. Noninvasive detection of coronary artery disease by myocardial imaging with thallium-201: the significance of pharmacologic interventions. Jpn Circ J 1981; 45:127-40.

88. Machecourt J, Denis B, Wolf JE, Comet M, Pellet J, Martin-No LP. Sensibilité et spécificité respective de la scintigraphie myocardique réalisée après injection de 201-TI au cours de l'efforts, après injection de dipyridamole et au repos: comparison chez 70 sujets coronarographies. Arch Mal Coeur 1981;74:147-56.

89. Huikuri HV, Korhonen UR, Airaksinen J, Ikaheimo MJ, Heikkla J, Takkunen JT. Comparison of dipyridamole-handgrip test and bicycle exercise test for thallium tomographic imaging. Am J Cardiol 1988;61:264-8.

90. Verani MS, Mahmarian JJ. Myocardial perfusion scintigraphy during maximal coronary artery vasodilation with adenosine. Am J Cardiol 1991;67:12D-17D.

91. Iskandrian AS, Heo J, Nguyen T, et al. Assessment of coronary artery disease using single-photon emission computed tomography with thallium-201 during adenosine-induced coronary hyperemia. Am J Cardiol 1991;67:1190-4.

92. Beer SG, Heo J, Iskandrian AS. Dipyridamole thallium Imaging. Am J Cardiol 1991;67:18D-26D.

N.B.: Tables I, II and III derived from Beer et al. [92].

12.
Cardiomyopathies:
Evaluation with radionuclide techniques

Introduction

In recent years radioactive tracers have been used more extensively in the care of patients with coronary artery disease (CAD), valvular lesions, intracardiac shunts and cardiomyopathies. Radionuclide techniques have achieved a role in cardiology equal in importance to electrocardiography, echocardiography and cardiac catheterization.

Several factors have contributed to the progress in nuclear cardiology. The first is the development of gamma scintillation cameras with better spatial resolution. The second is the availability of medically suitable radiopharmaceuticals which will selectively in the normal or injured myocardium. The third involves minicomputers and microprocessors which are nowadays fast, powerful and compact and allow the processing and storing of large volumes of data at a relatively low cost. Fourth, since radionuclide studies are noninvasive, they can easily be repeated and interventions can be studies at short term. At last, radionuclide studies provide information of cardiac function which can not be given with other diagnostic techniques. For example, recent research with cyclotron-produced radioisotopes, such as free fatty acids (FFA) labeled with carbon-11 or iodine-123, indicates that is possible to study regional myocardial metabolism and to differentiate diseases characterized by a decreased supply of blood from those characterized by an increased demand of substrate. Not only in CAD, but also in idiopathic cardiomyopathy, such studies may be valuable to improve out understanding of disease processes.

In this review, attention will be focused on the value of radionuclide techniques for the detection of cardiomyopathies, in particular hypertrophic cardiomyopathy. Before entering these issues, the currently available cardiovascular nuclear medicine procedures will be briefly discussed. Broadly speaking, the fall into two major categories: those concerned with the heart as a muscle and those concerned with the heart as a pump.

Cardiac instrumentation

The function of the gamma camera is to convert radioactivity into a pictorial representation. The current detection system consists of a collimator, one or more crystals, photomultiplier and an electronic circuit. The collimator is a device made of lead, which absorbs gamma rays (photons) traveling in a direction other than a straight line from the heart. The photons interact with the crystal(s) to produce visual light. The produced scintillations are concerted to an electronic signal by photomultiplier tubes. The electronic signals are computed as X, Y signals and visualized on an oscilloscope on the camera console as well as sent to a computer for subsequent data analysis.

The gammacamera is a stationary or mobile system, with a field of view from 18 to 40 diameter, positioned over the chest cage. One version of this, the single-probe detector or nuclear stethoscope, has a small field of view of about 5 cm, and is also rapidly gaining acceptance for monitoring of left ventricular function. The probe offers the advantage of true portability, decreased cost and enhanced detector sensitivity. However, only temporal information can be obtained (beat-to-beat analysis) but no information is provided (non-imaging probe).

Radiopharmaceuticals

Radionuclides have three main characteristics: (1) type of emission i.e. radiation of alpha, beta, gamma or positron (i.e. ß+) rays, (2) level of energy expressed in kiloelectron Volt (keV), and (3) physical and biological half-life. The ideal radionuclide for conventional cardiac evaluation should have the following properties: (1) 1 pure gamma emitting tracer with a photon energy of 100-200 keV, (2) a physical half-life of several hours to permit serial measurements over a short time period, (3) no pharmacologic effects which might affect physiological conditions, and (4) wide availability and low cost. So far, no currently used cardiac imaging agent meets all these requirements.

Regional myocardial blood flow

The most widely used tracer for the study of heart muscle is the radioisotope thallium-201 (half-life 72 hr, gamma emission 80 keV). After intravenous administration of 1.5 milliCuries (mCi), the initial distribution of thallium is related to the blood flow in myocardium. In normal persons, between 85% and 90% of the arterial concentration is extracted by ventricular muscle in a single passage. Since coronary blood flow is 4-5% of the cardiac output, it follows that about 3% of the injected amount will be taken up by the healthy myocardium. Decreased coronary blood flow and/or reduced cellular extraction results in the appearance of a decrease in thallium concentration i.e. cold spots on gamma camera images.

Abnormalities are classified as regional or diffuse, as for example in CAD or congestive cardiomyopathy (CCM) respectively. While it is clear that CAD is associated with the appearance of clear regional defects, a thin-walled dilated ventricle in which the thallium-201 is mostly uniformly distributed, is more likely to be noncoronary, but in such patients the ventricle is usually hypertrophied as indicated by the thickness of the ventricular walls on the thallium images. Although

216

useful information can be obtained from thallium images in the acute stage of myocardial infarction i.e. the site and size of the infarction, the most common indication is the detection of suspected CAD during exercise thallium scintigraphy. The patients are usually exercised on a treadmill with an intravenous line inserted into a dorsal hand vein (Fig. 1). A 12-lead electrocardiogram is obtained 3 min and patients exercise until the appearance of symptoms (angina or fatigue). The patients are injected with 1.5-2.0 mCi thallium-201 intravenously at maximum exercise and asked to continue the exercise for 30 sec during which time the thallium is effectively taken up by the heart muscle. Imaging starts preferably within 5 min after termination of the exercise with the use of a standard gammacamera interfaced with a nuclear medicine computer. We employ a low-energy all-purpose collimator with a 20% window around the 80 keV gammaline of thallium-201. Images of 6-8 min duration each are collected in the anterior, 45-degree and 70-degree left anterior oblique (LAO) positions (300.000 counts per image). The 3 projections are collected again 3-4 hr after the initial series of images without the need for an additional thallium injection. These late images are called delayed or redistribution images.

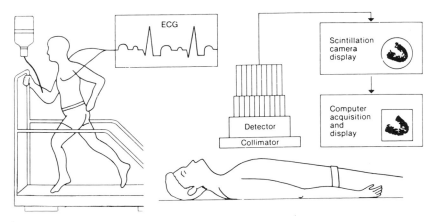

Figure 1
Exercise protocol for thallium scintigraphy. Patients are exercised according to the Bruce protocol until the appearance of symptoms (angina, fatigue). At maximal exercise 2 mCi thallium is intravenously administered. Thereafter multiple view scintigraphic imaging takes place and 2-4 hours later redistribution images are performed.

Image interpretation

Figure 2 schematically demonstrates the three ventricular views and the division of each projection into 3 segments. The 40- or 45-degree LAO view is often considered as the most important position, since this view provides the most optimal insight in the distribution of the 3 major coronary arteries. Adequate interpretation is achieved by visual comparison of the delayed and the exercise images. When both series of images are normal, it is very unlikely that the patient had CAD. However, in patients

217

with serious CAD transient defects can be observed (Fig. 3). A transient defect is defined as a defect in at least one segment on the exercise image associated with a normalization of thallium activity on the delayed image. This finding denotes reversible ischemia and is mostly consistent with a hemodynamically significant stenosis in the coronary artery that supplies the segment. A persistent defect is defined as a defect on both the initial and the delayed images. Such a defect in thought to represent myocardial scar due to old infarction. Until now, it has been demonstrated that thallium exercise scintigraphy is superior to exercise electrocardiography for the detection of patients with CAD. Both sensitivity and specificity are significantly higher for exercise thallium imaging [1].

Assessment of morphology

Apart from detection of CAD by the observation of regional defects, the thallium image can provide information of the configuration and size of the left ventricle. This information is useful for the appropriate determination of the various forms of cardiomyopathies. A thick-walled septum will very likely correspond with a hypertrophic cardiomyopathy, while a thin-walled left ventricle associated with a large cavity mostly goes along with a dilated cardiomyopathy.

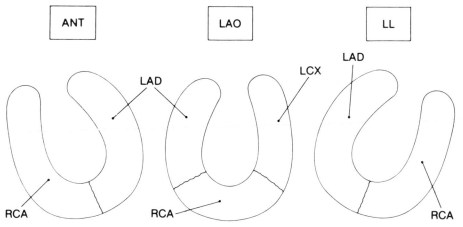

Figure 2
Schematic illustration of the myocardial segments analyzed on the thallium-201 images and the corresponding vascular beds. RCA = right coronary artery; LAD = left anterior descending coronary artery; LCX = left coronary artery; ANT = anterior; LAO 40 = 40-degree left anterior oblique; LL = left lateral

In normal circumstances, the right ventricle will not be visualized due to relatively less muscle mass and diminished blood supply compared to the left ventricle. However, under exercise conditions or with right ventricular hypertrophy the right ventricle may be observed on the thallium image.

Cardiac metabolism

Cardiac disease is at present most frequently diagnosed and treated in its final stage i.e. when structural or anatomical derangements have already developed. However, disease begins at the biochemical level and therapies are designed to terminate or reverse abnormal biochemical process, restore delivery of biochemical nutrients or supplement depleted ones. Any technique that provides biochemically specific information about the myocardium could play a vital role in the early diagnosis and management of human cardiac disease. This holds in particular for cardiomyopathies, since classification of primary cardiomyopathies is currently based on anatomic and functional abnormalities regardless of the underlying etiology. Biochemical studies will enhance our understanding of these disorders as well as aid in the development of effective treatment (Schelbert HR, Jpn Circ J 1986;50:1-29).

Although the interest for metabolism of the human heart dates from many years ago, it is only recently that radiolabeled FFA can be applied for noninvasive metabolic studies of the myocardium.

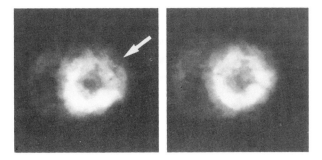

Figure 3
Exercise (left) and redistribution (right) thallium images in a patient with angina pectoris. After exercise, a prominent defect is seen in the posterolateral wall (arrow), while the distribution image 4 hr after thallium injection is normal. Coronary arteriography showed a significant lesion in the left circumflex coronary artery. The left anterior oblique view was taken.

FFA are preferred substrates for the normal myocardium and account for 70-80% of the energy production by the heart. In myocardial ischemia, there is an inhibition of FFA uptake in the myocardium, probably as a result of diminished coronary blood flow but also because of a shift to carbohydrate metabolism. FFA have been labeled with isotopes like carbon-11 (C-11) and iodine-123 (I-123). Since C-11 is a positron emitting radioisotope, special tomographic devices (positron cameras) are needed, which limit wide applicability of C-11-labeled fatty acids. Conversely, I-123 is an excellent radioisotope for gamma camera imaging (gamma energy 159 keV, half-life 13.3 hr). Initial results with FFA imaging I-123 labeled to hexadecanoic acid and to heptadecanoic acid) demonstrated that images are comparable to those obtained with thallium-201, Moreover, it has been shown that the metabolic turnover of FFA can be studied by the measurement of clearance rates from regional myocardium. In clinical studies it has been reported that significantly different clearance rates were measured between normally perfused, transient ischemic and acutely infarcted regions. With reference to clearance rates determined from normal regions (half-time values of about 25 min), we observed increased values in ischemic regions and decreased values in infarcted regions [2, 3]. These findings suggest a slow metabolic turnover of I-123-FFA in reversibly injured myocardium and a fast turnover in irreversible ischemic myocardium. In this way, the use of I-123-FFA may rapidly assess the nature of myocardial ischemia. As for cardiomyopathies, it has been shown that the determination of clearance rates in patients with CCM could be valuable. Twenty patients with CCM showed inhomogeneous tracer distribution and slow clearance rates suggesting altered FFA metabolism in diseased myocardial regions [4]. In an other study, 9 patients with CCM and 6 patients with hypertrophic cardiomyopathy (HCM) were evaluated with I-123-heptadecanoic acid [5]. Compared to controls, clearance rates were reduced (i.e. metabolic turnover) in both groups of patients. The reduction in uptake was however more pronounced in patients with CCM than in those with HCM. The interpretation of diminished uptake and decreased clearance of CCM and HCM is unclear at the present time.

The decrease in uptake may be caused by a disturbance of fatty acid transfer between extracellular binding sites on albumin whatever subcellular structure are involved. Regarding clearance, this may be reduced by a diminished demand for beta-oxidation or an alteration of the distribution of coenzyme A between the cytosol compartment and the intramitochondrial compartment. Also the carnitine shuttle across the mitochondrial membrane could be imcompetent, since it is supposed that the application of L-carnitine results in an improvement of fatty acid metabolism.

Whatever reason for the observed phenomenon, these data indicate the potential of I-123-FFA to provide insight in the pathophysiological and biochemical processes in patients with cardiomyopathies.

Cardiac function

Two techniques can be used for the assessment of cardiac function; (1) first-pass radionuclide angriography, and (2) multiple gated bloodpool scintigraphy. Usually for both methods technetium-99m (Tc-99m) is used as the imaging agent. The physical half-life of Tc-99m is 6 hr and its gamma energy 140 keV, ideally suited to current gamma cameras.

First-pass radionuclide angiography

With the first-pass technique, 15 mCi Tc-99m pertechnetate is rapidly injected in an antecubital vein as a compact bolus. The scintillation data of the first pass through the central circulation are accumulated by a multicrystal or single crystal camera. Complete mixing of the bolus is assumed to have occurred by the time the radionuclide enters the left ventricle. As a result, changes in radioactivity during the

220

ejection phase reflect proportional changes in chamber volume and are free of geometric assumptions. The efficacy of the first-pass method is dependent upon obtaining high count rates to assume statistical accuracy. The multicrystal camera provides a much higher count rate capacity than the currently available single crystal gamma cameras (max 500.000 versus max 90.000 counts per sec respectively).

A time-activity curve is generated over an area of interest over the ventricle. A typical left ventricular time-activity curve in characterized by cyclical fluctuations (peaks and valleys) in count rate. Each peak, or maximal ventricular activity, corresponds to end-diastole (ED) whereas each valley, or minimal activity, reflects end-systole (ES). These time-activity curves have to be corrected for noncardiac background activity, which can be determined by different empirically found methods.

The left ventricular ejection fraction (LVEF) is calculated by the summation of 4-5 cycles: ED-ES/ED. By choosing a region of interest over the right ventricle, the right ventricle EF can also reliably be determined by this technique. Qualitative information can be obtained by visual assessment of regional wall abnormalities of the right and left ventricle.

Gated blood pool imaging

With this technique, the cardiac blood pool is imaged after injection of a radionuclide which remains entirely in the intravascular space. This can be achieved by two methods: Tc-99m tagged to erythrocytes of the patient. At present, it is generally agreed that labeling of the erythrocytes provides a more stable tage, which is important when serial studies are desired. Imaging is mostly performed in the 45-degree LAO position for optimal separation of the right and left ventricle. With the use of a gamma camera and a computer system, scintillation data are recorded continuously in synchrony with the R-wave of the electrocardiogram. Data are recorded throughout the cardiac cycle and stored separately, depending on the relationship to each R-wave.

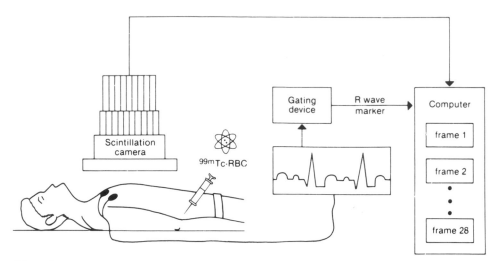

Figure 4
Equilibrium radionuclide angiocardiography or multiple gated cardiac blood pool imaging provides a means of assessing cardiac performance by synchronizing collection of scintillation data with electrocardiographic events (gating). Presently, the in-vivo labeling method is widely employed. First, the patient's own red blood cells (RBC) are "primed" with 5-15 mg of unlabeled stannous-pyrophosphate. Subsequently, after 15 minutes 20-30 mCi of technetium-99m is administered which then labels the red cells with high efficiency. The intravascular blood pool can now be visualized.

The RR interval is usually divided into 16 to 24 frames. Imaging is continued until 150.000-250.000 counts per frame are accumulated, which takes about 6 minutes. From these data, a time-activity curve can be generated over a region of interest over the left ventricle, which shows the activity accumulated over several hundred (300-500) cardiac cycles. The time-activity curve has to be corrected for background activity. The LVEF is then calculated by conventional equation and compares well with the ejection fraction obtained from contrast left ventriculography. Similar to the first-pass technique, visual inspection allows the assessment of regional wall motion abnormalities. However, the spatial resolution of conventional systems is not much less than 1 cm.

When we compare the first-pass technique with the gated blood pool scintigraphy, both techniques provide accurate data on cardiac function. Which technique to prefer depends on the expertise in the laboratory, the type of camera and specific clinical needs. An advantage of the gated blood pool technique is the possibility of data collection for several hours (4-6 hr) after tracer injection; serial measurements can be made after physiologic or pharmacologic intervention.

The assessment of LVEF during rest and exercise is probably the most widely used clinical application of the above-described techniques. Both the first-pass technique and the gate blood pool study are used to evaluate patients with suspected cardiac disease, although the gated blood pool has shown to be more feasible. Supine exercise gated blood pool scintigraphy can be carried out with the patient exercising on a special 'bicycle stress' table under the camera. At each level of the work load, data are acquired by the computer during a 2-min period. In a normal subject, LVEF will increase during exercise by the least 5%. In contrast, patients with significant CAD demonstrate generally an abnormal response on exercise: LVEF fails to increase or falls even to lower values, while very often regional wall abnormalities develop. However, one must realize that only regional wall abnormalities are specific for CAD, since a decrease in global LVEF can also occur in patients with valvular lesions and cardiomyopathies.

Congestive or dilated cardiomyopathy

Clinical findings of both right and left ventricular failure are characteristic of CCM. In general, the pathological findings are nonspecific; heart weight is increased, although ventricular dilation in excess of myocardial hypertrophy is often apparent. Apical thrombi are common in both ventricles and the coronary arteries demonstrate no significant lesions. Microscopic examination usually reveals diffuse interstitial fibrosis as well as foci of replacement fibrosis. Patients with CCM mostly have biventricular dysfunction. Typical examples are alcoholic and postpartem cardio-myopathy, and Chagas' disease. The left ventricle is more severely dilated than the right, and the LVEF is severely reduced (often less than 30%). Right ventricular dysfunction is related to both myocardial involvement and increased pulmonary artery pressure due to left ventricular failure. Wall motion is concentrically reduced, although the apical segment may be the akinetic or dyskinetic. The anterobasal segment and the basal septum show diminished wall motion in CCM, whereas these segments frequently show normal wall motion in ischemic heart disease.

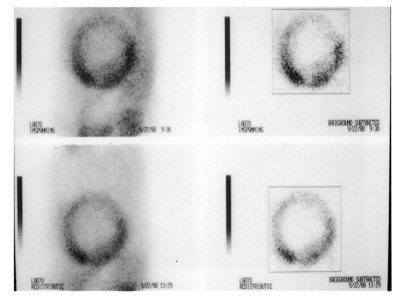

Figure 5
Thallium-201 scintigram of a patient with CCM. There is a homogeneous dilatation of the left ventricle both during exercise (upper images) and at rest (lower images)

223

Myocardial imaging with thallium usually demonstrates left ventricular dilation and either homogeneous or diffusely inhomogeneous (Fig. 5). Severe left ventricular dysfunction resulting from CAD and multiple myocardial infarctions has been called 'ischemic cardiomyopathy' and may have a picture indistinguishable from CCM. Bulkley et al. ([6] have reported the utility of thallium imaging and gated bloodpool scanning to make a distinction between ischemic cardiomyopathy and CCM. All patients with ischemic cardiomyopathy showed a defect on the thallium image involving more than 40% of the circumference of the left ventricular image in any projection. On the other hand, all but one patient with idiopathic CCM showed a defect of less than 20% of the left ventricular circumference in any projection. These findings are supported by the study of Saltissi et al [7], who clinically demonstrated that a defect size of more than 40% of the outer left ventricular perimeter strongly favoured an ischemic rather than a dilated cardiomyopathy. Fig. 6 shows the typical distribution patterns of metabolic tracers (I-123-FFA and C-11-FFA in patients with CCM.

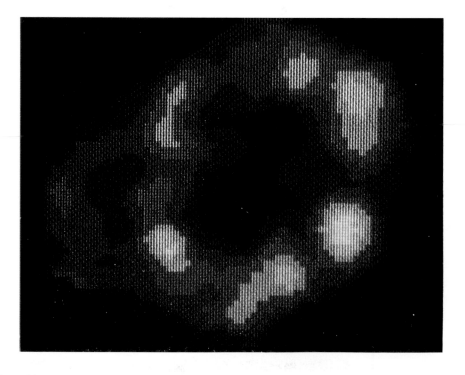

Figure 6A
Inhomogeneous metabolic tracer distribution in patients with congestive cardiomyopathy. Fig. 6A shows the inhomogeneous pattern in a patient studied with I-123 heptadecanoic acid.

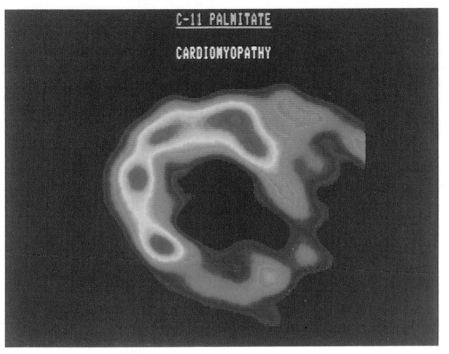

Figure 6B
Fig. 6B shows a similar pattern in a patient studies with C-11 palmitate. Note the dilated left ventricle in both patients. (From Ref. 4, Höck A, et al. J Nucl Ned 1983;24:22-8, and from Schelbert HR, Jpn Circ J 1986;50:1-29, respectively, with permission).

Also the gated blood pool scans proved to be useful in distinguishing both entities. Diffuse hypokinesis was associated with both forms of cardiomyopathies, but segmental wall abnormalities were more outspoken in the patients with ischemic cardiomyopathy. Moreover, right ventricular dilation was more striking in in the patients with idiopathic CCM.

Arreaza et al. [8] showed that radionuclide ventriculography could be useful to evaluate patients with Chagas' disease. Fourty-one patients with chronic Chagas' cardiomyopathy were studied, of whom 12 patients had congestive heart failure. Mean LVEF of these 12 patients was 28% and 9 patients showed diffuse hypokinesia of the left ventricle. From total-group results it was inferred that radionuclide angiography may distinguish the wall motion abnormalities of CAD from those of Chagas' origin.

Serial evaluation of LVEF and wall abnormalities with radionuclide angiography provides an objective method to monitor the effects of drug therapy. For example, in a patient with alcoholic cardiomyopathy one could easily evaluate an improvement in LVEF after withdrawal of alcohol intake and administration of diuretics and digitalis by serial radionuclide studies. On the other hand, it is possible to determine the deleterious effects of the potentially cardiotoxic agent doxorubicin (adriamycin). The treatment of malignant disease with adriamycin may result in congestive heart

225

failure. The gated blood pool scan showed this toxic cardiomyopathy to be of the congestive or dilated type [9]. Serial assessment of the left ventricular performance allowed identification of patients at risk for the development of congestive heart failure and of those who could receive therapy safely at substantially higher doses than those conventionally recommended.

Restrictive cardiomyopathy

Restrictive cardiomyopathy (RCM) is the least common class of cardiomyopathy outside the tropics. RCM simulates the findings of constrictive pericardial disease and shows normal-sized or small ventricles. It may be divided into two basic types of cardiomyopathy; (1) infiltrative RCM, such as amyloid disease, in which the left or both ventricular cavities are normal to decreased in size and the walls are normal to decreased in thickness, and (2) obliterative RCM, such as metastatic carcinoma, in which the involved ventricles are reduced in size and there is partial obliteration of one or both of the ventricular cavities.

Myocardial imaging with thallium may be helpful to depict increased mural thickness, as with amyloid disease, or regional myocardial defects, as with metastatic carcinoma. In case of leukemic infiltration, the myocardial image will display uniform thallium activity since the infiltration is usually homogeneous.

The gated blood pool scan is useful in distinguishing between CCM and RCM by depicting the sizes of the cardiac chambers [10]. In CCM all four chambers are dilated, whereas in RCM the ventricles are normal to reduced in size but the atria are dilated. In addition, the gated blood pool scan may differentiate between the infiltrative and the obliterative forms of RCM. In the infiltrative type, both ventricles are mostly normal or reduced in size, whereas in the obliterative type either or both ventricles are generally smaller than normal. However, since RCM is rare disease in Western countries, it is clear that radionuclide data on RCM are very scarce.

Hypertrophic cardiomyopathy

Hypertrophic cardiomyopathy (HCM) is characterized by left ventricular hypertrophy of unknown cause [11]. Hypertrophy is generally asymmetric, with the interventricular septum disproportionally thickened in comparison to the remainder of the left ventricular wall. HCM may be obstructive or non-obstructive. Left ventricular outflow obstruction is caused by hypertrophy of the anterior superior aspect of the interventricular septum and abnormal motion of the anterior leaflet of the mitral valve. Before the noninvasive techniques were developed, the diagnosis of HCM depended largely on accurate interpretation of physical findings.

Noninvasive imaging techniques have permitted the diagnosis of HCM with or without obstruction. Asymmetric hypertrophy (ASH) is easily documented by echocardiography and has been employed as a marker of HCM. However, although a septal-to-posterior wall radio of 1.3 or more is a sensitive indicator for HCM, it is not pathognomonic. For example, right ventricular hypertrophy may also lead to ASH. Systolic anterior motion (SAM) of the anterior mitral valve leaflet has been shown to correlate with the presence and the severity of the outflow obstruction; this finding may be used to distinguish between patients with and without obstruction. Similar to ASH, SAM is not pathognomonic for HCM and may occur in other forms of heart disease. In recent years, more attention has been focused on diastolic parameters. It has been shown that patients with HCM manifest abnormal diastolic dysfunction in terms of a prolonged relaxation-time index, impaired diastolic filling and increased chamber stiffness.

Both myocardial imaging with thallium-201 and the gated blood pool scan are helpful alternatives to the echocardiogram in the detection of HCM. Bulkley et al. [12] employed thallium imaging to evaluate the ratio of septal to posterior thickness in patients with HCM. ASH was observed in all 10 patients with HCM and confirmed in nine by cardiac catheterization. In addition, it was noted that the basal and midposterior were of equal thickness in patients with obstructive HCM, but that the basal wall was thinner than the midposterior wall inpatients with non-obstructive HCM. Three patients with chronic pulmonary hypertension has ASH on the thallium image, but in these patients the right ventricular free wall thickness was equal to the septal thickness, which is consistent with right ventricular hypertrophy.

Rubin et al. evaluated the presence of anginal symptoms in 10 patients with HCM by thallium exercise scintigraphy [13]. All 10 patients had normal coronary angiograms. In nine of the 10 patients thallium imaging revealed no significant perfusion defects and it was concluded that thallium exercise scintigraphy is a valuable method to rule out significant CAD in patients with HCM. Myocardial perfusion abnormalities are common with thallium-201 imaging in patients with hypertrophic cardiomyopathy. Persistent defects are mostly seen in patients with impaired systolic function, whereas reversible defects are usually noticed in patients with normal or supranormal left ventricular systolic function. Latest reports have indicated that the occurrence of reversible thallium-201 defects in patients with hypertrophic cardiomyopathy is yet highly indicative for the presence of myocardial ischemia.

The end-diastolic image of the gated blood pool scan in LAO view allows evaluation of the interventricular septal configuration. The appearance of the interventricular septum by gated scan not only depends on septal configuration but is also affected by the angle of view. In a shallow LAO view, the apical septum appears thickest, whereas in high oblique view the upper septum appears thickest. This phenomenon occurs because of the spiral geometry of the septum.

The most suited view, in which the septum appears most uniform from top to bottom is usually the 45-degree LAO view.

Pohost et al. [14] evaluated 12 patients with HCM by gated bloodpool scan and demonstrated in 11 patients (50%) disproportionate upper septal thickening. The middle or upper septum appeared thicker than the lower septum in any LAO projection. Moreover, 73% of the patients with HCM showed loss of the normal concavity on the left ventricular aspect of the septum. Although this flattening of the septum is a frequent finding in HCM, it is less specific than disporportionate upper septal thickening and can also be noticed in patients with aortic stenosis as well in normal subjects. The gated scan did also demonstrate obliteration of the left ventricular cavity and a circular defect in the left ventricular outflow tract. These abnormalities were best seen in the anterior and 45-degree LAO projection (Fig. 7).

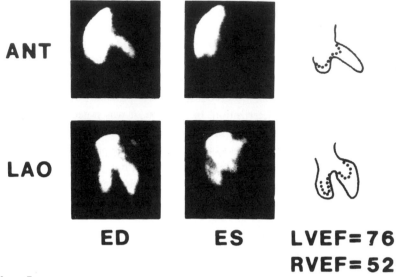

Figure 7
Radionuclide angiograms at rest in a patient with hypertrophic obstructive cardiomyopathy. The septum shows abnormal thickening both during end-diastole (ED) and end-systole (ES). Left ventricular wall motions is hyperdynamic with nearly complete cavity obliteration at systole. Left ventricular ejection fraction (LVEF) is markedly elevated at 0.76, while the RVEF is normal. ANT = anterior; LAO = 40-degree left anterior oblique. (From DS Berman and DT Mason. Clinical Nuclear Cardiology. Grune & Stratton. 1982 with permission).

Borer et al. studied 63 patients with HCM (40 with and 23 without obstruction) by rest and exercise gated bloodpool studies [15]. All 63 patients showed an elevated LVEF at rest compared to normal subjects. However, it was shown that during exercise LVEF was significantly more depressed in patients without obstruction compared to patients with obstruction. It was postulated that symptomatic patients without obstruction might benefit from inotropic therapy to support systolic function during exercise. In a recent study [16] Manyari et al. studied 19 patients with HCM and 20 control subjects by means of radionuclide angiography at rest and during exercise. The patients were divided into three groups according to their hemodynamic status; those without obstruction (five patients), those with latent obstruction (six patients), and those with obstruction at rest (eight patients). It was shown that the LVEF of the patients without obstruction were similar to those of the control both at rest and during exercise. In contrast, the LVEF of patients with latent and resting obstruction were supernormal at rest (more than 75%). Mean LVEF of patients with latent obstruction increased significantly with exercise, while mean LVEF of the patients with resting obstruction decreased significantly. It was concluded that radionuclide angiography is useful to distinguish between the three hemodynamic subgroups in patients with HCM, and that it may impairment of left ventricular systole not apparent at rest.

Bonow et al. studied 40 patients with HCM and used radionuclide angiography for the evaluation of left ventricular systolic function and diastolic filling, and for the effects of oral verapamil (Isoptin 320-480 mg/day) on the parameters [17]. All but one patient had normal or supernormal systolic function, but 28 patients (70%) showed evidence of diastolic dysfunction as indicated by a diminished peak filling rate and a prolonged time to peak filling rate (Fig. 8). Verapamil did not change the systolic function parameters, but improved diastolic function in 18 patients (40%). This study therefore showed that diastolic filling is abnormal in a high number of patients with HCM, and that verapamil normalizes or improves these abnormalities without altering systolic function.

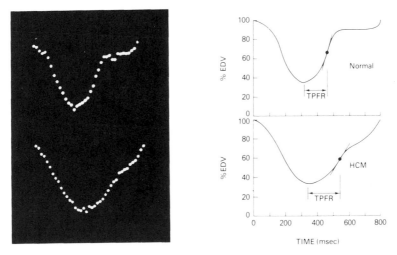

Figure 8
Time-activity curves from a normal volunteer (upper curve) and from a young patient with hypertrophic cardiomyopathy (HCM). The left panel shows the unretouched curves and the right panel depicts the schematic representations of the two curves. The patients with HCM has similar heart rate, ejection fraction and ejection time compared to the normal individual, but peak filling rate is reduced and time peak filling (TPFR) is prolonged. EDV = end-diastolic volume. From Bonow et al. [17 with permission]).

In a recent study [18], Bonow et al. confirmed these findings in 14 patients with HCM and used a nuclear stethoscope for the assessment of left ventricular systolic and diastolic function after intravenous administration of verapamil (0.17-0.72 mg/kg). It was concluded that the negative inotropic effects of intravenous verapamil are beneficial in HCM patients by decreasing left ventricular contractile function and by increasing left ventricular volume. The exact indications for the use of nifedipine

229

in hypertropic cardiomyopathy are not yet clear, although it may be more promising than verapamil because of its effects on improving ventricular filling. Diltiazem improves left ventricular relaxation and diastolic filling without altering left ventricular systolic function.

Conclusion

Radionuclide techniques provide useful information in determining the diagnosis, prognosis and therapeutic responses in patients with any of the several forms of cardiomyopathy. In patients with pulmonary congestive symptoms, radionuclide angiography may allow the differential diagnosis between those forms of cardiomyopathy in which diastolic dysfunction is the major problem and those forms in which the systolic dysfunction predominates.

Moreover, radionuclide angiography can be employed to rule out potential resectable left ventricular aneurysm, usually due to coronary artery disease in patients with congestive heart failure and suspected cardiomyopathy. The potential value of radionuclide angiography to determine the genesis of congestive symptoms in patients with suspected cardiomyopathy is exemplified by recent studies indicating that a variety of exercise-induced changes in left ventricular function can be found in patients with hypertrophic cardiomyopathy. Such patients commonly manifest pulmonary congestive symptoms, but radionuclide angiography indicates the presence of a normal or supernormal function while the patient is at rest. This finding, together with the appearance of septal hypertrophy and the presence of subnormal left ventricular filling rate, points strongly to a hemodynamic problem based on diastolic dysfunction and indicates the need for compliance-increasing therapy rather than inotropic support (calcium blocking agents versus conventional therapeutic approach, appropriate in patients with pulmonary vascular congestion).

Myocardial imaging with thallium is very helpful to distinguish myocardial dysfunction due to coronary artery disease from that caused congestive cardiomyopathy. Furthermore, thallium imaging may depict septal abnormalities in hypertrophic cardiomyopathy.

Research with labeled fatty acids in the field of cardiomyopathy is still in its infancy, but preliminary results are encouraging and stimulate further studies of biochemical disorders in cardiomyopathies.

Finally, although these radionuclide techniques can be quite helpful in the evaluation of patients with cardiomyopathy, application of other diagnostic modalities should be considered initially. These include electrocardiography, phonocardiography, and echocardiography. In the final analysis, the information provided by the appropriate noninvasive technique might establish the diagnosis and obviate the need of catheterization, angiography and myocardial biopsy. If invasive studies are required to establish the diagnosis of potentially treatable disease, serial imaging studies can be useful to follow the therapeutic effect of appropriate medical therapy.

References

1. Okada RD, Boucher CA, Strauss HW, Pohost GM. Exercise radionuclide imaging approaches to coronary artery disease. Am J Cardiol 1980;46: 1188-204.
2. Van der Wall EE, Den Hollander W, Heidendal GAK, Westera G, Majid PA, Roos JP. Dynamic myocardial scintigraphy with I-123 labeled free fatty acids in patients with myocardial infarction. Eur J Nucl Med 1981;6:383-9.
3. Van der Wall EE, Heidendal GAK, Den Hollander W, Westera G, Roos JP. Metabolic myocardial imaging with I-123-labeled heptadecanoic acid in patients with angina pectoris. Eur J Nucl Med 1981;6:391-6.
4. Höck A, Freundlieb C, Vyska K, Lösse B, Erbel R, Feinendegen LE. Myocardial imaging and metabolic studies with [17-I-123] iodoheptadecanoic acid in patients with idiopathic congestive cardiomyopathy. J Nucl Med 1983;24:22-8.
5. Dudczak R, Homan R, Zanganeh A, et al. Myocardial metabolic studies in patients with cardiomyopathy (CM). J Nucl Med 1983;24:P20(Abstract).
6. Bulkley BH, Hutchins GM, Bailey I, Strauss HW, Pitt B. Thallium 201 imaging and gated cardiac bloodpool scans in patients with ischemic and idiopathic congestive cardiomyopathy. A clinical and pathologic study. Circulation 1977;55:753-60.
7. Saltissi S, Hockings B, Croft DN, Webb-Peploe MM. Thallium-201 myocardial imaging in patients with dilated and ischaemic cardiomyopathy. Br Heart J 1981;46:290-5.
8. Arreaza N, Puigbo JJ, Acquatella, et al. Radionuclide evaluation of left-ventricular function in chronic Chagas cardiomyopathy. J Nucl Med 1983;24:563-7.
9. Gottdiener JS, Mathisen DJ, Borer JS, et al. Doxorubicin cardiotoxicity: assessment of late left ventricular dysfunction by radionuclide cineangiography. Ann Intern Med 1981;94:430-5.
10. Pohost G M, Fallon JT, Strauss HW. Radionuclide techniques in cardiomyopathy. In: Strauss HW, Pitt B (eds), Cardiovascular Nuclear Medicine, 1979, pp 326-39.
11. Van der Wall E. Hypertrophic obstructive cardiomyopathy. Evaluation of treatment by invasive and non-invasive methods. Thesis, Groningen, 1972.
12. Bulkley B H, Rouleau J, Strauss HW, Pitt B. Idiopathic hypertrophic subaortic stenosis: detection by thallium 201 myocardial perfusion imaging. N Engl J Med 1975;293:1113-6.
13. Rubin KA, Morrison J, Padnick MB, et al. Idiopathic hypertrophic subaortic stenosis: evaluation of anginal symptoms with thallium-201 myocardial imaging. Am J Cardiol 1979;44:1040-5.
14. Pohost GM, Vignola PA, McKusick KE, et al. Hypertrophic cardiomyopathy. Evaluation by gated cardiac bloodpool scanning. Circulation 1977;55:92-9.
15. Borer JS, Bacharach SL, Green MV, et al. Obstructive vs nonobstructive asymmetic septal hypertrophy: differences in left ventricular function with exercise. Am J Cardiol 1978;41:379-85.
16. Manyari DE, Paulsen W, Boughner DR, Purves P, Kostuk WJ. Resting and exercise left ventricular function in patients with hypertrophic cardiomyopathy. Am Heart J 1973;105:980-7.
17. Bonow RO, Rosing DR, Bacharach SL, et al. Effects of verapamil on left ventricular systolic function and diastolic filling in patients with hypertrophic cardiomyopathy. Circulation 1981;64:787-96.
18. Bonow RO, Ostrow HG, Rosing DR, et al. Effects of verapamil on left ventricular systolic and diastolic function in patients with hypertrophic cardiomyopathy: pressure-volume analysis with a non-imaging scintillation probe. Circulation 1983;68:1062-73.

13.
Clinical significance of silent ischemia and implications for treatment:
Role of radionuclide techniques

Summary

Radionuclide techniques have added substantial information to the detection and clinical significance of patients with silent ischemia. Noninvasive assessment of myocardial perfusion, metabolism, and wall motion have increased the knowledge of the pathophysiology of silent ischemia. Radioisotope techniques may provide information far beyond that obtained by electrocardiographic criteria alone. Whether patients with silent ischemia should be treated can only be inferred from indirect evidence suggested by preliminary trials. Only randomized controlled clinical trials will yield the definite answers as to the effects of treatment on clinical outcome.

Introduction

Silent ischemia has recently been demonstrated to be a common manifestation of ischemic heart disease. Defined as the objective evidence of myocardial ischemia without symptoms, silent ischemia has been estimated to occur in 2.5% of subjects without previous manifestations of coronary artery disease and in 25-75% of patients with significant coronary artery disease (1).

However, its precise clinical significance is still unclear and the treatment of silent ischemia remains the subject of much debate. This chapter reviews the most important clinical aspects of silent ischemia and the potential benefits of treatment of silent ischemia. Particularly, the role of radionuclide techniques in silent ischemia will be discussed.

SILENT ISCHEMIA: CLINICAL SIGNIFICANCE

Pathogenesis

Several mechanisms have been proposed for the pathogenesis of silent myocardial ischemia. These mechanisms include: 1) altered neural pathways, 2) insufficient ischemia to reach the anginal threshold, and 3) an abnormally high threshold of pain

(2). Cardiac transplant patients with surgical denervation of the heart at the time of implantation and diabetic patients with peripheral neuropathy are two important groups of patients who experience silent ischemia because of altered neurologic pathways. However, these patients may experience anginal equivalents such as dyspnea and therefore their angina may not be totally clinically silent. Insufficient ischemia to reach the anginal threshold has been shown in patients undergoing coronary angioplasty; after balloon occlusion of the coronary artery, chest pain is delayed for 20 to 30 seconds. Before the onset of chest pain cardiac contraction is reduced and typical electrocardiographic changes occur. The mechanism of an increased threshold of pain has been demonstrated by Falcone et al. (3) who suggested that higher baseline beta-endorphin plasma levels may play a role in the decreased sensitivity to pain in patients with silent ischemia.

Although all the above-mentioned mechanisms are correlated with the absence of symptoms, the exact mechanisms underlying silent ischemia are currently unresolved.

Means of detection and definitions

There are multiple means by which silent ischemia can be objectively documented. These means include: 1) electrocardiography, 2) two-dimensional echocardiography, 3) radioisotope techniques, and 4) heart catheterization.

Ad 1) For the detection of silent ischemia by electrocardiographic means, both ambulatory electrocardiographic monitoring and exercise electrocardiography are available. Regarding the superiority of either technique in detecting silent ischemia, Epstein et al. (4) have stated that continuous electrocardiographic monitoring to detect ischemia conveys little additional prognostic information over that obtained by exercise testing. As a result, exercise testing is most often used to uncover silent myocardial ischemia. There remains, however, a specific role for ambulatory electro-cardiographic monitoring in: a) patients who are unable to undergo exercise testing, b) patients with acute ischemic syndromes, or c) patients with a negative exercise test despite typical symptoms of myocardial ischemia.

Ad 2) Two-dimensional echocardiography may allow assessment of silent transient left ventricular wall motion abnormalities, both at rest and during physical (or dobutamine-induced) exercise.

Ad 3) Radionuclide techniques employ radioactive tracers to detect asymptomatic abnormalities in myocardial perfusion, metabolism and function both at rest and during exercise.

Ad 4) Heart catheterization allows the assessment of lactate accumulation during atrial pacing, the measurement of coronary sinus oxygen saturation, and the continuous monitoring of pulmonary, pulmonary capillary wedge, and left ventricular pressures in patients with silent ischemia.

Since most of the detection of silent ischemia has been performed with electrocardiographic means, especially with ambulatory Holter monitoring, the definition of silent ischemia has been based initially on electrocardiographic findings. Silent ischemia by Holter monitoring has been defined as ST-T segment depression of 1 mm for 1 minute separated from other ischemic episodes by 1 minute, the so-called "1x1x1 rule" (5). Later on, when it turned out that exercise electrocardiography provided at least as much information on the presence of silent ischemia, the conventional criteria for a positive exercise stress test have been used as well to define silent ischemia. Currently, after introduction of echocardiographic, radionuclide and catheterization techniques for the detection and follow-up of patients with silent ischemia, each modality has provided own specific criteria for the definition of silent ischemia.

Prognosis

Recent studies in patients with stable and unstable angina, and in patients following myocardial infarction have indicated a strong association between detectable silent ischemia and risk of adverse outcome (6-16). In all groups of patients, the presence of transient ischemia on exercise electrocardiography or during ambulatory electro-cardiographic monitoring identified a subgroup of patients at high risk for the development of subsequent unfavourable outcomes. In most studies, survival rates were similar among patients with and without angina. Patients with more than 2mm ST-T depression on exercise testing and/or patients with prolonged episodes of ischemia, ranging from 30 to more than 60 minutes in 24 hours appeared to have the most adverse outcomes. Although further studies in larger number of patients who are followed up prospectively are clearly needed to determine the precise independent role of silent ischemia, the data are strongly suggestive that the presence and duration of silent ischemia are important independent prognostic indicators.

Silent ischemia: role of radionuclide techniques

Although much of our current understanding of the prevalence, pathophysiology, and prognosis of silent ischemia comes from ambulatory electrocardiographic Holter monitoring and exercise electrocardiography, radionuclide imaging has added significant diagnostic and prognostic value to the documentation of silent ischemia (17,18).

Myocardial perfusion scintigraphy:thallium-201
The prevalence and significance of silent ischemia by thallium-201 perfusion scinti-graphy was addressed by several studies. Gasparetti et al. (19) studied 103 patients with symptom-limited exercise thallium-201 scintigraphy, of whom 59 (57%) of patients had no angina on exercise testing. Patients with silent ischemia and those with exercise-induced angina had comparable 1) exercise tolerance and hemody-

namics, 2) extent of arteriographic coronary artery disease, and 3) number of redistribution defects per patient. Using a radionuclide criterion for ischemia, patients were included who might not have been identified by exercise electrocardiography alone and patients were excluded with potentially false positive electrocardiographic responses. Furthermore, the thallium-201 data permitted the assessment of the extent of exercise-induced hypoperfused myocardium, which cannot be achieved by analysis of ST-T segment data alone. The authors concluded that the observed high prevalence of silent ischemia (57%) has important clinical implications because a substantial number of patients with silent ischemia might not have been identified by exercise electrocardiography alone. Koistinen et al. (20), using thallium-201 SPECT, showed a high prevalence of 9% of asymptomatic myocardial ischemia in diabetic patients versus 1.3% in a nondiabetic control group. Their results confirmed the relatively high prevalence of myocardial ischemia in diabetics. However, noninvasive screening of diabetics does not seem justified because of the low pretest probability.

Hecht et al. (21) used exercise thallium-201 single photon emission computed tomography (SPECT) to evaluate the extent of jeopardized myocardium in painful and silent ischemia. Angina pectoris was present historically in all 112 patients studied, but during the exercise studies only 28 patients reported anginal pain (prevalence of silent ischemia 75%). Similar amounts of ischemic myocardium on the thallium-201 scintigrams were observed in the two groups, indicating that both groups of patients were similar with respect to myocardium at risk.

Several authors have compared the clinical outcome of patients with silent ischemia and patients with typical angina (22-25). The Baltimore Longitudinal Study on Aging (22) showed that the prevalence of silent ischemia increases dramatically with age, reaching 15% in the ninth decade of life. An average 4.5 year follow-up in 407 asymptomatic volunteers revealed that 48% of subjects with concordant positive exercise electrocardiography and thallium-201 scintigrams developed clinical manifestations of coronary artery disease, including angina, infarction or cardiac death. However, 58% of all cardiac events occurred in patients with concordant negative thallium-201 scintigrams and exercise electrocardiography results. This study underscored the view that neither exercise electrocardiography nor thallium-201 scintigraphy is useful in screening asymptomatic subjects for coronary artery disease. Younis et al. (23) studied 107 patients with known asymptomatic coronary artery disease for 14 months after dipyridamole thallium-201 scintigraphy. It turned out that reversible and partially reversible perfusion defects were the only significant predictors of critical cardiac events, which were limited to death or myocardial infarction. Heller et al. (24) reviewed the exercise thallium-201 studies of 234 consecutive, unselected patients and correlated the results with 5-year clinical outcome. It was found that the incidence of major cardiac events was not significantly different between patients with or without angina at the time of exercise thallium-201 scintigraphy. Assey et al. (25), using thallium-201 exercise scintigraphy, reported an increased incidence of myocardial infarction in 27 patients with

236

silent ischemia compared to 28 patients with anginal pain during exercise. Silent ischemia was defined as the development of reversible thallium-201 perfusion defects in the absence of angina. Both groups had a similar amount of exercise-induced perfusion defects. They concluded that the presence of silent ischemia identified by thallium-201 scintigraphy is of prognostic value, independent of the extent of coronary artery disease and left ventricular ejection fraction.

Myocardial perfusion scintigraphy:rubidium-82

Selwyn et al. (26) showed a similar degree of myocardial perfusion defect by rubidium-82 positron emission tomography when patients with and without anginal pain were compared. The symptomatic patients had a higher double product and increased rubidium-82 uptake in the myocardial areas remote from the ischemia, suggesting that an increase in myocardial oxygen demand is important in eliciting angina at the time of myocardial ischemia. Deanfield et al. (27,28) demonstrated that silent ischemia precipitated by mental arithmetic and a cold pressor test resulted in decreased regional myocardial blood flow as assessed by rubidium-82 positron emission tomography. Furthermore, the heart rate at the onset of the cold pressor-provoked silent ischemia was significantly lower than that during exercise-induced ischemia.

These findings suggest that episodes of silent ischemia most likely result from a primary reduction in myocardial blood flow.

Myocardial metabolic imaging:iodine-123 phenyl pentadecanoic acid

Kahn et al. (29), in a study involving 45 patients using the metabolic tracer iodine-123 phenyl pentadecanoic acid and SPECT, reported that patients with exercise-induced silent ischemia showed at least as great an extent of ischemic myocardium as patients with painful exertional ischemia.

Radionuclide angiography

Radionuclide angiography has been successfully used to evaluate the clinical significance of silent ischemia. A radionuclide angiography study by Bonow et al (30) reported a 46% prevalence of silent ischemia in mildly symptomatic patients with angiographically proven coronary artery disease. Compared with the silent ischemia patients, the patients with angina in that study showed a significantly greater reduction in global left ventricular ejection fraction, despite similar degrees of coronary artery disease and resting left ventricular ejection fraction. Likewise, Iskandrian and Hakki (31) observed that patients with symptomatic coronary artery disease had worse exercise left ventricular function than those with asymptomatic coronary artery disease. In contrast, Cohn et al. (32), and recently Vassiliades et al. (33), found that similar amounts of myocardium were ischemic when radionuclide angiography was used to evaluate left ventricular function; the severity of exercise-induced global and regional left ventricular dysfunction was independent of the presence or absence of angina during exercise testing. Van der Wall et al. (34)

studied 42 patients following acute myocardial infarction by exercise radionuclide angiography. The presence of silent ischemia was based on electrocardiographic findings during the exercise test. The patients were categorized into two groups: 22 patients had typical angina and 20 patients had no symptoms during the test. There were no differences in global and regional left ventricular function between patients with and without anginal pain, indicating that silent ischemia does not represent a particular functional disease entity in patients after acute myocardial infarction. Rozanski et al. (35) used radionuclide angiography to assess the causal relation between acute mental stress and myocardial ischemia. Silent ischemia precipitated by mental stress was associated with an increase in systolic and diastolic blood pressures that was roughly equivalent to the increase seen with exercise-induced ischemia. These data suggest that, apart from a primary reduction in myocardial blood flow, increased myocardial oxygen demand may also play an important role in the pathophysiology of silent ischemia.

Several studies have addressed the clinical outcome of patients with silent left ventricular dysfunction. Breitenbucher et al. (36) conducted a 5-year follow-up study on 140 patients with documented ischemia and reported that the incidence of myocardial infarction was significantly greater in patients with silent ischemia than in patients with anginal pain. Of 140 patients who had a positive exercise radionuclide ventriculogram, defined as a 10% decrease or more in left ventricular ejection fraction, 84 (56%) patients did not experience angina during exercise. Of the 84 patients with silent ischemia, 12 (14%) had a subsequent myocardial infarction compared with 4 (7%) of 56% of the symptomatic group (P<0.05). Sudden death was noted in seven patients (8%) in the silent ischemia group compared with only one patient (2%) in the symptomatic group (P<0.05). The authors concluded that patients with silent ischemia have a less favourable prognosis than patients with anginal pain.

Kayden et al. (37) studied 12 patients following thrombolytic therapy prior to hospital discharge using an ambulatory ventricular function detector (VEST) positioned over the chest. Left ventricular function was monitored for 2 to 4 hours during routine activity and correlated with a simultaneously acquired electrocardiogram. Eight of 12 patients with silent left ventricular dysfunction suffered a cardiac event (unstable angina, myocardial infarction, sudden death), while 88% of ischemic episodes defined as a decrease of ejection fraction of 5% or more, were silent and unassociated with either chest pain or electrocardiographic changes. Thallium-201 scintigraphy was subsequently performed in 9 of 12 patients with transient left ventricular dysfunction. Reversible perfusion defects were found in only 2 of the 9 patients. Continuous left ventricular function monitoring may be more sensitive for the detection of silent ischemia and may provide important prognostic information beyond that obtained by electrocardiographic changes.

SILENT ISCHEMIA: IMPLICATIONS FOR TREATMENT

The treatment of silent ischemia remains a controversial issue. For a better understanding of the problem, several points need to be clarified. First, as has been stated previously, the presence of silent ischemia has to be based not only on electro-cardiographic shifts of the ST-T segment by Holter or exercise electrocardiography, but also on perfusion defects at thallium-201 exercise scintigraphy or on a decrease of global ejection fraction and the development of wall motion abnormalities at echocardiography or radionuclide angiography. Second, one has to realize that we are not simply treating 'silent ischemia' but patients with proven myocardial ischemia in the absence of symptoms, i.e. patients with functional abnormalities due to coronary artery disease without the occurrence of chest pain. In addition, most patients with silent ischemia also exhibit anginal symptoms. Third, the principal objective of treating patients with silent ischemia should be the improvement of prognosis, an issue that even in patients with symptomatic coronary artery disease -without myocardial infarction- has not been completely resolved. Until now, treatment of silent ischemia has mainly been focused on elimination of episodes of ischemia.

Rationale for treatment

Whether we should treat silent ischemia for reducing ischemic episodes seems a simple question if we assume that the pathological mechanisms of silent ischemia and angina are similar. Furthermore, since it has been shown that patients with silent ischemia have a prognosis similar to patients with anginal pain, it will be a logic issue that both conditions will respond to the same treatment. Several reports have already indicated that drugs that relieve angina can also suppress silent ischemia (38-40). Although silent ischemia can be treated with the standardly used antianginal agents, it is still far from certain that such treatment is necessary or justifies the extra cost it would require. Presently, only indirect evidence is available that active treatment of silent ischemia is beneficial. Until now, no one has compared the effects on mortality of an active anti-ischemic treatment with those of a placebo in a randomized, controlled, double-blind trial in patients with silent ischemia. Nevertheless, the current studies on treatment of silent ischemia show a convincing indirect rationale for its active treatment. In this section the most important therapeutic trials in patients with silent ischemia are reported.

Therapeutic trials

As previously mentioned, the main reason for treating patients with silent ischemia is to improve prognosis and the elimination of ischemia. Treatment should further be aimed at reduction of the "total ischemic burden", which is the sum of all painful and painless episodes of ischemia.
Several types of treatment are available for silent ischemia.

1) Reduction of risk factors

The first measure should be the elimination of coronary risk factors, a precaution whose advantages have been demonstrated clearly by the Multiple Risk Factor Intervention Trial (41). A reduction in elevated serum cholesterol levels suggested improved longevity in the Lipid Research Clinical Trial (42) The patients in these studies who had exercise-induced silent ischemia showed reduction of ischemic episodes when they took care of risk factors.

2) Nitrates

Nitrated are the most effective vasodilators with added properties of lowering preload and afterload. Several studies have reported beneficial effects of nitrates in patients with episodes of silent ischemia (43-49). Schang and Pepine (44) found that hourly sublingual administration of nitroglycerine markedly reduced the frequency of both symptomatic and asymptomatic ischemic episodes. Pepine et al. (45) observed that in patients with wall motion abnormalities on left ventriculography and with no associated pain, low-dose intravenous nitroglycerine could favourably reverse these changes. Shell et al. (46) and Schneeweis et al. (47) reported that transdermal nitroglycerine was very effective in suppression of episodes of silent ischemia. Distante et al. (48) showed that oral administration of isosorbide dinitrate was useful for treating symptomatic and asymptomatic episodes in patients with vasospastic angina. Feng et al. (49) found that oral isosorbide mononitrate was effective and well tolerated in postinfarction patients with silent ischemia. Efficacy of nitrates is enhanced by concomitant use of beta-blocking agents and calcium-antagonists (40).

3) Beta-blocking agents

Beta-blocking agents have been a clinical mainstay of long-term antianginal therapy for over 20 years. Beta-blockade significantly improves mortality and morbidity in at least the first two years after myocardial infarction, and has been proven to favourably influence the circadian rhythm of coronary events (50,51). Gottlieb et al. (52), in patients with unstable angina, showed that addition of propranolol to maximal nitrate and calcium-channel therapy resulted in fewer daily ischemic episodes compared to the patients with added placebo. Cohn et al. (53) demonstrated improved radionuclide left ventricular function with timolol and propranolol compared to baseline in patients with evidence of silent ischemia with exercise testing. In another study, Cohn et al (54) showed that long-acting propranolol abolished the circadian variation in silent ischemic episodes in patients with documented coronary artery disease. Willich et al. (55) determined the effects of metoprolol on silent ischemia and platelet aggregability in patients with proven coronary artery disease. Metoprolol decreased the number and duration of ischemic episodes, but the mechanism of action was not related to inhibition of platelet aggregation. Combination of beta-blocking agents with nitrates, calcium-antagonists and/or alpha-blocking agents may be effective by blunting the tendency of beta-blocking agents to increase vasomotor tone (40,56).

4) Calcium antagonists

Since silent ischemia may primarily be a problem of oxygen supply, i.e. increased vasomotor tone and vasoconstriction, therapy with calcium antagonists seems useful. Nifedipine has been studied in patients with episodes of silent ischemia with conflicting results regarding the drug's efficacy. Cohn et al. (57) treated patients with a combination of drugs in the nifedipine Total Ischemia Awareness Program (TIAP) study. Best results were seen after nifedipine was added to nitrates or beta-blocking agents in patients with either frequent or long episodes of silent ischemia. Mulcahy et al. (58) found in patients with proven coronary artery disease that nifedipine, unlike atenolol, had little effect on either the frequency or total duration of ischemic episodes, and did not alter the circadian distribution of ischemic episodes. The authors concluded that this finding is against the theory that ambulatory ischemia is mainly caused by alterations in coronary vasomotor tone. Deedwania et al. (59) showed that both nifedipine and atenolol were effective in reducing silent ischemic events, although atenolol proved to be more effective, particularly on the morning surge of silent myocardial ischemia. Frishman et al. (60) found that diltiazem reduced the number of episodes of silent ischemia in patients with chronic stable angina. Combination therapy with nifedipine provided no further advantage. Aoki et al. (61) observed that diltiazem prevented the development of exercise-induced thallium-201 perfusion defects in patients with vasospastic angina, of whom 64% were asymptomatic. Van der Wall et al. (62) showed that diltiazem had acute beneficial effects on asymptomatic ST segment depression and global and regional radionuclide left ventricular function in post-infarction patients with silent ischemia. As a result, diltiazem as monotherapy appears to be effective in the treatment of silent ischemic episodes both in patients with stable angina pectoris and in patients following myocardial infarction. (See Chapter 14).

5) Antiplatelet drugs

Transient acute decreases in coronary flow occur when platelet aggregates obstruct a stenotic segment of a coronary artery. Treatment with aspirin may eliminate these episodes. In general, aspirin is being used for the treatment of unstable angina and to prolong life in survivors of myocardial infarction. Mahony (63) showed in six patients with silent ischemia and documented coronary artery disease that aspirin decreased the number of episodes of myocardial ischemia in this patient population. This finding suggests that platelet aggregation is an important causative mechanism in silent ischemia.

6) Percutaneous transluminal coronary angioplasty

Coronary angioplasty has become a routine invasive procedure for the treatment of fixed discrete coronary artery stenoses. In most instances, balloon therapy has been shown successful in alleviation of ischemia. Tuczu et al. (64) showed that coronary angioplasty was a very good therapeutic option in patients who had documented coronary artery disease without symptoms. Anderson et al. (65) performed coronary angioplasty in patients with exercise-induced silent ischemia. Angioplasty achieved a very good primary success and was accompanied by low cardiac event rates and no deaths over several years of follow-up. Josephson et al. (66), using continuous electrocardiographic ambulatory monitoring, observed a reduction in silent ischemic episodes in patients following successful coronary angioplasty.

Hecht et al. (67) evaluated the occurrence of restenosis and the extent of ischemia in asymtomatic patients by tomographic thallium-201 exercise imaging following angioplasty (mean 6 months) and compared the results with symptomatic patients. They found that the thallium-201 imaging accurately identified restenosis in both symptomatic and asymptomatic patients, while the exercise electrocardiogram was inaccurate in detecting silent ischemia resulting from restenosis. The amount of ischemic myocardium did not differ in silent and symptomatic restenosis. Deligonul and colleagues (68) reported data from a large group of patients undergoing exercise testing approximately 30 days after apparently successful percutaneous transluminal coronary angioplasty. The presence of silent ischemia identified a subgroup at high risk for adverse events during follow-up.

7) Coronary artery bypass surgery

The prognosis of patients with documented coronary artery disease is determined primarily by the number of diseased vessels and by the left ventricular function (69). The effects of coronary artery bypass surgery have been impressive for over 20 years, particularly in patients with left main and three-vessel coronary artery disease. To determine whether coronary artery bypass surgery would prolong survival in patients with exercise-induced silent ischemia, Taylor et al. (70) were the first to demonstrate an increase in survival rate after successful treatment of patients with asymptomatic left main coronary artery disease from the Coronary Artery Surgery Study (CASS) registry. Also reported in the CASS registry by Weiner et al. (71,72) is the observation that surgically treated patients with three-vessel disease and left ventricular dysfunction have a substantial lower mortality than similar patients treated medically. Conversely, patients with unsuccessful grafts and/or incomplete revascularization procedures continued to demonstrate episodes of both symptomatic and silent myocardial ischemia (73).

Conclusion

Radionuclide techniques have considerably broadened our knowledge of the clinical significance of silent ischemia in patients with suspected and known coronary artery disease (74). The presence of abnormalities in myocardial perfusion, metabolism and wall motion in the absence of symptoms has accrued valuable information beyond that provided by asymptomatic electrocardiographic changes alone.

Whether silent ischemia should be treated is still unresolved (75). The sole reason for treatment of patients with silent ischemia is to improve prognosis. Although episodes of silent ischemia bear an adverse prognosis, it remains uncertain whether medical therapy or even invasive modalities will influence prognosis. Opinions regarding treatment have been crystallized into two extreme ends of the spectrum from "silent ischemia as silent killer" to "silent ischemia deserves silent treatment" (76). Several therapeutic modalities appear effective in reducing episodes of silent ischemia, but lacking are adequately controlled and randomized studies of this disorder. Until this information is available, we must continue to treat patients on the evidence currently present.

References

1. Cohn PF. Silent myocardial ischemia: classification, prevalence and prognosis. Am J Med 1985;79(Suppl 3A):2-6.
2. Maseri A, Chierchia S, Davies G, et al. Mechanisms of ischemic cardiac pain and silent myocardial ischemia. Am J Med 1985;(Suppl 3A)79:7-11.
3. Falcone C, Specchia G, Rondanelle R, et al. Correlation between beta-endorphin plasma levels and anginal symptoms in patients with coronary artery disease. J Am Coll Cardiol 1988;11:719-23.
4. Epstein SE, Quyyumi AA, Bonow RO. Current concepts: myocardial ischemia silent or symptomatic. N Engl J Med 1988;318:1038-43.
5. Weiner DA, Becker L, Bonow R. Report of group II: detection and diagnosis. Circulation 1987;75(suppl II):49-50.
6. Gottlieb SO, Weisfeldt ML, Ouyang P, Ellits ED, Gesternblith G. Silent ischemia predicts infarction and death during 2 years of follow-up of unstable angina. J Am Coll Cardiol 1987;10:756-60.
7. Quyyumi AA, Crake T, Wright C, Mockus L, Fox K. The role of ambulatory ST segment monitoring in the diagnosis of coronary artery disease: comparison with exercise testing and thallium scintigraphy. Eur Heart J 1987;8:124-29.
8. Rocco MB, Nabel EG, Campbell S, et al. Prognostic importance of myocardial ischemia detected by ambulatory monitoring in patients with stable coronary artery disease. Circulation 1988;78:877-84.
9. V Arnim TH, Gerbig HW, Krawietz W, Hofling B. Prognostic implications of transient -predomi- nantly silent- ischaemia in patients with unstable angina pectoris. Eur Heart J 1988;9:435-40.
10. Tzivoni D, Gavish A, Zin D, et al. Prognostic significance of ischemic episodes in patients with previous myocardial infarction. Am J Cardiol 1988;62:661-4.
11. Gottlieb SO, Gottlieb SH, Achuff SC, et al. Silent ischemia on Holter monitoring predicts mortality in high risk postinfarction patients. JAMA 1988;259:1030-5.
12. Mark DB, Hlatky MA, Califf RM, et al. Painless exercise ST deviation on the treadmill: long-term prognosis. J Am Coll Cardiol 1989;14:885-92.
13. Gottlieb SO, Weisfeldt ML, Ouyang P, Mellits ED, Gerstenblith G. Silent ischemia as a marker for early unfavourable outcome in patients with unstable angina. N Engl J Med 1986;314:1214-9.
14. Bonaduce D, Petretta M, Lanzillo T, et al. Prevalence and prognostic significance of silent myocardial ischaemia detected by exercise test and continuous ECG monitoring after acute myocardial infarction. Eur Heart J 1991;12:186-93.
15. Callaham PR, Froelicher VF, Klein J, Risch M, Dubach P, Fris R. Exercise-induced silent ischemia: age, diabetes mellitus, previous myocardial Infarction and prognosis. J Am Coll Cardiol 1989;14:1175-80.
16. Miranda CP, Lehmann KG, Lachterman B, Coodley EM, Froelicher VF. Comparison of silent and symptomatic ischemia during exercise testing in men. Ann Int Med 1991;114:649-56.
17. Gibson RS. Radionuclide diagnosis and assessment of acute myocardial infarction. Cardiovasc Clin 1989;20:155-72.
18. Dey HM, Soufer R. Efficacy of myocardial imaging in thrombolysis, risk analysis, and silent ischemia. Curr Opinion Cardiol 1990;5:795-802.
19. Gasperetti CM, Burwell LR, Beller GA. Prevalence of and variables associated with silent myocardial ischemia on exercise thallium-201 stress testing. J Am Coll Cardiol 1990;16:115-23.
20. Koistinen MJ. Prevalence of asymptomatic myocardial ischaemia in diabetic subjects. Br Med J 1990;301:92-5.

21. Hecht HS, Shaw RE, Bruce T, Myler RK. Silent ischemia: evaluation by exercise and redistribution tomographic thallium-201 myocardial imaging. J Am Coll Cardiol 1989;14:895-900.
22. Fleg JL, Gerstenblith G, Zonderman AB, et al. Prevalence and prognostic significance of exercise-induced silent myocardial ischemia detected by thallium scintigraphy and electrocardiography in asymptomatic volunteers. Circulation 1990;81:428-36.
23. Younis LT, Byers S, Shaw L, Barth G, Goodgold H, Chaitman BR. Prognostic importance of silent myocardial ischemia detected by intravenous dipyridamole thallium myocardial imaging in asymptomatic patients with coronary artery disease. J Am Coll Cardiol 1989;14:1635-41.
24. Heller LI, Tresgallo M, Sciacca RR, Blood DK, Seldin DW, Johnson LL. Prognostic significance of silent myocardial ischemia on a thallium stress test. Am J Cardiol 1990;65:718-21.
25. Assey ME, Walters GL, Hendrix GH, Carabello BA, Usher BW, Spann JW. Incidence of acute myocardial infarction in patients with exercise-induced silent myocardial ischemia. Am J Cardiol 1987;59:497-500.
26. Selwyn AP, Deanfield J, Shea M, et al. Different pathophysiology of painful and silent myocardial ischemia (Abstract). Circulation 1986;74(Suppl2):II57.
27. Deanfield JE, Shea M, Kennsett M, et al. Silent myocardial ischaemia due to mental stress. Lancet 1984;2:1001-104.
28. Deanfield JE, Shea M, Ribiero P, et al. Transient ST-segment depression as a marker of myocardial ischemia during daily life. Am J Cardiol 1984;54:1196-2000.
29. Kahn JK, Pippin JJ, Akers MS, Corbett JR. Estimation of jeopardized left ventricular myocardium in symptomatic and silent ischemia as determined by iodine-123 phenylpentadecanoic acid rotational tomography. Am J Cardiol 1989;63:540-44.
30. Bonow RO, Bacharach SL, Green MV, et al. Prognostic implications of symptomatic versus asymptomatic (silent) myocardial ischemia induced by exercise in mildly symptomatic and in asymptomatic patients with angiographically documented coronary artery disease. Am J Cardiol 1987;60:778-83.
31. Iskandrian AS, Hakki AH. Left ventricular function in patients with coronary heart disease in the presence or absence of angina pectoris during exercise radionuclide ventriculography. Am J Cardiol 1984;53:1239-43.
32. Cohn PF, Brown EJ, Wynne J, et al. Global and regional wall left ventricular ejection fraction abnormalities during exercise in patients with silent myocardial ischemia. J Am Coll Cardiol 1983;1:931-33.
33. Vassiliadis IV, Machac J, O'Hara M, T Sezhiyan T, Horowitz SF. Exercise-induced myocardial dysfunction in patients with coronary artery disease with and without angina. Am Heart J 1991;121:1403-8.
34. Van der Wall EE, Manger Cats V, Blokland JAK, et al. Silent ischemia after myocardial infarction: a particular functional disease entity? Eur Heart J 1989;10(Abstr Suppl):P280.
35. Rozanski A, Bairey CN, Krantz DS, et al. Mental stress and the induction of silent myocardial ischemia in patients with coronary artery disease. N Engl J Med 1988;318:1005-12.
36. Breitenbucher A, Pfisterer M, Hoffmann A, Burckhardt D. Long-term follow-up of patients with silent ischemia during exercise radionuclide angiography. J Am Coll Cardiol 1990;15:999-1003.
37. Kayden DS, Wackers FJTh, Zaret BL. Silent left ventricular dysfunction during routine activity after thrombolytic therapy for acute myocardial infarction. J Am Coll Cardiol 1990;15:1500-7.
38. Mulcahy D, Keegan J, Sparrow J, Park A, Wright C, Fox K. Ischemia in the ambulatory setting-the total ischemic burden: relation to exercise testing and investigation and therapeutic implications. J Am Coll Cardiol 1989;14:1166-72.
39. Frishman WH, Teicher M. Antianginal drug therapy for silent myocardial ischemia. Am Heart J 1987;114:140-7.
40. Deedwania PC, Carbajal EV. Prevalance and patterns of silent myocardial ischemia during daily life in stable angina patients receiving conventional antianginal drug therapy. Am J Cardiol 1990;65:1090-96.
41. Multiple Risk Factor Intervention Trial Research Group: Exercise electrocardiogram and coronary disease mortality in the multiple risk factor intervention trial. Am J Cardiol 1985;55:16-24.

244

42. Ekelund LG, Suchindran CM, McMahon RP, et al. Coronary heart disease morbidity and mortality in hypercholesterolemic men predicted from an exercise test: the lipid research clinics coronary primary prevention trial. J Am Coll Cardiol 1989;14:556-63.

43. Chatterjee K. Role of nitrates in silent myocardial ischemia. Am J Cardiol 1987;60:H18-H25.

44. Schang SJ, Pepine CJ. Transient asymptomatic ST-segment depression during daily activity. Am J Cardiol 1977;39:396-402.

45. Pepine CJ, Feldman RL, Ludbrook P, et al. Left ventricular dyskinesia reversed by intravenous nitroglycerin: a manifestation of silent myocardial ischemia. Am J Cardiol 1986;58:38B-42B.

46. Shell WE, Kivowitz CF, Rubins SB, See J. Mechanisms and therapy of silent myocardial ischemia: the effect of transdermal nitroglycerin. Am Heart J 1986;112:222-9.

47. Schneeweiss A, Marmor A. Transdermal nitroglycerin patches for silent myocardial ischemia during antianginal treatment. Am J Cardiol 1988;61:36E-38E.

48. Distante A, Maseri A, Severi S. Management of vasospastic angina at rest with continuous infusion of isosorbide dinitrate: a double crossover study in a coronary care unit. Am J Cardiol 1979;44:533-9.

49. Feng J, Feng XH, Schneeweiss A. Efficacy of isosorbide-5-mononitrate on painful and silent myocardial ischemia after myocardial infarction. Am J Cardiol 1990;65:32J-35J.

50. Imperi GA, Lambert CR, Coy K, et al. Effects of titrated beta blockade (metoprolol) on silent ischemia in ambulatory patients with coronary artery disease. Am J Cardiol 1987;60:519-24.

51. Khurmi NS, Bowles MJ, O'Hara MJ, Raftery EB. Effect of propranolol on indices of intermittent myocardial ischemia, assessed by exercise testing and ambulatory. ST-segment monitoring. Clin Cardiol 1986;9:391-7.

52. Gottlieb SO, Weisfeldt ML, Ouyang P, et al. Effect of the addition of propranolol to therapy with nifedipine for unstable angina pectoris: a randomized, double-blind, placebo-controlled trial. Circulation 1986;73:331-7.

53. Cohn PF, Brown EJ, Swinford R, Atkins H. Effects of beta blockade on silent regional left ventricular wall motion abnormalities. Am J Cardiol 1986;57:521-6.

54. Cohn PF, Lawson WE, Gennaro V, Brady D. Effects of long-acting propranolol on A.M. and P.M. peaks in silent myocardial ischemia. Am J Cardiol 1989;63:872-3.

55. Willich SN, Pohjola-Sintonen S, Bhatia SJS, et al. Suppression of silent ischemia by metoprolol without alternation of morning increase of platelet aggregability in patients with stable coronary artery disease. Circulation 1989;79:557-65.

56. Quyyumi AA, Wright C, Mockus L, et al. Effects of combined alpha and beta adrenoreceptor blockade in patients with angina pectoris: A double-blind study comparing labetalol with placebo. Br Heart J 1985;53:47-52.

57. Cohn PF, Vetrovec GW, Nesto R, et al. The nifedipine-total ischemia awareness program: a national survey of painful and painless myocardial ischemia including results of antiischemic therapy. Am J Cardiol 1989;63:534-9.

58. Mulcahy D, Keegan J, Cunningham D, et al. Circadian variation of total ischaemic burden and its alteration with anti-anginal agents. The Lancet 1988;1:755-9.

59. Deedwania PC, Carbajal EV, Nelson JR, Hait H. Anti-ischemic effects of atenolol versus nifedipine in patients with coronary artery disease and ambulatory silent ischemia. J Am Coll Cardiol 1991;17:963-9.

60. Frishman W, Charlap S, Kimmel B, et al. Diltiazem, nifedipine and their combination in patients with stable angina pectoris: effects on angina, exercise tolerance, and the ambulatory electrocardiographic St segment. Circulation 1988;77:774-86.

61. Aoki M, Koyanagi S, Sakai K, Irie T, Takshita A, Nakamura M, Nakagaki O. Exercise-induced silent myocardial ischemia in patients with vasospastic angina. Am Heart J 1990;119:551-6.

62. Van der Wall EE, Manger Cats V, Blokland JAK, et al. The effects of diltiazem on cardiac function in silent ischemia after myocardial infarction. Am Heart J 1989;118:655-61.

63. Mahony C. Effect of aspirin on myocardial ischemia. Am J Cardiol 1989;64:387-9.

64. Tuzcu EM, Nisanci Y, Simpfendorfer C, et al. Percutaneous transluminal coronary angioplasty in silent ischemia. Am Heart J 1990;119:797-801.

65. Anderson HV, Talley JD, Black AJR, Roubin GS, Douglas Jr JS, King III SB. Usefulness of coronary angioplasty in asymptomatic patients. Am J Cardiol 1990;65:35-9.

66. Josephson MA, Nademanee K, Intarachot V, et al. Abolition of Holter monitor-detected silent myocardial ischemia after percutaneous transluminal coronary angioplasty. J Am Coll Cardiol 1987;10:499-503.

67. Hecht HS, Shaw RE, Chin HL, Ryan C, Stertzer SH, Myler RK. Silent ischemia after coronary angioplasty: evaluation of restenosis and extent of ischemia in asymptomatic patients by tomographic thallium-201 exercise imaging and comparison with symptomatic patients. J Am Coll Cardiol 1991;17:670-7.

68. Deligonul U, Vandormael MG, Younis LT, Chaitman BR. Prognostic significance of silent myocardial ischemia detected by early treadmill exercise after coronary angioplasty. Am J Cardiol 1989;54:1-5.

69. Bruschke AVG, Buis B. Progression of coronary artery disease. Curr Opinion Cardiol 1987;2:996-1001.

70. Taylor HA, Deumite J, Chaitman BR, Davis KB, Killip T, Rogers WJ. Asymptomatic left main coronary artery disease in the coronary artery surgery study (CASS) registry. Circulation 1989;79:1171-9.

71. Weiner DA, Ryan TH, McCabe CH, et al. Comparison of coronary artery bypass surgery and medical therapy in patients with exercised-induced silent myocardial ischemia: a report from the coronary artery surgery study (CASS) registry. J Am Coll Cardiol 1988;12:595-9.

72. Weiner DA, Ryan TJ, McCabe CH, et al. The role of exercise-induced silent myocardial ischemia in patients with abnormal left ventricular function. A report from the coronary artery surgery study (CASS) registry. Am Heart J 1989;118:649-54.

73. Kaski JC, Sykora J, Rodriguez PL, et al. Asymptomatic episodes of ST-segment depression during ambulatory ECG monitoring disappear after successful bypass (Abstract). Clin Sci 1985;68(Suppl 11):P58.

74. Amsterdam EA. Silent myocardial ischemia: practical application of evolving concepts. J Am Coll Cardiol 1989;14:1173-4.

75. Meeter K, Fioretti P. Silent ischemia. Should its presence determine treatment? Neth J Cardiol 1990;3:63-5.

76. Shell WE. Silent ischemia: to treat or not. Am Heart J 1990;120:766-72.

14.

The effects of calcium antagonists on radionuclide function in patients with silent ischemia after myocardial infarction

Summary

Since silent ischemia may primarily be a problem of oxygen supply, i.e. increased vasomotor tone and vasoconstriction, therapy with calcium antagonists seems useful. Nifedipine has been studied in patients with episodes of silent ischemia with conflicting results regarding the drug's efficacy. When patients were treated with a combination of drugs, best results were seen after nifedipine was added to nitrates or beta-blocking agents in patients with either frequent or long episodes of silent ischemia. In patients with proven coronary artery disease it was shown that nifedipine, unlike atenolol, had little effect on either the frequency or total duration of ischemic episodes, and did not alter the circadian distribution of ischemic episodes. This finding is against the theory that ambulatory ischemia is mainly caused by alterations in coronary vasomotor tone. Diltiazem has been shown to reduce the number of episodes of silent ischemia in patients with chronic stable angina. Combination therapy with nifedipine provided no further advantage. In the following study we examined the efficacy of diltiazem in patients with evidence of silent ischemia after acute myocardial infarction.

Abstract

In a total group of 72 patients with an acute myocardial infarction, who underwent a maximal symptom-limited predischarge exercise test in conjunction with radionuclide angiography, 25 patients (35%) showed >1 mm asymptomatic ST-T segment depression during exercise. All 25 patients underwent repeated exercise radionuclide angiography two days later, 2 hours following oral intake of 120 mg diltiazem. Double product was not significantly different before and after diltiazem both at rest and during exercise. Maximal ST-T depression after diltiazem was reduced from 2.4 0.9 mm to 0.8 0.6 mm (p<0.01). Left ventricular ejection fraction at rest was before diltiazem 52.1±8.9% and after diltiazem 55.1±12.3% (pNS). During exercise, left ventricular ejection fraction improved after diltiazem from 42.8±12.1% to 49.1±10.8% (p<0.05). Regional wall motion score (1=normal, 2=hypokinetic, 3=akinetic, 4=dyskinetic) at rest before diltiazem was 9.9±2.3 and after diltiazem

9.0±1.9 (pNS). During exercise regional wall motion score improved after diltiazem from 5.9±1.3 to 4.2±1.2 (p<0.02). We conclude that diltiazem has acute beneficial effects on asymptomatic ST-T depression and on global and regional left ventricular function in post-infarction patients with silent ischemia.

Introduction

Previous studies have shown a prevalence of silent ischemia in post-infarction patients varying from 18-39% (1,2). Since in patients following myocardial infarction silent myocardial ischemia is a powerful predictor of subsequent mortality (3), attempts at diagnosis and treatment of silent myocardial ischemia appear to be justified in this subset of patients (4-6). In addition to ST-T segment changes observed during ambulatory electrocardiographic monitoring and exercise electrocardiograp hy, the occurrence of functional abnormalities during exercise radionuclide angiography have demonstrated to have an adverse prognostic value in asymptomatic patients (7-11). This holds in particular for patients after acute myocardial infarction, as in these patients prognosis is strongly related to left ventricular function during exercise (12). Regarding treatment of patients with silent ischemia, calcium-antagonists have been proposed as potential appropriate therapy (13-15). Accordingly, we designed the present study to determine the effects of the calcium-antagonist diltiazem on global and regional left ventricular function in patients with acute myocardial infarction and asymptomatic ST-T segment depression during exercise.

Patients and methods

A group of 72 consecutive patients, who underwent intracoronary thrombolysis for acute myocardial infarction, were exercised in conjunction with radionuclide angiography at predischarge. They had sustained a transmural myocardial infarction based on the presence of electrocardiographic Q-waves in conjunction with typical enzyme rise. The hospital course was uncomplicated in all patients. Silent ischemia was defined as >1 mm ischemic ST-T segment depression in any electrocardiographic lead on the predischarge radionuclide exercise test in the absence of chest pain. In case of development of silent ischemia, which occurred in 25 patients, the exercise radionuclide angiography test was repeated two days later, two hours following oral intake of 120 mg diltiazem.

Radionuclide angiography

The predischarge electrocardiographic stress test was in all patients performed in combination with radionuclide angiography. Radionuclide angiography was carried out with the use of a Toshiba 40A gamma camera. Red blood cells were labeled in vivo by intravenous injection of 750 MBq (20 mCi) technetium-99m. Preceding the

exercise studies, resting gated radionuclide angiograms were made both in the 40°
left anterior oblique (LAO) position with a 30° caudocranial tilt to provide optimal
separation of the left and right ventricle, and in 75° LAO position. Data were
collected in a matrix of 64 x 64 pixels. The resting studies were performed until a
total of 300.000 counts per frame (28 frames per RR-cycle). Thereafter the exercise
studies (maximal symptom-limited) were performed on an exercise table with a
bicycle ergometer. The starting workload was 50 watts and the exercise loads were
increased by 10 watt increments at one-minute intervals with a final stage of three
minutes. Reaching of the final stage was indicated by the development of angina or
exhaustion of the patient, who was then encouraged by the assistant physician to
complete the three minutes. The final stage was used for measuring the exercise left
ventricular ejection fraction (16 frames per cycle). For the exercise studies, only the
40° LAO view was used. Eight ECG leads were recorded and monitored
continuously throughout the study, namely six limb leads and two chest leads V2 and
V5 (V3 and V4 were omitted because of interference with the position of the gamma
camera). In the 25 patients who showed silent ischemia, the radionuclide studies
were repeated two days later and two hours following oral intake of a single dose of
120 mg diltiazem. In all cases the studies were carried out at the same hour as the
baseline radionuclide study and also care was taken for maintaining similar electrode
positions. Except for short-acting nitrates, no anti-anginal medication was allowed
between the two radionuclide studies. All other anti-anginal medication had been
discontinued at least two days before the baseline study.

Data analysis

The exercise electrocardiograms were analysed by two independent observers
blinded to prior treatment and patient identity. Asymptomatic horizontal ST-T
segment depression of >1 mm lasting for 0.08 s after the J-point in any lead was
considered evidence of silent ischemia. Both resting and exercise left ventricular
ejection fraction (LVEF) were determined by an automated edge detection progr am.
The lower limit of normal LVEF was considered to be 50% and an increase during
exercise of 5% or more in absolute values was considered as normal. Regional wall
motion score was visually assessed after dividing the left ventricle into seven
anatomical segments (with exercise only 3 segments were evaluated). Each segment
was graded on a four-point scale with 1 representing normal, 2 hypokinetic, 3
akinetic and 4 dyskinetic wall motion. Grading of segments was performed by two
independent observers unaware of the clinical findings. A total score for the left
ventricle was then obtained (normal score resting view = 7, normal score exercise
view = 3). Reversible ischemic changes in regional wall motion during exercise were
considered to be present in case of detoriation of preexistent resting wall motion
abnormalities in the infarcted area and/or the development of additional wall motion
abnormalities in noninfarcted segments.

Statistical analysis

Statistical analysis was performed with the paired Student's t test. A P value of <0.05 was considered significant. Data are presented as mean standard deviation.

Results

Twenty-five (35%) of our 72 patients met the electrocardiographic criteria for silent ischemia and therefore those patients underwent repeated exercise radionuclide angiography after diltiazem medication. Remarkably, there were no major differences in the site and extent of coronary artery disease between the patients with silent ischemia and those without asymptomatic ST-T segment depression.

Table I. Overall results in 25 patients with silent ischemia after myocardial infarction

	BASELINE	DILTIAZEM	P
Peak workload (% expected workload)	77±12	82±14	NS
Double product (min-1 x mmHg)			
rest	8890±1560	8670±970	NS
exercise	22960±2950	22400±2710	NS
ST-segment depression (mm)	2.4±0.9	0.8±0.6	<0.01
LVEF (%)			
rest	52.1±8.9	55.2±12.3	NS
exercise	42.8±12.1	49.1±10.8	<0.05
Regional wall motion score rest (7 segments; two views)	9.9±2.3	9.0±1.9	NS
rest (3 segments; one view)	4.2±1.6	4.1±1.5	NS
exercise (3 segments; one view)	5.9±1.3	4.2±1.2	<0.02

LVEF = left ventricular ejection fraction
P (diltiazem vs baseline)
two views = 40°LAO, 75°LAO; one view = 40°LAO

Table I shows the overall results in the silent ischemia group before and after treatment with diltiazem. Both peak workload and double product did not change significantly after diltiazem medication. The ST-T segment changes during exercise were favourably influenced by diltiazem and ST-T segment depression was significantly reduced after treatment with diltiazem (P< 0.01).

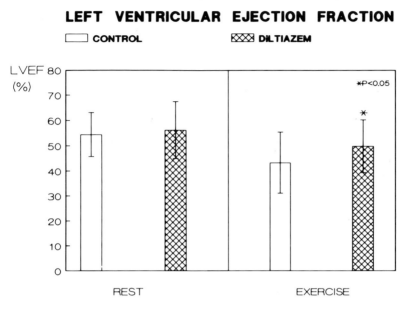

Figure 1
Left ventricular ejection fraction (LVEF) at rest and during exercise before (baseline) and after diltiazem.

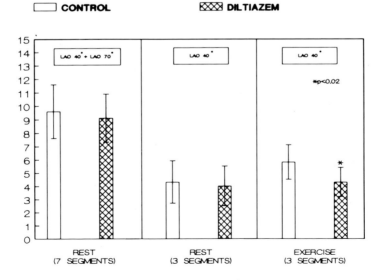

Figure 2
Regional wall motion score (RWMS) at rest and during exercise before (baseline) and after diltiazem.

Figures 1 and 2 show the LVEF response and the regional wall motion score during exercise after administration of diltiazem. Although exercise LVEF decreased both before and after diltiazem compared to resting LVEF, the change was less after diltiazem medication resulting in a significantly higher exercise LVEF after treatment compared to baseline exercise LVEF. With respect to individual LVEF responses during exercise, 18 patients showed an abnormal response at baseline (lack of increase in LVEF with 5% absolute units). After diltiazem only 10 patients showed an abnormal response and LVEF improved significantly ($P<0.05$). Regional wall motion abnormalities at rest were seen in 22 patients and did not change significantly after diltiazem. The wall abnormalities were invariably located in the area supplied by the infarct-related artery. During exercise all 25 patients showed changes in regional wall motion at baseline, whereas 16 patients showed these changes after diltiazem. The regional wall motion score improved significantly during exercise ($P<0.02$).

Discussion

Our study shows that the calcium-antagonist diltiazem exerts favourable effects on both global and regional exercise left ventricular function in patients with asymptomatic ST-T segment depression after myocardial infarction. The improved LVEF response was similar among patients with an abnormal resting LVEF ($<50\%$) and a normal LVEF. In addition, the development of ST-T segment depression was significantly less after treatment with diltiazem. Treatment of patients with silent ischemia appears indicated given the poor prognosis in patients with suspected and known coronary artery disease (3, 7-11, 16-22). In particular in patients after myocardial infarctiont the occurrence of reversible myocardial ischemia during exercise testing, whether or not it is accompanied by angina, identifies a subgroup of patients at high risk of future cardiac events and death (1-3,23). Weiner et al. (23) showed that in patients after infarction with silent ischemia the 7-year mortality was 24% in those who did not have surgery, which was nearly identical to the 7-year mortality of patients with angina (23%), and significantly higher than in patients with negative exercise tests (12%). Gottlieb et al . (1) studied 103 high-risk post-infarction patients with ambulatory electrocardiographic monitoring in the hospital. Painless ischemic ST-T segment depression was detected in 30 patients, 30% of whom died within 1 year compared to 11% of the patients without ischemic ST-T segment changes. In our study we used diltiazem because Frishman et al. (15) had shown a beneficial effect of diltiazem, in contrast to nifedipine, on exercise tolerance and anginal symptoms in patients with both stable angina and silent ischemia. In a recent study by Ghio et al. (24) the beneficial hemodynamic effects of diltiazem on left ventricular function in post-infarction patients were well established in 14 patients with a transmural infarction; it was shown that diltiazem favourably unloaded the left ventricle without concomitant depressant effects on myocardial contractility. Also in other studies diltiazem improved systolic function parameters in patients after myocardial infarction whether or not accompanied by impaired left ventricular function at rest (25-27). In addition, diltiazem favourably affects prognosis since it prevents reinfarction in a subset of post-infarction patients without overt congestive heart failure (28). In our study the patients were exercised 2 hours after a single oral dose of 120 mg. Previous studies had shown that diltiazem prolongs exercise time and reduces the frequency of anginal attacks already from 1 hour after oral admini-stration of 120 mg diltiazem and these effects correlated well with plasma diltiazem concentrations (29,30). Double product during exercise was not significantly changed by diltiazem. This finding was also reported by Petru et al. (31) and suggests improvement of coronary artery flow to ischemic myocardial areas after diltiazem. Increased coronary flow to the subendocard ium and border ischemic zones by diltiazem has been previously demonstrated in animal experiments (32,33). Also clinical studies sho wed that diltiazem increases coronary flow distal to a stenotic coronary artery (34,35). We did not evaluate the effects of diltiazem in patients without silent ischemia during exercise radionuclide angiography. In this way, the effects of diltiazem on ischemic parameters could have been compared in patients with and without silent ischemia. However, the patients without silent ischemia were similar in the extent of coronary artery disease, and they also showed similar LVEF responses and regional wall changes during exercise radionuclide angiography at baseline. These findings at least suggest that patients with silent ischemia post-infarction do not represent a particular functional disease entity needing a particular treatment regimen. Since prognosis is largely related to the extent of the disease (36), the indications for adequate therapeutical management in patients with silent ischemia are very likely the same as in patients with symptoms. Moreover, it has been shown that the drugs used to treat patients with symptomatic ischemia also reduce silent ischemia (14,19). We conclude that diltiazem has acute beneficial effects on asymptomatic ST-T depression and on global and regional left ventricular function during exercise in patients with silent ischemia after acute myocardial infarction.

References

1. Gottlieb SO, Gottlieb SH, Achuff SC, et al. Silent ischemia on Holter monitoring predicts mortality in high-risk postinfarction patients. JAMA 1988;259:1030-35.
2. Theroux P, Waters DD, Halphen C, Debaisieux J-C, Mizgala HF. Prognostic value of exercise testing soon after myocardial infarction. N Engl J Med 1979;301:341-45.
3. Bonaduce D, Petretta M, Lanzillo T, et al. Prevalence and prognostic significance of silent myocardial ischaemia detected by exercise test and continuous ECG monitoring after acute myocardial infarction. Eur Heart J 1991;12:186-93.
4. Cohn PF. Total ischemic burden: pathophysiology and prognosis. Am J Cardiol 1987;59:3C-6C.
5. Rozanski A, Berman DS. Silent myocardial ischemia II. Prognosis and implications for the clinical assessment of patients with coronary artery disease. Am Heart J 1987;114:627-38.
6. Selwyn AP, Ganz P. Myocardial ischemia in coronary disease. N Engl J Med 1988;318:1058-59.
7. Weiner DA, Ryan TJ, McCabe CH, et al. Significance of silent myocardial ischemia during exercise testing in patients with coronary artery disease. Am J Cardiol 1987;59:725-29.
8. Bonow RO, Bacharach SL, Green MV, Lafreniere RL, Epstein SE. Prognostic implications of symptomatic versus asymptomatic (silent) myocardial ischemia induced by exercise in mildly symptomatic and in asymptomatic patients with angiographically documented coronary artery disease.

Am J Cardiol 1987;60:778-83.

9. Nademanee K, Intarachot V, Josephson MA, Rieder D, Mody FV, Singh BN. Prognostic significance of silent myocardial ischemia in patients with unstable angina. J Am Coll Cardiol 1987;10:1-9.

10. Beller GA, Gibson RS. Sensitivity, specificity and prognostic significance of noninvasive testing for occult or known coronary artery disease. Prog Cardiovasc Dis 1987;29:241-70.

11. Breitenbücher A, Pfisterer M, Hoffmann A, Burckhardt D. Long-term follow-up of patients with silent ischemia during exercise radionuclide angiography. J Am Coll   Cardiol 1990;15:999-1003.

12. Gibbons RJ, Fyke F III, Clements IP, Lapeyre AC III, Zinsmeister AR, Brown ML. Noninvasive identification of severe coronary artery disease using exercise radionuclide angiography. J Am Coll Cardiol 1988;11:28-34.

13. Van der Wall EE, Manger Cats V, Blokland JAK, et al. The effects of diltiazem on cardiac function in silent ischemia after myocardial infarction. Am Heart J 1989;118:655-61.

14. Frishman WH, Teicher M. Antianginal drug therapy for silent myocardial ischemia. Am Heart J 1987;114:140-47.

15. Frishman WH, Charlap S, Kimmel B, Teicher M, Strom J. Diltiazem compared to nifedipine and combination treatment in stable angina. Clin Res 1986;34:398A (Abstract).

16. Coy KM, Imperi GA, Lambert CR, Pepine CJ. Silent myocardial ischemia during daily activities in asymptomatic men with positive exercise test responses. Am J Cardiol 1987;59:45-9.

17. Campbell S, Barry J, Rebecca GS, et al. Active transient myocardial ischemia during daily life in asymptomatic patients with positive exercise tests and coronary artery disease. Am J Cardiol 1986;57:1010-16.

18. Schroeder JS. Diagnostic and therapeutic considerations in silent myocardial ischemia. Am J Cardiol 1988;61:41F-47F.

19. Epstein SE, Quyyumi AA, Bonow RO. Myocardial ischemia - silent or symptomatic. New Eng J Med 1988;318:1038-43.

20. Mickley H, Pless P, Egstrup K, Rokkedal Neilsen J, Möller M. Silent ischemia is a predictor of severe angina pectoris after first myocardial infarction. Eur Heart J 1988;9 (suppl 1):314 (Abstract).

21. Van der Wall EE, Res JCJ, Van Eenige MJ, et al. Effects of intracoronary thrombolysis on global left ventricular function assessed by an automated edge detection technique. J Nucl Med 1986;27:478-83.

22. Res JCJ, Simoons ML, Van der Wall EE, et al. Long term improvement in global left ventricular function after early thrombolytic treatment in acute myocardial infarction. Br Heart J 1986;56:414-21.

23. Weiner DA, Ryan TJ, McCabe CH, et al. Comparison of coronary artery bypass surgery and medical therapy in patients with exercised-induced silent myocardial ischemia: a report from the coronary artery surgery study (CASS) registry. J Am Coll Cardiol 1988;12:595-99.

24. Ghio S, DeServi S, Ferrario M, Poma E, Bramucci E, Specchia AG. Acute haemodynamic effects of diltiazem in patients with recent Q-wave myocardial infarction. Eur Heart J 1988;9:740-45.

25. Boström P.-A, Lilja B, Johansson BW, Meier K. The effect of oral diltiazem on left ventricular performance in postinfarction patients. Clin Cardiol 1988;11:739-42.

26. Walsh EW, Porter CB, Starling MR, O'Rourke RA. Beneficial hemodynamic effects of intravenous and oral diltiazem in severe congestive heart failure. J Am Coll Cardiol 1984;3:1044-50.

27. Materne P, Lagrand V, Vandormael M, Colignon P. Kulbertus HE. Hemodynamic effects of intravenous diltiazem with impaired left ventricular function. Am J Cardiol 1984;54:733-7.

28. The Multicenter Diltiazem PostInfarction Trial research group. The effect of diltiazem on mortality and reinfarction after myocardial infarction. N Eng J Med 1988;319:385-92.

29. Hossack KEF, Bruce RA, Ritterman JB, Kusumi F, Trimble S. Divergent effects of diltiazem in patients with exertional angina. Am J Cardiol 1982;49:538-46.

30. Chaitman BR, Wagniart P, Pasterna A, et al. Improved exercise tolerance after propranolol, diltiazem or nifedipine in angina pectoris: comparison at 1, 3 and 8 hours and correlation with plasma drug concentration. Am J Cardiol 1984;53:1-9.

31. Petru MA, Crawford MH, Sorensen SG, Chaudhuri TK, Levine S, O'Rourke RA. Short- and long-term efficacy of high-dose oral diltiazem for angina due to coronary artery disease: a placebo-controlled, randomized, double-blind crossover study. Circulation 1983;68:139-47.

32. Franklin D, Millard RW, Nagao T. Responses of coronary collateral flow and dependent myocardial mechanical function to the calcium antagonist diltiazem. Chest 1980;78(suppl I):200-4.

33. Bache RJ, Dymek DJ. Effect of diltiazem on myocardial blood flow. Circulation 1982;65(suppl I):19-26.

34. Dash H, Copenhaver GL, Ensminger S. Improvement in regional wall motion and left ventricular relaxation after administration of diltiazem in patients with coronary artery disease. Circulation 1985;72:353-63.

35. Vigorito C, Giordano A, De Caprio L, et al. Regional coronary hemodynamic effects of diltiazem in man. Am Heart J 1988;116:799-805.

36. Bruschke AVG, Kolsters W, Kolsters W, Landmann J. The anatomic evolution of coronary artery disease demonstrated by coronary arteriography in 256 nonoperated patients. Circulation 1981;63:527-32.

254

15.
What's new in cardiac imaging

Summary

Currently, nuclear cardiology techniques can not only be employed for detecting, localizing and sizing the extent of myocardial damage, but can also be used in combination with exercise or pharmacologic stress for detecting residual myocardial ischemia and thereby determining prognosis. New radionuclides have emerged that allow greater accuracy and feasibility for distinguishing viable from irreversible injury in patient with myocardial infarction, in particular after reperfusion therapy. A variety of new imaging approaches has been proposed, both with gamma- and positron-emitting tracers. This chapter will address the most important new cardiac imaging agents and the latest developments with the currently used tracers.

I. MYOCARDIAL PERFUSION SCINTIGRAPHY

Thallium-201 revisited

A major topic of interest at the current time is the value of 24-hour delayed imaging (1) and, in particular, reinjection of thallium-201 at rest following redistribution (2). Conventional exercise/redistribution thallium-201 imaging may overestimate the extent of infarction because it has been shown that seemingly persistent defects may fill in on 24-hour delayed images or after reinjection, indicating residual myocardial viability in presumed necrotic areas. Dilsizian et al. (2) demonstrated improved or normal thallium-201 uptake after reinjection in 49% of apparently fixed defects, observed at redistribution. This phenomenon is of major interest in patients after myocardial infarction, as in this group of patients one wishes to know whether the infarcted tissue is completely necrotic or still contains viable, potentially jeopardized, myocardial cells. This may have important implications for further patient management in terms of a more conservative approach in case of a definite necrotic area versus a more aggressive approach in case of remaining viable myocardial tissue (See Section Metabolic imaging).

To circumvent the radiophysical limitations of thallium-201 (low gamma-emission of 80 keV, long half-life of 72 hours), technetium-99m labeled isonitrile complexes have been developed by E.I Du Pont de Nemours & Co. The technetium-99m labeled isonitriles consist of lipophilic cationic technetium-99m complexes. Technetium-99m methoxy-isobutyl-isonitrile (technetium-99m SestaMIBI, Cardiolite®) exhibits the best biological properties for clinical implications. Due to the short half-life of 6 hours, dosages up to 10 times as much as thallium-201 can be administered, resulting in better counting statistics. Similar to thallium-201, technetium-99m SestaMIBI accumulates in the myocardium predominantly according to myocardial blood flow. Although the first-pass myocardial extraction of technetium-99m SestaMIBI is less efficient than that of thallium-201, the relative myocardial uptakes of both tracers are similar under physiologic flow conditions. In contrast to thallium-201, it has a slow washout with minimal myocardial redistribution. These features make technetium-99m SestaMIBI more suitable for SPECT imaging, and allow more flexibility in the time for starting the imaging procedure following tracer injection (3) (Fig. 1).

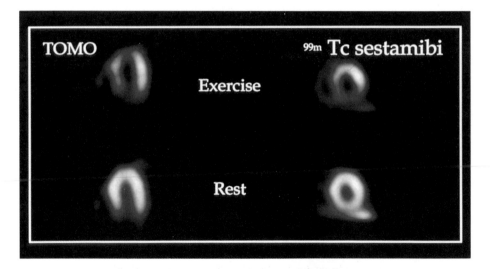

Figure 1
Short-axis Tc-99m SestaMIBI scintigram of a patient with exercise-induced angina. The upper image (exercise) shows a defect in the inferoseptal area which completely fills in at rest lower image). Coronary arteriography revealed a proximal 95% (lesion in a dominant right coronary artery. (Courtesy of H. Larkin, Du Pont de Nemours International S.A., with permission).

The tracer is particularly useful in patients with acute myocardial infarction for the immediate assessment of myocardial salvage in the reperfused regions without any delay in administration of thrombolytic therapy (4). Performing subsequent comparative studies after repeat injections, e.g. 1 to 4 days later, the zone of hypoperfusion representing the final infarct can be identified and compared to the perfusion defect of the initial risk zone (5). Wackers et al. (6) showed that a reduction of greater than 30% in defect size was highly predictive of patency, while the majority of patients with less than a 30% decrement in defect size on delayed imaging had an occluded infarct-related artery. This observation is important because at present there are few reliable noninvasive methods that predict successful reperfusion. In the future, technetium-99m SestaMIBI may be more effective than thallium-201 for predischarge assessment in patients after myocardial infarction because it will enable simultaneous assessments of exercise ejection fraction and exercise myocardial perfusion. The predischarge routine of the future may well incorporate a first-pass analysis of ventricular function at rest, a delayed gated tomographic assessment of the size of the perfusion defect, and the performance of the first-pass and gated tomographic procedures with exercise.

In patients with suspected coronary artery disease, it has been shown that the planar imaging results of exercise technetium-99m were comparable to those obtained with thallium-201. For technetium-99m SestaMIBI, both a stress-rest sequence and a rest-stress sequence have been proven suitable protocols, although a rest-stress sequence may be preferable when using a same-day protocol.

Technetium-99m SQ30, 217

Another isonitrile agent, technetium-99m SQ30, 217 (Cardiotec®), a boronic adduct of technetium oxime (BATO), is a neutral lipophilic flow agent characterized by high myocardial extraction and rapid clearance kinetics. The myocardial first-pass retention fraction of this agent averages 90% in an open-chested canine model. Clearance of the tracer occurs in a biexponential manner with 67% of retained activity clearing with a halftime of 2.3±0.6 minutes. An advantage of this agent is that it would allow repeated flow determinations within short time intervals. Hendel et al. (7) described the initial use of technetium-99m teboroxime in 30 patients using a rapid dynamic planar imaging technique. Delayed postexercise images obtained 5 to 10 minutes after exercise demonstrated rapid disappearance of exercise-induced defects noted on the initial (0 to 5 minutes) postexercise views. Performing an exercise study with technetium-99m teboroxime could permit detection of ischemic heart disease within 10 minutes after tracer injection (Fig. 2). Iskandrian et al. (8) reported a close (89%) agreement for technetium-99m teboroxime and thallium-201 in patients with coronary artery disease, both on planar and tomographic images. The image quality was improved by shorter acquisition times, the upright position of the patient in planar imaging, and appropriate filtering for the tomographic images.

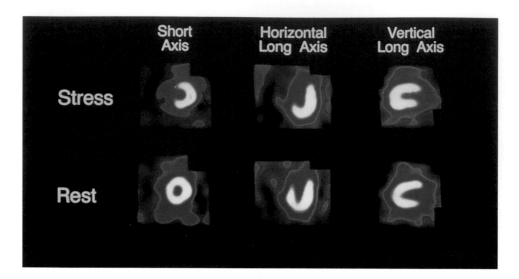

Figure 2
Tomographic Tc-99m teboroxime scintigram of a patient with typical angina. The stress images show perfusion defects in the anteroseptal areas. The resting images are normal indicating revesible ischemia. At coronary arteriography a 90% stenosis proximal to the septal branch of the left anterior descending coronary artery was found. (Courtesy of Ph. Leaver, Squibb Diagnostics, with permission).

Rubidium-82

Currently, rubidium-82 represents the most practical flow marker for assessing myocardial perfusion. Gould et al. (9) were the first to show that the generator-produced positron-emitter rubidium-82 (half-life 76 seconds) provided an accurate diagnosis of myocardial perfusion and flow reserve in patients with coronary artery disease. Williams et al. (10) examined the use of rubidium-82 in the coronary care unit and clinical laboratory for detection of perfusion defects due to myocardial infarction. They studied 22 patients with myocardial infarction and the rubidium-82 images showed similar sensitivity and specificity as for the thallium-201 images.

Nitrogen-13 ammonia

Ammonia labeled with the positron-emitter nitrogen-13 (half-life 10 minutes) has been successfully used to image relative myocardial flow under either physiologic and pharmacologic conditions. The use of nitrogen-13 ammonia requires an on-site cyclotron, and its extraction by myocardial tissue is dependent both on flow and on metabolic trapping catalyzed by glutamine synthetase. Krivokapich et al. (11)

258

performed rest and exercise studies in normal volunteers using nitrogen-13 ammonia and they found that an average blood flow reserve of 2.2 with exercise correlated well with invasively established values. It was concluded that nitrogen-13 ammonia may be used for determining absolute flows in patients with coronary artery disease.

Oxygen-15 water

In contrast to rubidium-82 and nitrogen-13 ammonia, which show a nonlinear extraction at high flow rates, water labeled with the positron-emitter oxygen-15 (half-life 2 minutes, need for on-site cyclotron) is an ideal, freely diffusible, perfusion tracer with an almost linear relation of extraction to blood flow. In normal volunteers, Bergmann et al. (12) showed that oxygen-15 water allowed the measurement of absolute myocardial blood flow. To validate this approach in patients before and after coronary angioplasty, Walsh et al. (13) noticed a significant change in regional myocardial flow reserve following successful angioplasty. This finding demonstrates the utility of positron-emission tomography with oxygen-15 water to assess the effects of interventions on flow and on flow reserve.

Copper-62 (II) pyruvaldehyde bis(N-4-methylthiosemicarbazone

Copper-62 (II) pyruvaldehyde bis(N-4-methylthiosemicarbazone) (copper-62-PTSM) is a new generator-produced positron tracer under development with a high myocardial extraction (14). Further clinical testing and validation is needed.

II. MYOCARDIAL INFARCT-AVID SCINTIGRAPHY

Imaging of acute myocardial infarction with infarct-avid imaging agents allows definition of the zone of acute myocardial necrosis as an area of increased radioactivity ("hot spot"). A number of agents has been used, such as technetium-99m pyrophosphate and more recently indium-111 labeled antimyosin.

Technetium-99m pyrophosphate revisited

Technetium-99m pyrophosphate was first introduced as a means of diagnosing acute myocardial infarction in 1974, and proved to be highly sensitive for the clinical diagnosis of acute infarct (15). Technetium-99m pyrophosphate forms a complex with calcium deposited in damaged myocardial cells. As myocardial uptake is flow dependent, the uptake is poor in the centre of low flow areas of a large infarct, where the uptake is predominantly epicardial. In experimental studies it was shown that technetium-99m pyrophosphate infarcts larger than 3 grams can be visualized by in vivo imaging (16). Especially right ventricular infarction can be easily diagnosed as reported by Braat et al. (17). The timing of the technetium-99m pyrophosphate study is of critical importance, and best results have been obtained 24-72 hours post-infarction by which ideally any intervention to salvage myocardium should have taken place (18). Although the sensitivity of pyrophosphate imaging is high, the specificity is rather low since a number of different disease processes show radio-isotope accumulation by the myocardium. Positive images have been observed in patients with myocardial trauma, ventricular aneurysm, and after radiation therapy. Additionally, the uptake of technetium-99m pyrophosphate in skeletal structures may restrict the proper interpretation of infarct size.

Although these disadvantages have prevented the wide use of technetium-99m pyrophosphate in clinical practice, recent studies have illustrated again its use in patients with acute myocardial infarction. Hashimoto et al. (19) performed early technetium-99m pyrophosphate tomographic imaging, and showed that positive images were very adequate in sizing myocardial infarction soon after coronary reperfusion as early as eight hours after the onset of infarction. In another recent study, Takeda et al. (20) reported that technetium-99m pyrophosphate and indium-111 antimyosin antibody scintigraphy appeared to be comparable methods for infarct detection.

Indium-111 antimyosin

The development of easily applicable infarct-avid agents, that provide scintigrams which become abnormal within shorter periods with closer correlation between tissue uptake and severity of necrosis, is extremely important. Radiolabeled indium-111 antimyosin is a monoclonal antibody that binds to cardiac myosin exposed upon cell death. Maximal uptake occurs in regions of lowest flow, and mostly in necrotic areas (Fig. 3). The first application of radiolabeled antimyosin antibodies for in vivo imaging of myocardial infarction was performed by Khaw et al. (21).

Infarct size in grams can be calculated from transaxially reconstructed, normalized, and background corrected indium-111 antimyosin tomographic images (22). By performing dual-isotope tomographic imaging with indium-111 monoclonal antibodies and thallium-201, infarct size and percentage of infarcted myocardium can be estimated accurately (23). Furthermore, the antimyosin images can be then superimposed on the perfusion images to distinguish between viable and necrotic tissue.

Not only for detection of myocardial necrosis, but also for assessment of prognosis indium-111 antimyosin has proven to be valuable. Follow-up for evaluation of major cardiac events was conducted in a large multicenter study to relate the extent of antimyosin uptake to the major event rate (24). The incidence of cardiac events ranged from 5-8% in patients with negative or minimally positive scans, up to an event rate of about 40% in patients with extensive myocardial uptake of antimyosin. In a subsequent study, Johnson et al. (25) showed in 42 infarct patients that a mismatch pattern between thallium-201 defects and antimyosin uptake (i.e. regions with neither thallium-201 nor antimyosin uptake) identified patients at further ischemic risk.

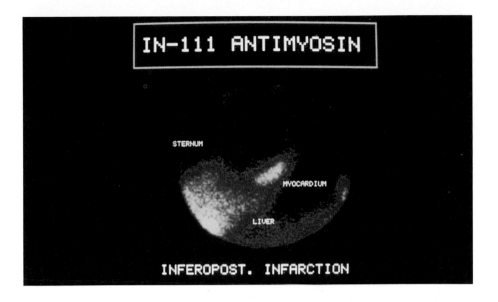

Figure 3
Planar In-lll antimyosin scintigram of a patient with an acute inferoposterior wall infarction. There is clear accumulation of tracer activity in the inferior wall. Note also increased activity in the liver. (From: B. van Vlies, Thesis 1989, Amsterdam; Courtesy of W. van Prooyen, Centocor BV, with permission).

Van Vlies et al. (26), in patients following reperfusion therapy, showed that the level and extent of indium-111 antimyosin uptake could predict improvement of left ventricular wall motion.

Drawbacks of indium-111 antimyosin are the blood pool contamination and interference from liver activity with indium-111, its suboptimal imaging characteristics (gamma-emission 170 and 247 keV, half-life 68 hours), and the late moment of reliable infarct definition at approximately 48 hours after infarction.

Apart from the use of indium-111 antimyosin in acute myocardial infarction, several studies have reported on the value of antimyosin antibodies in the evalation of myocarditis and heart transplant rejection. Carrio et al. (27) studied patients with suspected myocarditis and they noticed a high myocardial uptake (heart/lung uptake ratio of 2), suggesting a considerable incidence of ongoing cell damage despite a small proportion of positive right ventricular endomyocardial biopsies. Ballester-Rodes et al. (28) analyzed the patterns of myocyte damage after transplantation in 21 patients 24, 48, and 72 hours after indium-111 antimyosin administration. Differences in heart-to-lung ratio between absent and moderate rejection were significant. Dec et al. (29) showed that a normal indium-111 antimyosin scintigram is associated with a very low rate (8%) of myocarditis on endomyocardial biopsy in patients with dilated cardiomyopathy and clinically suspected myocarditis. This finding may prompt reconsideration of the need for biopsy in such patients.

III. METABOLIC IMAGING

Scintigraphy with radiolabeled metabolic substrates has become available for noninvasive studies of the normal and diseased myocardium. Metabolic imaging provides insight into the in-vivo myocardial biochemistry and may assist in guiding and evaluating therapeutic interventions for acute ischemic states.

Carbon-11 palmitate, Fluorine-18 deoxyglucose

Radioactive tracers derived specifically for imaging on the basis of their known biologically activity have been studied extensively. Positron-emitters as carbon-11 palmitate (half-life 20 minutes) and fluorine-18 deoxyglucose (half-life 108 minutes), and the single photon agents radioiodinated free fatty acids and their analogs, are suitable for assessing infarct size and viable myocardial tissue (30,31). Positron-emission tomography is valuable in delineating areas with reversible and irreversible injury, in assessing the feasibility of surgical revascularization, coronary angioplasty, or thrombolysis with respect to potentially salvageable tissue (32). The potential benefits of interventions could be evaluated more precisely in patients after myocardial infarction with advanced coronary disease and severely impaired ventricular function. Clinical studies in infarct patients showed that areas with persistent thallium-201 perfusion defects have evidence of remaining metabolic activity in 47% of regions when studied with positron emission tomography, indicating overestimation of irreversible injury (33). The implication, derived from this finding, is that in areas with perfusion defects, if glucose activity remains, the region is viable (mismatch pattern); conversely, if such activity is absent, the area is likely to be infarcted or necrotic (match pattern). In case of remaining viability, patients are more likely to benefit from therapeutical interventions than patients with definite necrotic myocardial areas. Although the assessment of a mismatch pattern is unique to positron imaging, remaining myocardial viability can also be assessed by reinjection of thallium-201 immediately following the performance of the redistribution images. However, Tamaki et al. (34) recently showed that, by comparing thallium-201 to fluorine-18 deoxyglucose, thallium-201 still underestimates the extent of tissue viability. At present, fluorine-18 deoxyglucose seems to be the best accepted radionuclide indicator of viable tissue.

Iodine-123 fatty acids

Metabolic imaging has also been performed with single-photon radiopharmaceuticals using radioiodinated free fatty acids. These can be imaged by both planar and tomographic techniques. Van der Wall et al. (35) demonstrated regionally decreased uptake of I-123 labeled heptadecanoic in patients with acute myocardial infarction. In addition, altered fatty acid metabolism based on abnormal clearance rates was demonstrated in the infarcted regions. Van Eenige et al. (36) demonstrated that myocardial time-activity curves, using monoexponential curve fitting (plus a constant), allow the appreciation of fatty acid oxidation and storage. Visser et al. (37), in acute infarct patients, showed restored fatty acid metabolism in myocardial areas that were successfully reperfused. Hansen et al. (38), using iodine-123 phenyl-pentadecanoic acid (IPPA) and tomographic imaging, reported that this compound was suitable for identifying abnormalities in myocardial metabolism. IPPA was at least as sensitive as thallium-201 for detecting coronary artery disease using tomographic imaging and exercise testing, and provides imaging not only on coronary flow but on metabolic activity of myocardium and may thus be useful in identification of hibernating myocardium. Ugolini et al. (39), in patients with dilated cardiomyopathy, observed a more heterogeneous distribrution of fatty acid uptake and a rapid myocardial clearance.

Carbon-11 acetate

Carbon-11 acetate has emerged as a metabolic tracer capable of assessing metabolic activity, myocardial oxygen consumption, and viability independent of the metabolic environment (Fig. 4).

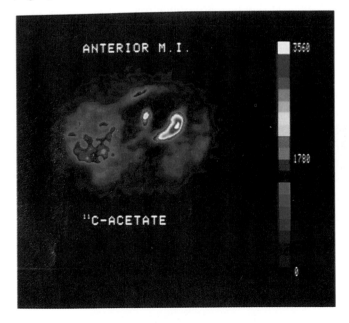

Figure 4
Tomographic image with the positron emitter C-11 acetate of a patient with an anterior wall infarction, refecting oxygen metabolism. There is a metabolic defect in the anterior wall. (From Bergmann et al., Washington University, St. Louis Mo, USA, with permission).

Armbrecht et al. (40) showed a very close correlation between carbon-11 acetate clearance kinetics and myocardial oxygen consumption independent of glucose-loaded or fasting states. Buxton et al. (41) showed decreased myocardial oxygen consumption using carbon-11 acetate together with enhanced fluorine-18 deoxyglucose accumulation early after reperfusion in a canine model. This was initially accompanied by regional wall motion abnormalities which returned to normal 24 hours later after resumption of myocardial oxygen consumption. Walsh et al. (42) showed a significant difference in regional myocardial oxygen consumption estimated from carbon-11 acetate in normal human myocardium compared with areas of myocardial infarction. The clearance of carbon-11 acetate was 6% of that in normal tissue within 48 hours of myocardial infarction and was unchanged 7 days later. The use of carbon-11 acetate may broaden our knowledge of regional myocardial viability in the near future.

Fluorine-18 misonidazole

A new class of imaging agents, misonidazole derivatives, has been developed as tracers of tissue hypoxia and these compounds are selectively retained in hypoxic myocardial tissue. Fluorine-18 misonidazole diffuses across the cell membrane and undergoes enzymatic reduction yielding a reactive enzyme radical. When oxygen is present the compound is regenerated and diffuses out of the cell. In case of absence of oxygen, the reduced fluorine-18 misonidazole remains in the cell. Shelton et al. (43) observed in dogs a significant retention of fluorine-18 misonidazole in ischemic myocardium within 3 hours after occlusion ($23\pm8\%$) versus $12\pm7\%$ and $5\pm2\%$ after 6 or >24 hours respectively (retention in normal myocardium $2\pm1\%$). As marked tracer retention occurred only early after induction of ischemia, this agent holds promise for the noninvasive identification of jeopardized but salvageable myocardium, and may be useful in enhancing the understanding of the basic role of myocardial hypoxia in cardiac disease and its response to treatment.

IV. NEURONAL IMAGING AGENTS

The new ability to noninvasively mapping the distribution of sympathetic nerves may provide important insights into mechanisms whereby an imbalance in sympathetic activity may relate to clinical disorders. The noninvasive characterization of the cardiac sympathetic nervous system by radionuclide imaging techniques provides important pathophysiological information in various cardiac disease states. Imaging of the neuronal pathways may delineate the mechanisms by which neural discharge affects arrhythmogenesis and sudden cardiac death.

Iodine-123 metaiodobenzylguanidine

Iodine-123 metaiodobenzylguanidine (MIBG) can be used to depict adrenergic innervation of the heart. Kline et al. (44) were the first to demonstrate the value of iodine-123 MIBG for imaging the catecholamine stores of the myocardium. Focal denervation produced regional diminished uptake of iodine-123 MIBG (45). In an experimental study in dogs, Dae et al. (46) showed that combined iodine-123 MIBG and thallium functional maps display the regional distribution of sympathetic innervation. Stanton et al. (47) reported that, by comparing iodine-123 MIBG and thallium-201, regional sympathetic denervation occurs in patients after myocardial infarction. Henderson et al. (47) observed reduced retention of iodine-123 MIBG in patients with congestive cardiomyopathy because of increased clearance of iodine-123 MIBG.

Carbon-11 hydroxyephedrine

Also positron-emitting radiopharmaceuticals specific for sympathetic neurons have been developed. The myocardial distribution of carbon-11 hydroxyephedrine proved to be homogeneous throughout the normal heart, with a myocardial to blood pool ratio exceeding 5 to 10 minutes after radioisotope administration. Schwaiger et al. (49) studied patients with recent cardiac transplants and they observed that uptake of carbon-11 hydroxyephedrine was 82% less than in normal subjects.

Fluorine-18 dopamine

Goldstein et al. (50), in an experimental study, used a precursor of norepinephrine, fluorine-18 dopamine, and they noticed that this positron-emitter can be used to visualize sites of sympathetic innervation and to examine cardiac sympathetic function. (Fig. 5)

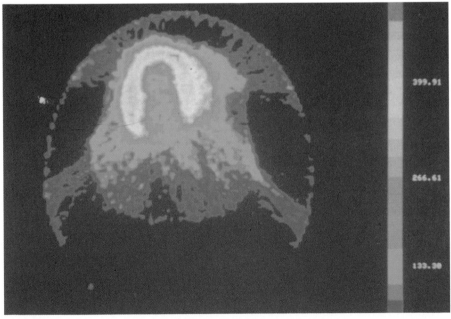

Figure 5
Tomographic image with the positron emitter F-18 fluorodopamine of a canine heart. The sympathetic innervation of the heart is clearly visualized. (From Ref. 50, Goldstein et al., Circulation 1990;81:1606-21, with permission).

Conclusion

Radionuclide imaging with both gamma- and positron-emitting tracers remains a field with a huge perspective in nuclear cardiology. This holds in particular for imaging of myocardial tissue abnormalities. Radionuclide angiography has reached a phase of consolidation: gold-195m is already 10 years old, and tantalum and iridium are struggling to find clinical acceptance. New tracers for myocardial perfusion have been developed, but evaluation of tissue disorders is no longer restricted to the visualization of myocardial perfusion only. Nowadays, imaging of cardiac metabolism, noninvasive detection of infectious disease of the myocardial cell, and visualization of the sympathetic system of the heart has become a clinical reality.

References

1. Kiat H, Berman DS, Maddahi J, et al. Late reversibility of tomographic myocardial thallium-201 defects: an accurate marker of myocardial viability. J Am Coll Cardiol 1988;12:1456-63.
2. Dilsizian V, Rocco T, Freedman NMT, Leon MB, Bonow RO. Enhanced detection of ischemic but viable myocardium by the reinjection of thallium after stress-redistribution imaging. N Engl J Med 1990:323: 141-6.
3. Verzijlbergen JF, Cramer MJ, Niemeyer MG, Ascoop CAPL, Van der Wall EE, Pauwels EKJ. ECG-gated and static Technetium-99m-SESTAMIBI planar myocardial perfusion imaging; a comparison with Thallium-201 and study of observer variabilities. Am J Physiol Imaging 1990;5:60-7 .
4. Santoro GM, Bisi G, Sciagrá R, et al. Single photon emission computed tomography with technetium-99m hexakis 2-methoxyisobutyl isonitrile in acute myocardial infarction before and after thrombolytic treatment: assessment of salvaged myocardium and prediction of late functional recovery. J Am Coll Cardiol 1990;15:301-14.
5. Kayden DS, Mattera JA, Zaret BL, Wackers FJTh. Demonstration of reperfusion after thrombolysis with technetium-99m isonitrile myocardial imaging. J Nucl Med 1988;29:1865-7.
6. Wackers FJ, Gibbons RJ, Verani MS, et al. Serial quantitative planar technetium-99m isonitrile imaging in acute myocardial infarction: efficacy for noninvasive assessment of thrombolytic therapy. J Am Coll Cardiol 1989;14:861-72.
7. Hendel RC, McSherry B, Karimeddini M, Leppo JA. Diagnostic value of a new myocardial perfusion agent, Teboroxime (SQ 30,217), utilizing a rapid planar imaging protocol: preliminary results. J Am Coll Cardiol 1990;16:855-61.
8. Iskandrian AS, Heo J, Nguyen T, Mercuro J. Myocardial imaging with Tc-99m teboroxime: technique and initial results. Am Heart J 1991;121:889-94.
9. Gould KL, Goldstein RA, Mullani NA, et al. Noninvasive assessment of coronary stenoses by myocardial perfusion imaging during pharmacologic coronary vasodilatation. VIII. Clinical feasibility of positron cardiac imaging without a cyclotron using generator-produced rubidium-82. J Am Coll Cardiol 1986;7:775-89.
10. Williams KA, Ryan JW, Resnekov L, et al. Planar positron imaging of rubidium-82 for myocardial infarction: a comparison with thallium-201 and regional wall motion. Am Heart J 1989;118: 601-10.
11. Krivokapich J, Smith G, Huang S-C, et al. N-13 ammonia myocardial imaging at rest and with exercise in normal volunteers. Circulation 1989;30:1328-37.
12. Bergmann S, Herrero P, Markham J, Weinheimer C, Walsh M. Noninvasive quantitation of myocardial blood flow in human subjects with oxygen-15-labeled water and positron-emission tomography. J Am Coll Cardiol 1989;14:639-52.
13. Walsh M, Geltman E, Steele R, et al. Augmented myocardial perfusion reserve after coronary angioplasty quantified by positron-emission tomography with labeled water. J Am Coll Cardiol 1990;15:119-27.
14. Shelton ME, Green MA, Mathias CJ, Welch MJ, Bergmann SR. Assessment of regional and renal blood flow using copper-PTSM and positron emission tomography. Circulation 1990:82:990-7.

15. Willerson JT, Parkey RW, Stokely EM, et al. Infarct sizing with technetium-99m stannous pyrophosphate scintigraphy in dogs and man; relationship between scintigraphic and precordial mapping estimates of infarct size in patients. Cardiovasc Res 1977;11:291-6.

16. Stokely EM, Buja M, Lewis SE, et al. Measurement of acute myocardial infarcts in dogs with 99m-Tc-stannous pyrophosphate scintigrams. J Nucl Med 1976;17:1-5.

17. Braat SH, Brugada P, De Zwaan C, Coenegracht JM, Wellens HJJ. Value of electrocardiogram in diagnosing right ventricular involvement in patients with an acute inferior wall myocardial infarction. Br Heart J 1983;49:368-72.

18. Olson HG, Lyons KP, Butman S, et al. Validation of technetium-99m stannous pyrophosphate myocardial scintigraphy for diagnosing acute myocardial infarction more than 48 hours old when serum creatine kinase-MB has returned to normal. Am J Cardiol 1983;52:245-51.

19. Hashimoto T, Kambara H, Fudo T, et al. Early estimation of acute myocardial infarct size soon after coronary reperfusion using emission computed tomography with technetium-99m pyrophosphate. Am J Cardiol 1987;60:952-7.

20. Takeda K, LaFrance ND, Weisman HF, Wagner HN, Becker LC. Comparison of indium-111 antimyosin antibody and technetium-99m pyrophosphate localization in reperfused and nonreperfused myocardial infarction. J Am Coll Cardiol 1991;17:519-26.

21. Khaw BA, Beller GA, Haber A, Smith TW. Localization of cardiac myosin antibody in myocardial infarction. J Clin Invest 1976;58:439-46.

22. Antunes ML, Seldin DW, Wall RM, Johnson LL. Measurement of acute Q-wave myocardial infarct size with single photon emission computed tomography imaging of indium-111 antimyosin. Am J Cardiol 1989;63:777-83.

23. Johnson LL, Lerrick KS, Coromilas J, et al. Measurement of infarct size and percentage myocardium infarcted in a dog preparation with single photon computed tomography, thallium-201 and indium 111-monoclonal antimyosin Fab. Circulation 1987;76:181-90.

24. Johnson LL, Seldin DW, Becker LC, et al. Antimyosin imaging in acute transmural myocardial infarctions: results of a multicenter clinical trial. J Am Coll Cardiol 1989;13:27-35.

25. Johnson LL, Seldin DW, Keller AM, et al. Dual isotope thallium and indium antimyosin SPECT imaging to identify acute infarct patients at further ischemic risk. Circulation 1990;81:37-45.

26. Van Vlies B, Baas J, Visser CA, et al. Predictive value of indium-111 antimyosin uptake for improvement of left ventricular wall motion after thrombolysis in acute myocardial infarction. Am J Cardiol 1989;64:167-71.

27. Carrio I, Berna L, Ballester M, et al. Indium-111 antimyosin scintigraphy to assess myocardial damage in patients with suspected myocarditis and cardiac rejection. J Nucl Med 1988;29:1893-900.

28. Ballester-Rodes M, Carrio-Gasset I, et al. Patterns of evolution of myocyte damage after human heart transplantation detected by indium-111 monoclonal antimyosin. Am J Cardiol 1988;62:623-7.

29. Dec GW, Palacios I, Yasuda T, et al. Antimyosin antibody cardiac imaging: its role in the diagnosis of myocarditis. J Am Coll Cardiol 1990;16:97-104.

30. Ter-Pogossian MM, Klein MM, Markham J, Roberts R, Sobel BE. Regional assessment of myocardial metabolic integrity in vivo by positron-emission tomography with C-11-labeled palmitate. Circulation 1980;61:242-55.

31. Sochor H, Schwaiger M, Schelbert HR, et al. Relationship between Tl-201, Tc-99m (Sn) pyrophosphate and F-18 2-deoxyglucose uptake in ischemically injured dog myocardium. Am Heart J 1987;114:1066-77.

32. Bergmann SR, Lerch RA, Fox KAA, et al. Temporal dependence of beneficial effects of coronary thrombolysis characterized by positron tomography. Am J Med 1982;73:573-81.

33. Brunken R, Schwaiger M, Grover-McKay M, Phelps ME, Tillisch J, Schelbert HR. Positron emission tomography detects tissue metabolic activity in myocardial segments with persistent thallium perfusion defects. J Am Coll Cardiol 1987;10:557-67.

34. Tamaki N, Othani H, Yamashita K, et al. Metabolic activity in the areas of new fill-in after thallium-201 reinjection: comparison with positron emission tomography using fluorine-18-deoxyglucose. J Nucl Med 1991;32:673-8.

35. Van der Wall EE, Den Hollander W, Heidendal GAK, Westera G, Majid PA, Roos JP. Dynamic scintigraphy with I-123 labelled free fatty acids in patients with myocardial infarction. Eur J Nucl Med 1981;6:383-9.

36. Van Eenige MJ, Visser FC, Duwel CMB, Karreman AJP, Van Lingen A, Roos JP. Comparison of 17-iodine-131 heptadecanoic acid kinetics from externally measured time-activity curves and from serial myocardial biopsies in an open-chest canine model. J Nucl Med 1988;29:1934-42.

37. Visser FC, Westera G, Van Eenige MJ, Van der Wall EE, Heidendal GAK, Roos JP. Free fatty acid scintigraphy in patients with successful thrombolysis after myocardial infarction. Clin Nucl Med 1985;10;35-9.

38. Hansen CL, Corbett JR, Pippin JJ, et al. Iodine-123 phenylpentadecanoic acid and single photon emission computed tomography in identifying left ventricular regional metabolic abnormalities in patients with coronary heart disease: comparison with thallium-201 myocardial tomography. J Am Coll Cardiol 1988;12:78-87.

39. Ugolini V, Hansen CL, Kulkarni PV, Jansen DE, Akers MS, Corbett JR. Abnormal myocardial fatty acid metabolism in dilated cardiomyopathy detected by iodine-123 phenylpentadecanoic acid and tomographic imaging. Am J Cardiol 1988;62:923-8.

40. Armbrecht J, Buxton D, Schelbert HR. Validation of {1-11C}acetate as a tracer for noninvasive assessment of oxidative metabolism with positron-emission tomography in normal, ischemic, postischemic, and hyperemic canine myocardium. Circulation 1990;81:1584-605.

41. Buxton D, Schwaiger M, Mody F, et al. Regional abnormality in oxygen consumption in reperfused myocardium assessed with {1-11C}acetate and positron-emission tomography. Am J Cardiac Imaging 1989;3:276-87.

42. Walsh MN, Geltman EM, Brown MA, et al. Noninvasive estimation of regional myocardial oxygen consumption by positron-emission tomography with carbon-11 acetate in patients with myocardial infarction. J Nucl Med 1989;30:1798-808.

43. Shelton M, Hwang D-R, Herrero P, Walsh M. In vivo delineation of myocardial hypoxia during coronary occlusion using fluorine-18 fluoromisonidazole and positron-emission tomography: a potential approach for identification of jeopardized myocardium. J Am Coll Cardiol 1990;16:477-85.

44. Kline RC, Swanson DP, Wieland DM, et al. Myocardial imaging in man with I-123 metaiodobenzyl-guanidine. J Nucl Med 1981;22:192-32.

45. Minardo JD, Tuli MM, Mock BH, et al. Scintigraphic and electrophysiological evidence of canine myocardial sympathetic denervation and reinnervation produced by myocardial infarction or phenol application. Circulation 1988;78:1008-19.

46. Dae MW, O'Connell JW, Botvinick EH, et al. Scintigraphic assessment of regional cardiac adrenergic innervation. Circulation 1989;79:634-44.

47. Stanton MS, Tuli MM, Radtke NL, et al. Regional sympathetic denervation after myocardial infarction in humans detected noninvasively using I-123-metaiodobenzylguanidine. J Am Coll Cardiol 1989;14:1519-26.

48. Henderson EB, Kahn JK, Corbett JR, et al. Abnormal I-123 metaiodobenzylguanidine myocardial washout and distribution may reflect myocardial adrenergic derangement in patients with congestive cardiomyopathy. Circulation 1988;78:1192-9.

49. Schwaiger M, Kalff V, Rosenspire K, et al. Evaluation of sympathetic nervous system in human heart by positron-emission tomography. Circulation 1990;82:457-64.

50. Goldstein DS, Chang PC, Eisenhofer G, et al. Positron emission tomographic imaging of cardiac sympathetic innervation and function. Circulation 1990;81:1606-21.

16.
Guidelines for clinical use in nuclear cardiology

Introduction

The use of radioactive tracers in clinical cardiology has become a routine procedure in the diagnosis and management of patients with cardiac disease. Since the role of nuclear cardiology has become increasingly important amongst other diagnostic techniques, the cardiac radionuclide imaging procedures need further refinement and require continued investigation to prove or disprove their clinical utility. Accordingly, it is considered important to define the current usefulness of these procedures and to provide recommendations for today cardiac imaging. This chapter includes a description of cardiac instrumentation, the most common procedures, the clinical utilities, and the appropriate recommendations.

This report is divided into five different sections:

 I. Instrumentation
 II. Nuclear cardiology procedures
III. Clinical indications
IV. Imaging protocols
 V. Personnel and equipment facilities

I. INSTRUMENTATION

Radionuclide cardiac imaging is performed with a gamma camera connected with a computer. The camera is used to convert the radiation distribution into a pictorial representation, called the scintigram. This image can be displayed on an oscilloscope or can be stored in a computer memory for further data analysis.
The currently used gamma detectors can be divided into:

A.   *Conventional gamma cameras*
     1) single crystal camera (Anger camera),
     2) multicrystal camera,
     3) non-imaging probe (nuclear stethoscope)

B.   *Specially dedicated gamma cameras*
      1) Single photon emission computed tomography (SPECT),
      2) Positron camera (Positron emission tomography, PET)

ad A. *Conventional gamma cameras*

The single crystal camera is most widely used in clinical cardiology and technically adequate for providing most of the clinically important nuclear cardiology information such as myocardial perfusion scintigraphy and radionuclide angiography. The multicrystal gamma camera is a more sensitive device than the single type camera and is therefore very well suited for first pass radionuclide angiography. A modification of the gamma camera involves the use of a nuclear probe or nuclear "stethoscope", which is a small high-sensitivity device but generates no images. Although initially advocated as a promising tool, its clinical utility has still to be determined.

ad B. *Specially dedicated gamma cameras*

The SPECT camera generates cross-sectional tomographic images of the heart by two different approaches, 1) longitudinal tomography, and 2) transaxial tomography. The longitudinal approach (with for instance the seven pinhole collimator) views the heart from a limited number of angles, but this technique has currently no wide application. With the transaxial approach the camera rotates at least 180° around the patient and multiple images will be obtained at different angles relative to the heart. Its clinical experience is rather large but its definite role has to be established.

The positron (PET) camera is a less widely available and rather expensive type of multicrystal camera, and is mostly used as a research tool. The PET camera employs one or more rings of detectors arranged around the patient and it detects only positron (positive electron) emitting radioactive tracers. It has been shown a very valuable device for the detection and quantitative analysis of regional changes in coronary blood flow and myocardial metabolism. Until now, no clinical cardiology studies have been performed with positron emission tomography in the Netherlands. In the future, the University Hospital of Groningen will start with clinical cardiac PET evaluations.

II. NUCLEAR CARDIOLOGY PROCEDURES

Broadly speaking, radionuclide cardiology techniques fall into two major categories: those concerned with the heart as a muscle and those concerned with the heart as a pump. However, with the extension of these techniques and the development of new radioactive tracers, a lot of different approaches have become possible for the study of cardiac muscle and function. Since a variety of different names has been used for identification of each of the procedures, two special reports (1,2) by the International Task Force Committee on Nuclear Cardiology have been appeared in recent years. In both reports extensive guidelines have been proposed.

In our report the most important issues raised by the International Committee are described and additional information based on our own experience will be provided. The most commonly used procedures in today cardiac imaging are:

A.   **Radionuclide angiography (RNA)**
1. First pass RNA
2. Equilibrium RNA

B.   **Myocardial scintigraphy**
1. Myocardial perfusion scintigraphy
2. Myocardial infarct-avid scintigraphy
3. Myocardial metabolic imaging
4. Miscellaneous procedures

ad A. **Radionuclide angiography**

RNA techniques are used for the noninvasive evaluation of cardiac function. Two RNA techniques can be used; 1) First pass RNA, and 2) Equilibrium RNA. Usually for both methods technetium-99m (Tc-99m) is used as the imaging agent. Its physical half-life is 6 hours and its gamma-energy of 140 keV, ideally suited to current gamma cameras.

1)   *First pass RNA*

With the first pass technique 550-750 MegaBecquerel (MBq, = 15-20 milliCurie, mCi) Tc-99m pertechnetate (or other Tc-99m compounds) is injected intravenously as a compact bolus. Subsequently, the radioactivity is measured during the first pass of the tracer through the central circulation as it moves into the right atrium, right ventricle, pulmonary artery, lungs, left atrium, and left ventricle. Data are collected for approximately 20-30 seconds. By the generation of time-activity curves one can reliably determine left and right ventricular ejection fraction (LVEF, RVEF) based on changes in radioactivity over time (4-5 RR intervals). In particular, RVEF can adequately be determined since there is no overlap of left ventricular blood pool activity as in the equilibrium approach. Furthermore, the first pass approach is very well suited for left to right shunt detection and for qualitative assessment of regional wall motion abnormalities. First pass RNA can be performed both at rest and during exercise. The efficacy and reliability of the first pass method depend on obtaining sufficiently high count rates to assure statistical reliability and therefore best results are obtained with a multicrystal high-sensitivity camera.

2)   *Equilibrium RNA*

The equilibrium technique uses Tc-99m labeled to red cells and the cardiac blood pool can be imaged for several hours after administration. Data are recorded in synchrony with the R-wave of the electrocardiogram and, using the multiple gated acquisition approach, every cardiac cycle is divided into 16-28 frames. Several hundred cycles are summed up for an imaging interval ranging from 2-15 minutes. From these data a time-activity curve can be generated over the left ventricle and LVEF can be determined. The equilibrium technique can be applied both at rest and during exercise, and also allows the evaluation of changes in regional wall motion during exercise.

ad B. **Myocardial scintigraphy**

Myocardial scintigraphy techniques are usually employed for the evaluation of muscle cell viability using tracers that are either markers of perfusion and/or metabolism, or concentrate within necrotic myocardial cells.

1) *Myocardial perfusion scintigraphy*

Myocardial perfusion scintigraphy is a unique aspect of nuclear cardiology for imaging of regional myocardial blood flow distribution. Thallium-201 (Tl-201, 80 keV, half-life 72 hours) is currently the radionuclide of choice. After intravenous injection of 55-75 MBq (1.5-2 mCi) Tl-201 distributes in proportion to regional blood flow. Tl-201 is extracted by viable myocardium and within 10 minutes an adequate myocardial image can be obtained. Myocardial infarction or ischemia may be diagnosed by the visually estimated findings of absent or diminished tracer uptake (cold spot) in regional myocardial areas. Tl-201 is particularly useful in combination with the electrocardiogram during a standard symptom-limited exercise test for the detection of transient exercised-induced ischemia. This is based on redistribution of Tl-201 which results in disappearance of defects at rest after exercise-induced scintigraphic perfusion defects. Comparison of the exercise scintigrams and the resting (redistribution) images taken 3-4 hours later may show, a) absence of defects (normal scan), b) filling in of defects (transient ischemia), or c) persistence of defects (prior myocardial infarction without additional ischemia). Apart from visual assessment, quantitative analysis of Tl-201 distribution, including washout kinetics provides additional information of abnormal flow in individual coronary arteries. Unfortunately, not all radionuclide imaging laboratories operate quantitative analysis since its clinical value is still in dispute.

A slightly different approach using TI-201 scintigraphy is pharmacologic stress with intravenous dipyridamole in patients unable to exercise. Compared to standard exercise testing, pharmacologic stress with dipyridamole shows similar results.

The relatively poor resolution of Tl-201 has led to a search for a Tc-99m labeled perfusion agent. A rather new agent is Tc-99m-hexakis-methoxy-isobutyl-isonitrile (SestaMIBI, Cardiolite[R]) that localizes in the myocardium similar to Tl-201, but lacks redistribution after exercise-induced ischemia. This means that an additional injection at rest is necessary for the assessment of transient ischemia. Advantages of Tc-99m labeled SestaMIBI are its optimal gamma-energy (140 keV) and the potential of tomographic studies with SPECT. Until now, clinical studies have been performed with promising results but it has certainly not replaced Tl-201 for myocardial perfusion imaging.

A new compound is Tc-99m labeled Teboroxime (Cardiotec[R]) which has shown promising initial results for perfusion imaging of the myocardium. Clinical validation has to be awaited.

2) *Myocardial infarct-avid scintigraphy*

At present, two radiopharmaceuticals can be employed for imaging necrotic myocardial areas in patients with myocardial infarction. One such tracer is Tc-99m pyrophosphate which localizes in zones with recently infarcted myocardium (hot spot). The best visualization of infarcted regions occurs 48 to 72 hours after the acute event, which reduces the clinical value of this agent.

A more recently developed tracer involves the indium-111 tagged specific monoclonal antibody against cardiac myosin (Myoscint[R]), which shows maximal accumulation in necrotic areas 18 to 24 hours after the acute event. This agent may also be useful for the early detection of cardiac rejection after heart transplantation. Although very promising in relatively small patient studies, large-scale clinical studies must be performed to prove the value of Indium-III antimyosin in the acute clinical setting. Particularly, the additional merits have to be proven over other diagnostic approaches.

3) *Myocardial metabolic imaging*

Radiolabeled free fatty acids with the gamma-emitter iodine-123 (159 keV, half-life 13.2 hours) have been used for myocardial imaging and for assessment of cardiac metabolism by the external measurement of fatty acid kinetics expressed in myocardial turnover rates. Although excellent images have been obtained, the kinetics are not well understood which makes the use of radioiodinated fatty acids currently still a research tool. Therefore, the clinical value of these gamma-emitting tracers has yet to be determined and more is expected from the positron-emitting metabolic tracers.

4) *Miscellaneous procedures*

Other radionuclide techniques that have been applied to the cardiovascular system are; a) assessment of regional myocardial blood flow after intracoronary injection of xenon-133 or krypton-81m, b) thrombus imaging with indium-111 radiolabeled platelets, c) imaging with gallium-67 for detection of myocarditis. Their clinical value is not totally proven and these studies remain experimental.

III. Clinical indications (Table I)

Table 1 Clinical value of standard nuclear cardiology techniques.

	Perfusion scintigraphy		Radionuclide Angiography			
	Tl-201		First Pass Tc-99m		Equilibrium Tc-99m-RBC	
	Rest	Ex	Rest	Ex	Rest	Ex
Unstable Angina	+	-	+	-	+	-
Acute Myocardial Infarction	+	-	+	-	+	-
Coronary Artery Disease	+	+++	+	+++	+	+++
Valvular Heart Disease	+	+	+	+	++	+++
Cardiomyopathies	+	+	+	+	+++	+++
Congenital Heart Disease	+	+	++	+	+	++

Tl-201 = Thallium-201   Tc-99m = Technetium-99   Tc-99m-RBC = Technetium-99 labeled to red blood cells   Ex = Exercise, - = does not apply, + = limited value, ++ = useful but other techniques are useful as well, +++ = very useful

A) *Unstable angina*

The use of radionuclide techniques in the diagnosis of unstable angina is limited because they must be applied during chest pain and compared with studies without chest pain. Therefore, logistic problems prevent wide applicability of the imaging techniques in unstable angina.

B) *Acute myocardial infarction*

The clinical use of radionuclide imaging in the diagnosis of acute myocardial infarction is limited. Segmental Tl-201 perfusion defects occur in 100% of patients within 6 hours after the acute event, but the sensitivity of the test declines when the images are made later than 6 hours. Moreover, a positive test does not distinguish between acute ischemia, acute infarction, or old infarction. Only in case of a nondiagnostic electrocardiogram or when the diagnosis is doubtful, Tl-201 imaging can be a useful adjunct for diagnosing acute myocardial infarction.

The use of RNA offers a valuable tool for the assessment of complications associated with acute myocardial infarction, such as diminished left or right ventricular function or the detection of a (pseudo)aneurysm. This may have important implications for patient management in the acute phase. The radionuclide techniques have also a major impact on the prognosis after myocardial infarction since the prognosis is predominantly determined by the extent of residual ischemia and by residual left ventricular function. The results of Tl-201 exercise scintigraphy before discharge have substantial predictive value for the occurrence of early and late cardiac events. Also RNA at rest and during exercise may be valuable tests additional to the standard predischarge exercise test, since LVEF at rest and the response to exercise are important prognostic indicators.

C) *Coronary artery disease*

The major and most important application of the radionuclide techniques is the evaluation of patients with suspected coronary artery disease.

The combination of exercise electrocardiography with the radionuclide techniques provides optimal diagnostic and, in particular, prognostic information. Based on Bayes' theorem, the predictive value of a test depends on the prevalence of disease (pretest likelihood of disease). The prevalence is determined by gender, age, and symptoms and can be estimated from specially designed tables (3). Since the tests provide maximal additional information in a population with a disease prevalence of 50%, the techniques are of greatest value in populations with a pretest likelihood in the range of 30-70%. In practical terms, the tests are of most benefit in middle-aged patients with atypical angina, but they have reduced value in elderly patients with typical angina or in young patients with non-anginal chest pain. Exercise radionuclide studies should always be considered in symptomatic patients with abnormal resting electrocardiograms and/or equivocal ST-T wave abnormalities during exercise. Overall sensitivity and specificity of the radionuclide techniques in combination with the exercise electrocardiogram are substantially higher than of the exercise electrocardiogram alone.

The prediction of the extent of coronary artery disease is difficult since only the artery that becomes hemodynamically most compromised during exercise will show scintigraphic abnormalities. On the other hand, Tl-201 scintigraphy has been found useful for the detection and location of individual coronary artery stenoses. The sensitivity is high (80-90%) in particular for stenoses of the left anterior descending and right coronary artery. The assessment of the severity of the individual stenosis may be important in patients to undergo elective angioplasty and in whom the functional significance of the stenosis is important to know. Radionuclide techniques are very helpful to evaluate long-term follow-up after myocardial revascularization. In patients following thrombolysis, angioplasty, or venous bypass surgery, Tl-201 exercise scintigraphy can be used to evaluate the therapeutic effects or to define the ischemic segments of the left ventricle in case of recurrent symptoms. Also exercise RNA provides useful information on cardiac function after interventional procedures, but detailed segmental analysis is limited since only single projections are obtained during exercise.

Apart from interventional procedures, also the effects of various forms of medical therapy can be assessed with radionuclide imaging techniques.

D) *Valvular heart disease*

Both first pass and equilibrium RNA provide a means to reliably evaluate right and left ventricular function in patients with valvular heart disease. They have also been used to assess the severity of aortic or mitral regurgitation by measuring regurgitant fraction based on differences in stroke counts of the left and right ventricle. However, difficulties in separating counts from enlarged ventricles and atria restricts the accuracy of the method and makes RNA of limited value for adequate quantitative assessment. Serial determinations of LVEF can be used as a guideline for the decision about timing of valve repair in patients with aortic regurgitation, but still no consensus has been reached about the clinical significance of an abnormal ejection fraction response to exercise.

E) *Myocarditis and Cardiomyopathies*

In patients suspected of myocarditis RNA is very useful for the detection of left and right ventricular dysfunction. In particular, serial radionuclide angiography is valuable for detecting reduced left ventricular function in patients treated with Adriamycin which is potentially toxic to myocardial tissue.

The diagnosis of dilated cardiomyopathy can be very well established by radionuclide angiography. Usually a global biventricular dysfunction is observed although left ventricular function is mostly more compromised.

Tl-201 scintigraphy can be used to distinguish between congestive and ischemic cardiomyopathy, since the former shows inhomogeneous Tl-201 uptake and the latter demonstrates large defects of 40% or more of the left ventricular circumference on the Tl-201 scintigrams.

In patients with hypertrophic cardiomyopathy the RNA technique may provide important information by showing a hypercontractile left ventricle with an abnormally high LVEF, and a hypertrophied interventricular septum. Also diastolic function can be evaluated by observing the left ventricular volume curve, and the effects of therapeutic agents on diastolic function can be assessed.

F) *Congenital heart disease*

First pass RNA allows identification and quantitation of left to right shunts. Left to right shunts result in high levels of radioactivity in the right ventricle or the lungs, and the resultant time-activity curves obtained from different compartments can be used to localize the level of the shunt. Left to right shunts can be quantitated using the ratio of the pulmonary to systemic flow from the time-activity curve over the right lung. Since the diagnosis is based on delayed pulmonary transit, other clinical causes of pulmonary transit delay (valvular heart disease, congestive heart failure) have to be excluded.

Right to left shunts can be qualitatively assessed by early visualization of activity in the left ventricle or in the aorta.

The use of Tl-201 scintigraphy in valvular heart disease is very limited and may only be appropriate in case of suspected concomitant coronary artery disease.

In general, radionuclide techniques are no first-choice methods for demonstrating intracardiac shunts.

IV. IMAGING PROTOCOLS

Protocol Tl-201 exercise scintigraphy

There is a general agreement on a standard protocol for myocardial perfusion scintigraphy with Tl-201. The patients are usually exercised on a treadmill or a bicycle ergometer with an intravenous line inserted into a dorsal hand vein. Long-acting antianginal medication should be discontinued at least 48 hours before the test provided the condition of the patient allows such a regimen. Also food intake before the test should be kept to a minimum. A 12-lead electrocardiogram, modified according to Mason-Likar, is obtained every minute and patients exercise until the appearance of symptoms (angina or fatigue). Next criteria for discontinuation of the exercise are the occurrence of hypotension and/or the development of malignant arrhythmias. The patients are injected with a bolus of 55-75 MBq (1.5-2.0 mCi) Tl-201 intravenously at maximal exercise and asked to continue the exercise for 30 seconds during which time the Tl-201 is effectively taken up by the myocardium. Imaging starts preferably within 5 minutes after termination of the exercise with the use of a standard gamma camera interfaced with a nuclear medicine computer. A low-energy high-sensitivity collimator is employed with a 20% window around the 80 keV energy peak of Tl-201. Images of 6-8 minutes duration each are collected in the anterior, 35° and 70° left anterior oblique (LAO) positions. Routinely, 500.000 counts per image are collected with a maximal acquisition time of 8 minutes per projection. The 3 projections are collected again 3-4 hours after the initial series of images without the need for an additional thallium injection. These late images are called delayed or redistribution images. Between the exercise and redistribution images the patient is asked to refrain from substantial meals and to preferably limit his intake to soft drinks.

Reinjection

Recently, it has been demonstrated that reinjection of Tl-201 following the acquisition of the redistribution images may show additionally filling in of seemingly persistent defects. This finding indicates that some areas that were presumed to be necrotic still contain viable tissue. Since this may have important consequences for patient management, it is our policy to follow a standard reinjection procedure in all patients referred for Tl-201 exercise scintigraphy. The excess radiation dose (0.5 mCi, 18 MBq) is largely compensated by improved diagnosis and subsequent better management strategy.

Interpretation of data

Interpretation of the Tl-201 scintigrams is usually performed by visual analysis of the analogue images and requires a lot of expertise. The results are commonly interpreted as follows: 1) normal = uniform distribution of activity throughout the left ventricular wall, whereby decrease in apical activity of similar extent on both the postexercise scan and the redistibution scan is considered normal, 2) ischemia = reversible perfusion defect, and 3) infarction = nonreversible or persistent perfusion defect. Typically, the three-view scintigrams are divided into seven different segments. The segments are graded according to intensity of perfusion with 1) normal Tl-201 activity, 2) diminished activity, and 3) absence of activity (normal score = 7). Apart from myocardial segment analysis, enhanced lung uptake is taken into consideration as a sign of severe coronary artery disease with left ventricular dysfunction.

Quantitative analysis of the images and washout kinetics may improve the diagnostic value of the test and is considered to be more objective. Abnormally slow washout in the absence of a visually apparent defect also indicates regional ischemia. However, quantitative analysis is not unanimously accepted due to the time-consuming procedure and its controversial additional value in clinical practice. Accordingly, each laboratory should develop its own standards based upon its own clinical setting and protocols, and determine its own way of appropriate analysis.

Protocol dipyridamole infusion testing

In patients who are unable to achieve predicted maximal heart rate during bicycle or treadmill exercise testing, it is necessary to dispose of alternate exercise methods for detecting coronary artery disease. Dipyridamole (Persantin[R]) infusion testing has been proven to offer a safe and reasonable alternative (4). The patient is administered 0.14 kg intravenous dipyridamole per kg bodyweight per minute during 4 minutes in a large antecubital vein. Two minutes after completion of the administration of dipyridamole, 75 MBq (2 mCi) Tl-201 is administered intravenously as a bolus. During the first 30 minutes blood pressure, heart rate, and the electrocardiogram are registered every minute. In case of occurrence of serious angina pectoris and/or symptomatic hemodynamic changes, 125-250 mg aminophylline is administered intravenously as an antidote. Ten minutes after Tl-201 injection, myocardial imaging is started in the three standard projections. After 3-4 hours the redistribution scintigrams are obtained in similar projections. At present, dipyridamole Tl-201 scintigraphy is preceded by mild exercise (30 Watts) if such is possible for the patient. This approach inproves the quality of the images.

Protocol first pass and equilibrium RNA

With the first pass technique 550-750 MBq (15-20 mCi) is intravenously injected as a compact bolus. The study is usually performed in the anterior or 30° right anterior oblique position for optimal temporal and anatomical separation of right atrium, right ventricle, and left ventricle. Data collection is started as soon as the bolus enters the superior vena cava, and is terminated after passing of activity through the left ventricle. Acceptable count rates can be obtained from the right ventricle, but count rates from the left ventricle are generally suboptimal. A conventional gamma camera can still be used, but more satisfying results are obtained with a multicrystal camera, which has an increased count rate capability. Therefore, equilibrium studies are more widely used in clinical practice. In some laboratories, the equilibrium technique is routinely preceded by the first pass technique.

With the equilibrium technique, the in-vivo labeling method is nowadays widely employed. First, the patients own red blood cells (RBC) are "primed" with 5-15 mg intravenously injected unlabeled stannous-pyrophosphate. Subsequently, after 15 minutes 750 MBq (20 mCi) Tc-99m pertechnetate is administered, which then labels the red cells with high efficiency and the intravascular blood pool can be visualized. A high sensitivity collimator is employed with a 20% window around the 140 keV energy peak of Tc-99m.

At rest, studies are acquired until a total of 300.000 counts per frame (usually 28 frames per RR-cycle) has been collected which takes about 7 to 15 minutes. Imaging at rest should be performed in at least two, preferably in three or four separate positions. In general the 40° and 70°LAO position is used. The assessment of LVEF during rest and exercise is probably the most widely used clinical application of the RNA techniques. Both the first pass technique and the equilibrium study are used to evaluate patients with suspected cardiac disease, although the equilibrium has shown to be more feasible. Supine exercise equilibrium scintigraphy can be carried out with the patient exercising on a special bicycle stress table under the camera. After the resting studies have been performed the same 40°LAO projection is used during exercise with a caudal tilt of at least 10°, so that the right and left ventricle can be viewed separately. A restraining harness is used to minimize patient motion under the camera during exercise. Preceding the test, the maximal expected workload is estimated from specially designed tables based on gender, weight and length of the patient. If possible, long-acting anginal medication should be discontinued at least 48 hours before the test. Exercise loads are increased stepwise by 25 Watt increments at three-minute intervals until the patient experiences symptoms of angina, dyspnea, or fatigue of sufficient severity to limit further exercise or until the patients develops severe hypotension or malignant arrhythmias. At each level of the work load, data are acquired by the computer during a two-minute period. The used high-sensitivity collimator allows the collection of maximal 150.000 counts per frame (16 frames per RR-cycle) within two minutes, which is sufficient for the evaluation of the exercise studies. Alternatively, the exercise loads can also be increased by 10 Watt increments at one-minute intervals with a final stage of three minutes; in that case only information during maximal exercise is obtained. Electrocardiographic leads are recorded and monitored continuously throughout the study.

Interpretation of data

Similar to Tl-201 exercise scintigraphy each laboratory should determine its own protocols and normal values. However, it has been attempted to reach a world-wide consensus on the normal range of LVEF and RVEF at rest and during exercise. For this purpose, pooled data of 1200 normal subjects from 28 leading centres in the field of nuclear cardiology was analysed (5). Based on these data, the following limits of normal have been almost ubiquitously accepted.

Weighted mean normal values for LVEF at rest are 62.3±6.1% (±1SD) with a lower limit of normal of 50% and for RVEF 52.3±6.2% with a lower limit of normal of 40%. During exercise, a normal increase for both LVEF and RVEF has been accepted to be 5% or more over a normal resting value. Subgroup analysis of results at rest reveals no significant differences regarding selection of normal subjects (based on normal catheterization findings versus normal volunteers with low probability of disease), age or sex. Data on reproducibility and variability show that RNA can be considered as a reliable method today.

Regional wall motion is best assessed from the cine display. The left ventricle is subdivided anatomically into multiple segments according to standard definitions. While quantitative methods for analysis of regional wall motion do exist, standardized visual analysis of the entire equilibrium study also provides relevant semi-quantitative data. The left ventricle as visualized in two views is divided into 7 anatomic segments. Each segment is graded on a four-point scale with 1 being normal, 2 hypokinetic, 3 akinetic and 4 dyskinetic. A total score for the left ventricle then is derived (normal score = 7). Various regional abnormalities may be detectable only in a single position as a result of overlap of segments or chambers. For example inferior and posterior wall regional abnormalities, including aneurysms, only may be apparent in the 70°LAO position. Particularly for the inferior wall, the 40°LAO position often may be misleading or incorrect because of overlap of the apical region. Also right ventricular motion can be adequately evaluated by cine display.

Although no world-wide consensus has been obtained for quantitative measurements of regional wall motion, yet two methods have been applied for measuring regional LVEF. Basically, one method divides the ventricle into radial sectors while the other divides it into rectangular segments bordering the major and minor axes of the left ventricle. Both methods yield similar results. With the rectangular method, normal ejection fraction is 0.66±0.13 in the anteroseptum, 0.85±0.12 in the apex, and 0.74±0.16 in the inferoposterior segment. Regional LVEF measurements are reproducible and useful in studies that require quantitative measurements of wall motion, such as before and during drug therapy.

Regurgitation fraction

In patients without aortic or mitral regurgitation, the left-to-right ventricular stroke index is 1.15 ± 0.15. The ratio is greater than one in normal patients because the right ventricular stroke volume is under-estimated owing to overlapping of the right atrium on the right ventricle. In patients with mitral or aortic regurgitation, the ratio is greater than 1.35. There is good agreement between the stroke-volume index and qualitative angiographic estimates of regurgitation. The limitations of applying the regurgitation index are that:1) right-sided regurgitation should not be present, 2) global LVEF should be greater than 30%, and 3) there should be good separation of the right atrium from the right ventricle. There is always some overlap of the right atrium on the right ventricle and this problem may be more severe with significant right atrial enlargement.

V. PERSONNEL AND EQUIPMENT FACILITIES

Specific guidelines for personnel and equipment facilities have been reported by the Nuclear Medicine Study Group (6). These guidelines have been prepared for persons who either provide or use optimal resources for radioactive tracer studies of the heart and circulation.

Physician

The performance of cardiac radionuclide procedures requires both cardiological and nuclear medical skills. In some instances individual physicians will have combined experience and expertise in both aspects of nuclear cardiology; these individuals can assume total responsibility for the patient and the study. In other instances close cooperation between cardiological and nuclear medicine specialists will be essential for optimal patient care and optimal quality control. In order to maintain optimal quality control a general nuclear laboratory should perform a minimum of 500 nuclear cardiology studies per year. This number rises to 1000 studies in a dedicated nuclear cardiology laboratory. Also data analysis and interpretation should be part of the quality control i.e. the combined presence of a nuclear medicine physician and a cardiologist is a first prerequisite for proper evaluation of the data.

Location and Space

Nuclear cardiological procedures will mostly be performed in a general nuclear medicine facility capable of providing a broad range of diagnostic studies. Larger nuclear medicine units will contain several types of procedure rooms. These rooms will include physiological testing instrumentation; they may be used for thallium-201 myocardial scintigraphy as well as for equilibrium and/or first pass studies.

Equipment

Essential equipment in a nuclear cardiology facility includes, apart from a computer and a gamma camera, facilities for electrocardiographic monitoring and exercise testing equipment. The proper use of personnel radiation monitors, area monitors and dose calibrators belongs to the competency of the nuclear medicine department. Equipment maintenance has to be performed by a specially trained nuclear technologist. Also internal methods for quality control and dose measurements of the used radiopharmaceuticals must be accomplished by trained nuclear technologists.

Electrocardiographic Monitor
For monitoring a patient at rest or during physiological and pharmacological interventions, a multichannel (3 or more channels) electrocardiogram is recommended. The ECG monitor is connected to both the console and strip-chart recorder. The console should contain a persistence digital oscilloscope with three channels to be used by the physician both for the study and for the monitoring safety of the performance.

Exercise Testing Equipment
An exercise table with a bicycle ergometer is used for exercise RNA studies. The table should be immobile during exercise, and the patient should be well stabilized on the table. The bicycle should permit variable work loads, and variable positions for the patient. Equipment for upright exercise can be used for first pass RNA and Tl-201 exercise studies.
Tl-201 exercise scintigraphy can both be performed on a bicycle ergometer and on a treadmill. It is usually easier to stress the patient to maximum capacity during treadmill exercise. Alternatively, an upright bicycle ergometer with a variable work load can be used (and is required with a first pass RNA). With equilibrium RNA, exercise can be performed in any position from upright to supine. For patients with pulmonary disease or heart failure, exercise is more comfortable in a semi-sitting or sitting position.
An emergency cart must be available for resuscitation. The cart should contain all routine equipment and drugs necessary for cardiopulmonary resuscitation. Supplies should be arranged in an orderly, easily accessible manner with a visible, on-cart directory to the various medications. A defibrillator must be close at hand when physiological and/or pharmacological exercise testing are performed. An emergency call button or telephone should be available in the room so that additional help can be summoned. A well-trained physician should of course survey the exercise test.

Radionuclide dosage

Presently, there are no specific guidelines available which define precisely the maximal permissible activity or dose which can administered to a patient for diagnostic nuclear cardiology procedures. Rather, the approach advocated is to keep the total dose as low as possible, while allowing for the acquisition of reliable diagnostic results. In terms of serial studies, the risk benefit ratio of individual study should be the predominant factor determining whether or not a given examination should be performed. Furthermore, the radiation burden of a diagnostic nuclear procedure should be put into perspective relative to other radiologic procedures being performed, specially coronary arteriography. In these latter radiologic procedures, the radiation exposure to critical organs such as bone marrow and thyroid, will be substantially higher for the comparable nuclear studies. Although guidelines exist in some countries for radioactive drugs used for research, there are no accepted guidelines for the total number of clinically indicated studies involving routine radionuclides that can be administered over a period of time. In general, the goal should be to achieve the maximal diagnostic or therapeutic information with the minimal total dose. The number of studies that can be performed must be determined by the clinical question to be answered and the overall risk benefit ratio.

References

1. Zaret BL, Battler A, Berger HJ, Bodenheimer MM, Borer JS, Brochier M, Hugenholtz PG, Neufeld HN, Pfisterer ME. Report of the Joint International Society and Federation of Cardiology/World Health Organization Task Force on Nuclear Cardiology. Circulation 1984;70:768A-81A.
2. O'Rourke RA, Chatterjee K, Dodge HT, Fisch C, Levine H, Pohost GM, Resnekov L. Guidelines for Clinical Use of Cardiac Radionuclide Imaging. Circulation 1986;74:1469A-82A.
3. Diamond GA, Forrester JS. Analysis of probability as an aid in the clinical diagnosis of coronary artery disease. N Engl J Med 1979;300:1350-8.
4. Laarman GJ. Thallium-201 myocardial scintigraphy after dipyridamole infusion. Thesis, Leiden, 1988.
5. Pfisterer ME, Battler A, Zaret BL. Range of normal values for left and right ventricular ejection fraction at rest and during exercise assessed by radionuclide angiography. Eur Heart J 1985;6: 647-55.
6. Adelstein SJ, Holman BL, Wagner HN, Zaret BL. Optimal resources for radioactive tracer studies of the heart and circulation. Circulation 1984;70: 524A-36A.

SOURCES

Chapter 1. In: Coronary Circulation (Eds. Spaan JAE, Bruschke AVG, Gittenberger-de Groot AC). Martinus Nijhoff Publishers, Dordrecht, The Netherlands, 1987:140-55.
(Co-authors: Pauwels EKJ, Bruschke AVG)

Chapter 2. In: Noninvasive Imaging of Cardiac Metabolism (Ed. van der Wall EE. Martinus Nijhoff Publishers, Dordrecht, The Netherlands, 1987:39-59.

Chapter 3. In: Cardiac Imaging (Ed. Visser CA). Proceedings of a symposium, Academic Medical Center. Rodopi Publishers, Amsterdam, The Netherlands, 1987:117-38.

Chapter 4. Parts of text derived from: Slide Series I, Nuclear Cardiology, Cardiovascular IV-10, 1985, (Co-author: Wackers FJT), and from Slide Series II, Thallium-201 Exercise Scintigraphy, Cardiovascular IV-12, 1989. (Co-authors: Laarman GJ, Wackers FJT) Postgraduate Medical Services. Boehringer Ingelheim.

Chapter 5. Neth J Cardiol 1990;3:67-81.
(Co-authors: Prpic H, Blokland JAK, Pauwels EKJ, Bruschke AVG)

Chapter 6. Neth J Cardiol 1989;2:89-98.

Chapter 7. Am Heart J 1991;121:1203-20.
(Co-authors: de Roos A, van Voorthuisen AE, Bruschke AVG)

Chapter 8. Eur J Nucl Med 1990;17:83-90.
(Co-authors: Niemeyer MG, de Roos A, Bruschke AVG, Pauwels EKJ)

Chapter 9. Angiology (in press).
(Co-authors: Niemeyer MG, Pauwels EKJ, van Dijkman PRM, Blokland JAK, de Roos A, Bruschke AVG)

Chapter 10. Current Opinion in Cardiology 1987;2:1051-7.

Chapter 11. To be published.
(Co-authors: Niemeyer MG, Pauwels EKJ, Bruschke AVG)

Chapter 12. In: Recent Views On Hypertrophic Cardiomyopathy (Eds. van der Wall E, Lie KI). Martinus Nijhoff Publishers, Dordrecht, The Netherlands, 1985:33-51.

Chapter 13. Eur Heart J (in press).
(Co-authors: Pauwels EKJ, Bruschke AVG)

Chapter 14. Am Heart J 1989;118:655-61.
(Co-authors: Manger Cats V, Blokland JAK, Bosker HA, Arndt JW, Pauwels EKJ, Bruschke AVG)

Chapter 15. Diagnostic Imaging International 1991;3:30-6.
(Co-authors: Pauwels EKJ, Bruschke AVG)

Chapter 16. Neth J Cardiol 1988;1:45-52.
(Coauthors: Braat S, Visser FC, Blokland JAK, van Kroonenburgh MJPG, Bruschke AVG, Ascoop CAPL)